Systems Thinking and Models in Public Health

Systems Thinking and Models in Public Health

Editors

Philippe J. Giabbanelli
Andrew Page

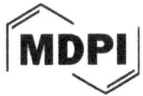

Basel • Beijing • Wuhan • Barcelona • Belgrade • Novi Sad • Cluj • Manchester

Editors
Philippe J. Giabbanelli
Department of Computer
Science & Software Engineering
Miami University
Oxford
United States

Andrew Page
Translational Health Research
Institute
Western Sydney University
Penrith
Australia

Editorial Office
MDPI
St. Alban-Anlage 66
4052 Basel, Switzerland

This is a reprint of articles from the Special Issue published online in the open access journal *Systems* (ISSN 2079-8954) (available at: www.mdpi.com/journal/systems/special_issues/STMPH).

For citation purposes, cite each article independently as indicated on the article page online and as indicated below:

Lastname, A.A.; Lastname, B.B. Article Title. *Journal Name* **Year**, *Volume Number*, Page Range.

ISBN 978-3-7258-0744-4 (Hbk)
ISBN 978-3-7258-0743-7 (PDF)
doi.org/10.3390/books978-3-7258-0743-7

© 2024 by the authors. Articles in this book are Open Access and distributed under the Creative Commons Attribution (CC BY) license. The book as a whole is distributed by MDPI under the terms and conditions of the Creative Commons Attribution-NonCommercial-NoDerivs (CC BY-NC-ND) license.

Contents

About the Editors vii

Preface ix

Philippe J. Giabbanelli and Andrew Page
Systems Thinking and Models in Public Health
Reprinted from: *Systems* 2024, 12, 101, doi:10.3390/systems12030101 1

Ateekh Ur Rehman, Yusuf Siraj Usmani, Syed Hammad Mian, Mustufa Haider Abidi and Hisham Alkhalefah
Simulation and Goal Programming Approach to Improve Public Hospital Emergency Department Resource Allocation
Reprinted from: *Systems* 2023, 11, 467, doi:10.3390/systems11090467 4

Narjes Shojaati and Nathaniel D. Osgood
Evaluating the Impact of Increased Dispensing of Opioid Agonist Therapy Take-Home Doses on Treatment Retention and Opioid-Related Harm among Opioid Agonist Therapy Recipients: A Simulation Study
Reprinted from: *Systems* 2023, 11, 391, doi:10.3390/systems11080391 23

Yuan Tian, Jenny Basran, James Stempien, Adrienne Danyliw, Graham Fast and Patrick Falastein et al.
Participatory Modeling with Discrete-Event Simulation: A Hybrid Approach to Inform Policy Development to Reduce Emergency Department Wait Times
Reprinted from: *Systems* 2023, 11, 362, doi:10.3390/systems11070362 40

Jianjun Zhang, Jingru Huang, Tianhao Wang and Jin Zhao
Dynamic Optimization of Emergency Logistics for Major Epidemic Considering Demand Urgency
Reprinted from: *Systems* 2023, 11, 303, doi:10.3390/systems11060303 71

Ruhao Ma, Fansheng Meng and Haiwen Du
Research on Intelligent Emergency Resource Allocation Mechanism for Public Health Emergencies: A Case Study on the Prevention and Control of COVID-19 in China
Reprinted from: *Systems* 2023, 11, 300, doi:10.3390/systems11060300 91

Eileen Goldberg, Cindy Peng, Andrew Page, Piumee Bandara and Danielle Currie
Strategies to Prevent Suicide and Attempted Suicide in New South Wales (Australia): Community-Based Outreach, Alternatives to Emergency Department Care, and Early Intervention
Reprinted from: *Systems* 2023, 11, 275, doi:10.3390/systems11060275 112

Narjes Shojaati and Nathaniel D. Osgood
An Agent-Based Social Impact Theory Model to Study the Impact of In-Person School Closures on Nonmedical Prescription Opioid Use among Youth
Reprinted from: *Systems* 2023, 11, 72, doi:10.3390/systems11020072 123

Pei Shan Loo, Anaely Aguiar and Birgit Kopainsky
Simulation-Based Assessment of Cholera Epidemic Response: A Case Study of Al-Hudaydah, Yemen
Reprinted from: *Systems* 2022, 11, 3, doi:10.3390/systems11010003 143

Janet Michel, David Evans, Marcel Tanner and Thomas C. Sauter
Identifying Policy Gaps in a COVID-19 Online Tool Using the Five-Factor Framework
Reprinted from: *Systems* **2022**, *10*, 257, doi:10.3390/systems10060257 163

Wen-Yi Chen
On the Relationships among Nurse Staffing, Inpatient Care Quality, and Hospital Competition under the Global Budget Payment Scheme of Taiwan's National Health Insurance System: Mixed Frequency VAR Analyses
Reprinted from: *Systems* **2022**, *10*, 187, doi:10.3390/systems10050187 173

Mariam Abdulmonem Mansouri, Leandro Garcia, Frank Kee and Declan Terence Bradley
Systems-Oriented Modelling Methods in Preventing and Controlling Emerging Infectious Diseases in the Context of Healthcare Policy: A Scoping Review
Reprinted from: *Systems* **2022**, *10*, 182, doi:10.3390/systems10050182 198

About the Editors

Philippe J. Giabbanelli

At nationally ranked American universities, Dr. Giabbanelli has developed and delivered a range of courses on predictive modeling and health, including machine learning, network science, computational epidemiology, artificial intelligence, and virtual worlds. He has taught at all levels, from introductory programming courses to data structures, algorithms, and graduate-level seminars. His research focuses on developing and applying artificial intelligence tools to support population health interventions. This has resulted in over 130 publications of which the quality has been recognized in several ways, including six best paper awards and nominations, and the 2022 Annual Outstanding Faculty Research Award from the College of Engineering and Computing at Miami University, where he is currently a tenured faculty member. Dr. Giabbanelli is actively involved in scientific leadership as editor for five journals, lead editor of several special issues, or track/program/general chair at international ACM or IEEE conferences.

Andrew Page

Dr. Andrew Page is a Professor and Chair of Epidemiology at the Translational Health Research Institute. He has extensive research experience in epidemiology, psychology, and public health, with particular interests in the study of suicide and mental health, the social determinants of health, injury prevention, breast cancer screening, and maternal and child health. Dr. Page also has interests in the application of systems science and simulation approaches to epidemiological evidence in order to inform policy and health service decision–support tools. Dr. Page is also the Director of the Master of Epidemiology program in the School of Medicine.

Preface

Systems thinking and modeling have been essential approaches to identifying the drivers of health outcomes and analyzing their complex interrelationships, paving the way to interventions that improve outcomes while minimizing unintended consequences. These methods support interdisciplinary teams in representing and navigating complex systems, thus asking essential 'what-if' questions and serving numerous other goals, from guiding data collection efforts to comparing the perspectives of stakeholders or validating theories. This volume features methodological innovations and applications for several determinants and key global health priority areas.

Priority determinants include, but are not limited to, social determinants (e.g., health inequalities), climate change (through its impact on health), behavioral factors, and facets of the healthcare system ranging from primary services to secondary prevention (i.e., screening and case-finding) and tertiary cases (e.g., treatment optimization, resource allocation). Systems thinking and modeling can shed light on how such determinants ultimately shape health outcomes and/or the cost-effectiveness of an intervention. The contributions of this volume touch on several determinants, collectively providing a comprehensive overview of the challenges and applications of systems thinking to public health.

This volume will benefit researchers in the fields of public health, systems thinking or modeling. The content is accessible to early-career researchers, such as graduate students, who may choose specific chapters within their areas of interest as part of identifying open challenges to inspire their own research.

Philippe J. Giabbanelli and Andrew Page
Editors

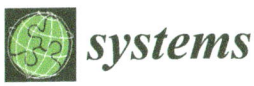

Editorial

Systems Thinking and Models in Public Health

Philippe J. Giabbanelli [1,*] and Andrew Page [2]

1. Department of Computer Science & Software Engineering, Miami University, Oxford, OH 45056, USA
2. Translational Health Research Institute, Western Sydney University, Penrith, NSW 2751, Australia
* Correspondence: giabbanelli@gmail.com

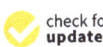

Citation: Giabbanelli, P.J.; Page, A. Systems Thinking and Models in Public Health. *Systems* **2024**, *12*, 101. https://doi.org/10.3390/systems12030101

Received: 10 March 2024
Accepted: 14 March 2024
Published: 16 March 2024

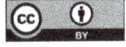

Copyright: © 2024 by the authors. Licensee MDPI, Basel, Switzerland. This article is an open access article distributed under the terms and conditions of the Creative Commons Attribution (CC BY) license (https://creativecommons.org/licenses/by/4.0/).

In responding to population health challenges, epidemiologists want to identify causal associations between an exposure (e.g., tobacco smoking) and disease (e.g., lung cancer) so we can intervene to improve human health. In epidemiology, these kinds of 'causal' questions are addressed by comparing exposed and unexposed groups to identify individual component causes (or 'risk factors') of disease. This counterfactual approach aims to hold everything constant except the factor of interest and, if successfully achieved, this can tell us if 'X causes Y'. However, a focus on single risk factors necessarily overlooks the complexity and multifactorial nature of most health outcomes, particularly chronic disease outcomes. The causes of disease can operate at the macro or micro level, across the life course, and they are also inextricably intertwined with social, economic and political environments. The single 'risk factor' approach to understanding disease outcomes is limited in the face of this complexity [1–3]. Similarly, demonstrating that an intervention works in a highly controlled study setting does not necessarily mean that it will work in the same way when implemented in a dynamic population in the presence of these other complex determinants of disease.

There are alternative methods that explicitly characterize and model complex systems, and epidemiologists and public health practitioners are increasingly working in multidisciplinary groups to apply these methods to capture the complexity and dynamics of human populations and systems. Computational simulation and systems thinking—approaches used extensively in other disciplines such as ecology, engineering and computer science to guide decision making and priorities resources—can capture the dynamics and complex determinants of disease. These approaches use a combination of existing primary data sources, evidence from the literature, stakeholder engagement and dynamic hypothesis testing to better characterize how an exposure or an intervention is likely to affect disease outcomes in populations. Several reviews have highlighted the strong interest in applying systems thinking and modeling to public health [4–6].

Models allow the testing of 'what if' scenarios and can be used to determine a course of action more efficiently than by a typical 'trial-and-error' approach to the implementation and evaluation of population health interventions. Framed as 'decision support tools', models can help local and national decision makers determine where best to target investments and with what intensity so that the impact of limited resources can be optimized [7–9]. The greatest value of computational simulation is achieved when it is embedded in the program evaluation cycle and used not only as a decision support tool for policy or service planning, but also to prospectively support implementation, monitoring and evaluation. These tools can help identify data collection priorities, realistic targets for impact and important indicators for evaluating progress against those targets.

We present a series of articles that demonstrate the importance of systems thinking and the use of computational simulation models to address public health questions. The articles in this issue address a diversity of contemporary topics in public health, and also demonstrate how public health problems can be examined using a range of complementary modelling approaches, including system dynamics models, agent based models, and discrete event simulation models.

Shojaati and Osgood [Contribution 1] and Shojaati et al. [Contribution 2] investigate models of community-based management of opioid use and its impact on treatment retention and opioid-related harm [Contribution 2], and also the impact of social influence and social networks on illicit opioid use among young people during and after periods of school closures using agent based models [Contribution 1]. A series of articles focus on health services use, in particular emergency department (ED) use and hospital admissions, including the modeling of patient flow and wait times [Contribution 3], the optimisation of limited healthcare resources [Contributions 4–7], and the benefits of using systems thinking approaches to inform the implementation of triage and referral systems [Contribution 8]. Goldberg et al. [Contribution 9] present findings from a system dynamics model of suicidal behaviour, and investigate the potential impacts of combinations of population and health service interventions to prevent suicide and attempted suicide. Loo et al. [Contribution 10] also use system dynamics modeling to historically evaluate the prevention and management of cholera outbreaks in Yemen.

The central importance of participatory approaches involving stakeholders and model users is also highlighted in this Special Issue, in terms of understanding the system and in the design, parameterization and implementation of models for decision support in public health [Contributions 3, 8, 9]. Co-design and consultation is key for tools to have policy and planning relevance [Contribution 11]. This is explicitly demonstrated by Tian et al. [Contribution 3] in the development and use of a multi-criteria framework to identify and prioritize interventions to reduce ED wait times. The authors provide a rich description of the processes related to involving stakeholders in prioritization of model scope and refining the model thanks iterative feedback with stakeholders. Finally, we also include a scoping review of emerging infectious disease (EID) in the wake of the COVID-19 pandemic [Contribution 12], which emphasises the ongoing importance of ensuring that our analytic approaches are informed by current evidence. In this review, Mansouri et al. [Contribution 12] describe the types of systems-oriented approaches that have been used to investigate EIDs. The authors emphasize the importance of the quality, geographic specificity, and timeliness of data needed.

Author Contributions: P.J.G. and A.P. worked together throughout the entire editorial process of this Special Issue. They reviewed, edited, and finalized this manuscript. All authors have read and agreed to the published version of the manuscript.

Funding: This research received no external funding.

Conflicts of Interest: The authors declare no conflict of interest.

List of Contributions

1. Shojaati, N.; Osgood, N.D. An Agent-Based Social Impact Theory Model to Study the Impact of In-Person School Closures on Nonmedical Prescription Opioid Use among Youth. *Systems* **2023**, *11*, 72.
2. Shojaati, N.; Osgood, N.D. Evaluating the impact of increased dispensing of opioid agonist therapy take-home doses on treatment retention and opioid-related harm among opioid agonist therapy recipients: A simulation study. *Systems* **2023**, *11*, 391.
3. Tian, Y.; Basran, J.; Stempien, J.; Danyliw, A.; Fast, G.; Falastein, P.; Osgood, N.D. Participatory Modeling with Discrete-Event Simulation: A Hybrid Approach to Inform Policy Development to Reduce Emergency Department Wait Times. *Systems* **2023**, *11*, 362.
4. Chen, W.-Y. On the Relationships among Nurse Staffing, Inpatient Care Quality, and Hospital Competition under the Global Budget Payment Scheme of Taiwan's National Health Insurance System: Mixed Frequency VAR Analyses. *Systems* **2022**, *10*, 187.
5. Ma, R.; Meng, F.; Du, H. Research on Intelligent Emergency Resource Allocation Mechanism for Public Health Emergencies: A Case Study on the Prevention and Control of COVID-19 in China. *Systems* **2023**, *11*, 300.

6. Rehman, A.U.; Usmani, Y.S.; Mian, S.H.; Abidi, M.H.; Alkhalefah, H. Simulation and Goal Programming Approach to Improve Public Hospital Emergency Department Resource Allocation. *Systems* **2023**, *11*, 467.
7. Zhang, J.; Huang, J.; Wang, T.; Zhao, J. Dynamic Optimization of Emergency Logistics for Major Epidemic Considering Demand Urgency. *Systems* **2023**, *11*, 303.
8. Michel, J.; Evans, D.; Tanner, M.; Sauter, T.C. Identifying Policy Gaps in a COVID-19 Online Tool Using the Five-Factor Framework. *Systems* **2022**, *10*, 257.
9. Goldberg, E.; Peng, C.; Page, A.; Bandara, P.; Currie, D. Strategies to Prevent Suicide and Attempted Suicide in New South Wales (Australia): Community-Based Outreach, Alternatives to Emergency Department Care, and Early Intervention. *Systems* **2023**, *11*, 275.
10. Loo, P.S.; Aguiar, A.; Kopainsky, B. Simulation-Based Assessment of Cholera Epidemic Response: A Case Study of Al-Hudaydah, Yemen. *Systems* **2022**, *11*, 3.
11. Freebairn, L.; Rychetnik, L.; Atkinson, J.-A.; Kelly, P.; McDonnell, G.; Roberts, N.; Whittall, C.; Redman, S. Knowledge mobilisation for policy development: implementing systems approaches through participatory dynamic simulation modelling. *Health Res. Policy Syst.* **2017**, *15*, 83.
12. Mansouri, M.A.; Garcia, L.; Kee, F.; Bradley, D.T. Systems-oriented modelling methods in preventing and controlling emerging infectious diseases in the context of healthcare policy: A scoping review. *Systems* **2022**, *10*, 182.

References

1. Contu, P.; Breton, E. The application of the complexity theory to public health interventions: A review of the literature. *Eur. J. Public Health* **2020**, *30* (Suppl. S5), ckaa166.461. [CrossRef]
2. Heitman, K.R. Reductionism at the dawn of population health. *Syst. Sci. Popul. Health* **2017**, 9–24.
3. Barbrook-Johnson, P.; Castellani, B.; Hills, D.; Penn, A.; Gilbert, N. Policy evaluation for a complex world: Practical methods and reflections from the UK Centre for the Evaluation of Complexity across the Nexus. *Evaluation* **2021**, *27*, 4–17. [CrossRef]
4. Carey, G.; Malbon, E.; Carey, N.; Joyce, A.; Crammond, B.; Carey, A. Systems science and systems thinking for public health: A systematic review of the field. *BMJ Open* **2015**, *5*, e009002. [CrossRef] [PubMed]
5. McGill, E.; Er, V.; Penney, T.; Egan, M.; White, M.; Meier, P.; Whitehead, M.; Lock, K.; de Cuevas, R.A.; Smith, R.; et al. Evaluation of public health interventions from a complex systems perspective: A research methods review. *Soc. Sci. Med.* **2021**, *272*, 113697. [CrossRef] [PubMed]
6. Bagnall, A.M.; Radley, D.; Jones, R.; Gately, P.; Nobles, J.; Van Dijk, M.; Blackshaw, J.; Montel, S.; Sahota, P. Whole systems approaches to obesity and other complex public health challenges: A systematic review. *BMC Public Health* **2019**, *19*, 8. [CrossRef] [PubMed]
7. Jit, M.; Cook, A.R. Informing Public Health Policies with Models for Disease Burden, Impact Evaluation, and Economic Evaluation. *Annu. Rev. Public Health* **2023**, *45*. [CrossRef] [PubMed]
8. Rutter, H.; Savona, N.; Glonti, K.; Bibby, J.; Cummins, S.; Finegood, D.T.; Greaves, F.; Harper, L.; Hawe, P.; Moore, L.; et al. The need for a complex systems model of evidence for public health. *Lancet* **2017**, *390*, 2602–2604. [CrossRef] [PubMed]
9. Mabry, P.L.; Marcus, S.E.; Clark, P.I.; Leischow, S.J.; Méndez, D. Systems science: A revolution in public health policy research. *Am. J. Public Health* **2010**, *100*, 1161–1163. [CrossRef] [PubMed]

Disclaimer/Publisher's Note: The statements, opinions and data contained in all publications are solely those of the individual author(s) and contributor(s) and not of MDPI and/or the editor(s). MDPI and/or the editor(s) disclaim responsibility for any injury to people or property resulting from any ideas, methods, instructions or products referred to in the content.

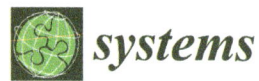

Article

Simulation and Goal Programming Approach to Improve Public Hospital Emergency Department Resource Allocation

Ateekh Ur Rehman [1,*], Yusuf Siraj Usmani [1], Syed Hammad Mian [2], Mustufa Haider Abidi [2] and Hisham Alkhalefah [2]

1 Department of Industrial Engineering, College of Engineering, King Saud University, Riyadh 11421, Saudi Arabia; yusmani@ksu.edu.sa
2 Advanced Manufacturing Institute, King Saud University, Riyadh 11421, Saudi Arabia; smien@ksu.edu.sa (S.H.M.); mabidi@ksu.edu.sa (M.H.A.); halkhalefah@ksu.edu.sa (H.A.)
* Correspondence: arehman@ksu.edu.sa

Abstract: Efficient and effective operation of an emergency department is necessary. Since patients can visit the emergency department without making an appointment, the emergency department always treats a lot of critical patients. Moreover, the severity of the ailment determines which patients should be prioritized. Therefore, the patients are greatly impacted as a consequence of longer waiting times caused primarily by incorrect resource allocation. It frequently happens that patients leave the hospital or waiting area without treatment. Certainly, the emergency department's operation can be made more effective and efficient by examining its work and making modifications to the number of resources and their allocation. This study, therefore, investigates the emergency department of a public hospital to improve its functioning. The goal of this research is to model and simulate an emergency department to minimize patient wait times and also minimize the number of patients leaving the hospital without service. A comprehensive simulation model is developed using the Arena simulation platform and goal programming is undertaken to conduct simulation optimization and resource allocation analysis. Hospital management should realize that all resources must be prioritized rather than just focusing on one or two of them. The case scenario (S3) in this study that implements goal programming with variable weights yields the most favorable results. For example, it is observed in this instance that the number of patients leaving the system without service drops by 61.7%, and there is also a substantial drop in waiting times for various types of patients.

Keywords: simulation Arena; emergency department; hospital; resource allocation; goal programming

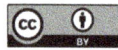

Citation: Rehman, A.U.; Usmani, Y.S.; Mian, S.H.; Abidi, M.H.; Alkhalefah, H. Simulation and Goal Programming Approach to Improve Public Hospital Emergency Department Resource Allocation. *Systems* **2023**, *11*, 467. https://doi.org/10.3390/systems11090467

Academic Editors: Philippe J. Giabbanelli and Andrew Page

Received: 3 August 2023
Revised: 29 August 2023
Accepted: 1 September 2023
Published: 8 September 2023

Copyright: © 2023 by the authors. Licensee MDPI, Basel, Switzerland. This article is an open access article distributed under the terms and conditions of the Creative Commons Attribution (CC BY) license (https://creativecommons.org/licenses/by/4.0/).

1. Introduction

The healthcare sector has recently undergone substantial transformations. As a result, hospitals as evolving systems must constantly adapt to meet the needs of the modern healthcare system. Hospitals must not only innovate to deliver superior treatment at a cheaper price, but also boost administrative reliability and effectiveness. Healthcare modeling and simulation is one such contemporary technique which can offer a number of benefits, such as lowering expenditures and improving patient satisfaction [1–4]. In any hospital, an emergency department is a critical section because it cares for patients around the clock. The patients in the emergency department have to undergo various phases [5] such as arrival registration, data retrieving, triage assignment, nurse assignment, doctor evaluation, imaging, and laboratory tests, planning treatment, follow-up for the availability of inpatient beds, and physicians, and finally release or admittance. It is also evident that any emergency department process delays at a specific phase build pressure on the systems and their resources. Thus, simulation along with an optimization tool is an ideal approach that can be adopted by hospital management to enhance the working of the emergency department. Therefore, the goal of this work is to combine simulation with the multi-objective goal programming technique to minimize the waiting times of the patients visiting the emergency department. A simulation model of an emergency department from a public hospital (King Khaled University Hospital, KKUH, Riyadh) in Saudi Arabia is developed and analyzed using the Arena® Simulation Software, version 16.2 (Rockwell Automation). Subsequently, Arena's OptQuest tool is deployed to run multiple simulation scenarios created by the goal programming approach. Certainly, when simulation and goal programming are integrated, it is possible to take advantage of the unique benefits of both approaches and exploit their full potential. For example, in this work, the simulation model records and replicates patient movement, while goal programming accomplishes several objectives across a spectrum of opposing requirements. The objective of this research is also to assist hospital administration in better understanding patient movement so that they can make informed and better decisions in an emergency department. The seriousness of the case determines which patients should be prioritized while treating both critical and non-critical patients. A department's ability to function properly depends on the assigned number of doctors, nurses, beds, etc. The financial burden on a hospital cannot be unfairly increased by increasing the amount of resources, and, on the other hand, patients would suffer if there were to be fewer resources available. It is thus emphasized that there is a necessity of identifying an adequate number of resources and their allocation. Additionally, it has been noted that patients frequently leave hospitals or waiting rooms unsupervised and do not return to the same facility when waiting periods are great. Hence, the appropriate assignment of resources would also minimize the waiting times and thus the number of patients leaving the queue untreated. The details of resources, distinct entities, and their interactions and flow within the model; relevant data collection; model initialization; and goal programming model, the various performance measures and an approach to find an optimal solution that satisfies those targets are presented here, in the following sections and sub-sections.

2. Background

The application of simulation to research various elements of hospital operations has a long history in the scientific community. Indeed, academics and researchers have effectively used simulation and other mathematical-based approaches to address an array of hospital-related issues [6–13]. For instance, Chouba et al. [14] built a simulation model of the emergency department and minimized patient average waiting time. They stated that the quality of treatment could be improved by making optimal use of the resources, which, according to the authors, are a key component. Similarly, Feng et al. [15] observed that due to the hindered access to medical supplies, optimizing resource allocation to reduce patient lengths of stay and unnecessary expenses is imperative. The research findings of Storrow et al. [16] proposed and demonstrated the value of an efficient healthcare simulation model. They suggested reducing the time for implementing emergency services and the response time using the established modeling approaches. Indeed, multiple health and medical domains utilized simulations, and in the past decade, numerous simulation approaches have caught the interest of many healthcare academicians [17]. As reported by Bahari and Asadi [18], the optimal combination of resources must be determined to solve real case studies by applying the simulation and decision-making models with more than one objective. Furthermore, Yeh and Lin [19] used a simulation for minimizing patient queue time in an emergency department as well as provided the use of multi-criteria decision-making for enhancing patient care and staffing in the hospital administration of the Show-Chwan Memorial Hospital in central Taiwan. Subsequently, Oddoye et al. [20] estimated the ideal staffing needs for the medical assessment units and reduced system inefficiencies to optimize the flow of patients.

Recent developments have seen the use of hybrid modeling, operations research, integrated methodologies, and participatory approaches in addition to more conventional techniques. This is due to the fact that using sophisticated modeling techniques or a reliable forecasting system are essential for implementing superior management strategies that maximize resource utilization, cut costs, and boost consumer trust [21]. For example, by taking into account actual emergency department data, Tabar and Zeil [22] created a forecasting model to effectively simulate the consequences of special events on emergency department visits. A simulation approach based on agent-based modeling and exhaustive search was reported by Cabrera et al. [23] to formulate a decision support system for hospital emergency department. They aimed to assist the authorities in establishing guidelines that could enhance emergency department operations. Similarly, as a nurse scheduling strategy, Rerkjirattikal et al. [24] proposed scheduling optimization tools to make an effective nurse shift rotation schedule considering both personal choices for working shifts and day-off assignments and the equitable distribution of the workload. Castanheira-Pinto et al. [25] also emphasized the relevance of simulation and optimization tools for comprehending and efficiently enhancing the operations of any complicated system. They established a simulation methodology to accomplish the desired benchmarks for emergency departments in public hospitals. They devised a number of alternative scenarios using the data collected from the hospital's database in order to maximize the intricate operations of the emergency department.

Numerous research works also combined optimization models with discrete-event simulation to streamline staffing levels and shorten the average length of stay for patients [26–30]. Hybrid simulation is certainly becoming more popular as healthcare systems have grown more sophisticated and multifaceted [31,32]. Due to complicated systems and large amounts of data, it is difficult for an isolated simulation model to effectively make appropriate decisions. Moreover, studies reveal that the most popular method of developing hybrid simulation models in healthcare is the combination of discrete event simulation with system dynamics [33]. A hybrid modeling approach based on forecasting and real-time simulation introduced by Harper and Mustafee [34] was useful to reduce emergency department overcrowding. The approach used seasonal ARIMA time-series forecasting and could be useful for policymakers, clinicians, and managers at the regional level who are responsible for managing emergency department operational performance. The research study of Tang et al. [35] also described a simulation model to capture a large emergency department's operation and assess the impact of a COVID-19-like disease on the throughput of an emergency department. In another similar study [36], an optimization model was implemented to identify optimal physician staffing levels for minimizing the combined cost of patient wait times, handoffs, and physician shifts in a hospital emergency department. Likewise, Doudareva and Carter [37] and Mustafee et al. [38] developed discrete event simulation models of emergency departments to diagnose bottlenecks and evaluate performance improvement approaches. A research study by Harper and Mustafee [39] proposed the use of participatory design research methodology for the development of real-time simulation models in healthcare. The methodology emphasized model usefulness and usability using iterative cycles of development and evaluation. Prabhu et al. [40] also explored the impact of delays resulting from the imaging process and bundling the imaging orders on patient flow in the emergency department using discrete event simulation. The results showed that bundling imaging orders can also reduce patient time in the emergency department. Apart from reducing patient waiting time, evaluating staff strength and overcrowding, etc., simulation models have also been utilized by researchers for emergency department evacuation, logistics optimization, layout design, etc. [41–43].

It has been repeatedly demonstrated in the literature that simulation modeling is the most effective method for enhancing the performance of any complicated system. Researchers in the healthcare industry have frequently utilized it to increase the effectiveness and efficiency of their particular departments. These improvements have mostly been focused on decreasing patient wait times and raising patient satisfaction by properly scheduling and distributing resources. The need for combining a simulation model with an optimization tool has also been underlined by the researchers as a way to improve the efficacy of the simulations. However, it seems that there are fewer works than anticipated that integrate simulation with optimization. This work is intended to move in that direction by combining goal programming with a simulation model to increase patient satisfaction in an emergency department of a public hospital. Thus, the following sections describe patient flow in the hospital under consideration, its simulation model, and the application goal programming.

3. Simulation Model

The Arena simulation software is employed to build the desired model. The patient flow in the KKUH's emergency department as seen in Figure 1 is studied by this simulation model. Furthermore, the input analyzer in Arena is used to create distributions by fitting probability distribution functions to the data. The developed simulation model and the optimization OptQuest model are available at the online repository Zenodo at https://doi.org/10.5281/zenodo.8209820 (accessed on 10 August 2023). The details of resources, process flow, data related to arrival and service rates, model initialization, performance measures adopted are discussed here, below.

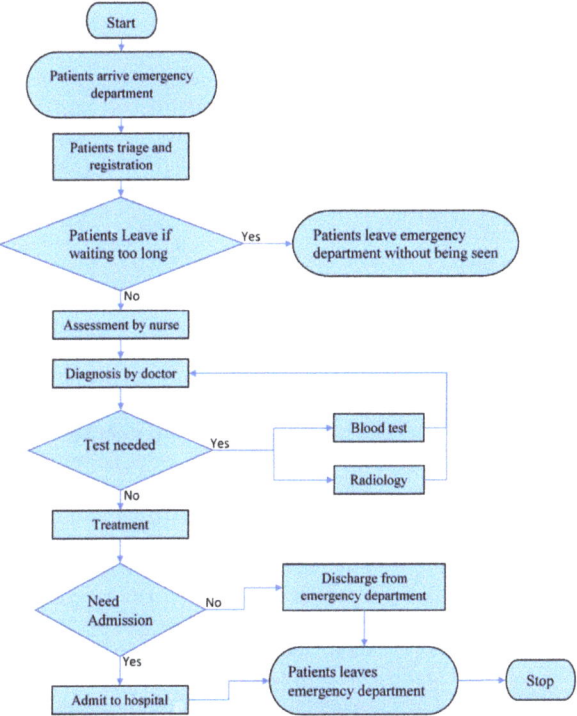

Figure 1. Patient flow diagram in the emergency department.

3.1. Process Flow

The model operation starts with the arrival of the patient at the triage and registration desk. The triage nurse assesses the severity of the case, assigns the triage level to the patient, and performs registration. The process of sorting patients at a medical facility to receive medical care based on severity of injury or illness after their arrival and assigning priorities is called the triage process. The triage system at KKUH has five levels, as described below.

- Level 1—Resuscitation: life-threatening.
- Level 2—Emergent: could become life-threatening.
- Level 3—Urgent: not life-threatening.
- Level 4—Less urgent: not life-threatening.
- Level 5—Non-urgent: needs treatment when time permits.

The patient has to wait for the availability of bed and nurse. Once they are assigned, each patient is called for a primary checkup. After that, the patient as an entity moves to the doctor for discussion and consultation. Based on the triage level and discussion, the patient is assigned a treatment strategy and laboratory tests if desired. Following the doctor's diagnosis, the patient has two options: either they undergo the test or receive immediate treatment. If the patient receives the test recommendation, there are, again, two possibilities: either they have a single test or multiple tests. If the patient has to take the tests, the treatment begins only after the results are known. The patient is either admitted to the inpatient department or discharged from the emergency department following their treatment. For further treatment, the patients which need to be admitted are required to wait till the availability of bed in an inpatient department. The bed remains occupied in the emergency department till the patient is moved upwards. The process flow established in the Arena for KKUH's emergency department is presented in Figure 2.

In Figure 2, patients quit the system after waiting for a certain period of time. With an increase in waiting times, the number of patients leaving the system keeps rising. Therefore, it is crucial to reduce waiting times through efficient scheduling and resource allocation in order to reduce the number of patients leaving the system and serve the greatest possible number of patients.

3.2. Resources

Considering the various phases that the patients have to undergo in the emergency department, doctors and nurses are regarded as resources. The distinct entities are defined for the doctor and nurse to perform interactions within the model. Each entity takes a set of resource states as it flows in the model; these states are waiting, assessment, evaluation, and treatment. After the nurse evaluates the patient, the doctor must be consulted to discuss the treatment strategy. In the developed model, each shift has consulting doctors. The doctor's job is to either treat patients or issue orders (such as for laboratory or radiology testing). This, in turn, determines the patient's course of action, including the decision of whether to pursue direct medical treatment, laboratory testing, radiography, or a combination of both tests before treatment. The doctor attends to patients who have the highest triage score on a high-priority basis and vice versa. Similarly, the model has two types of nurses, including triage and bedside nurses. Triage nurses perform initial assessment to determine a patient's urgency and establish a priority ranking based on that urgency or criticality. On the contrary, prior to the patient being seen by a doctor, bedside nurses perform a secondary evaluation of the patient. Additionally, bedside nurses participate in radiology tests and laboratory blood testing for high-priority patients. Also, they collaborate with doctors to determine the future course of action of a treatment plan. The emergency department is set to operate in three shifts. The following Table 1 lists the various resources that are currently allocated during each shift.

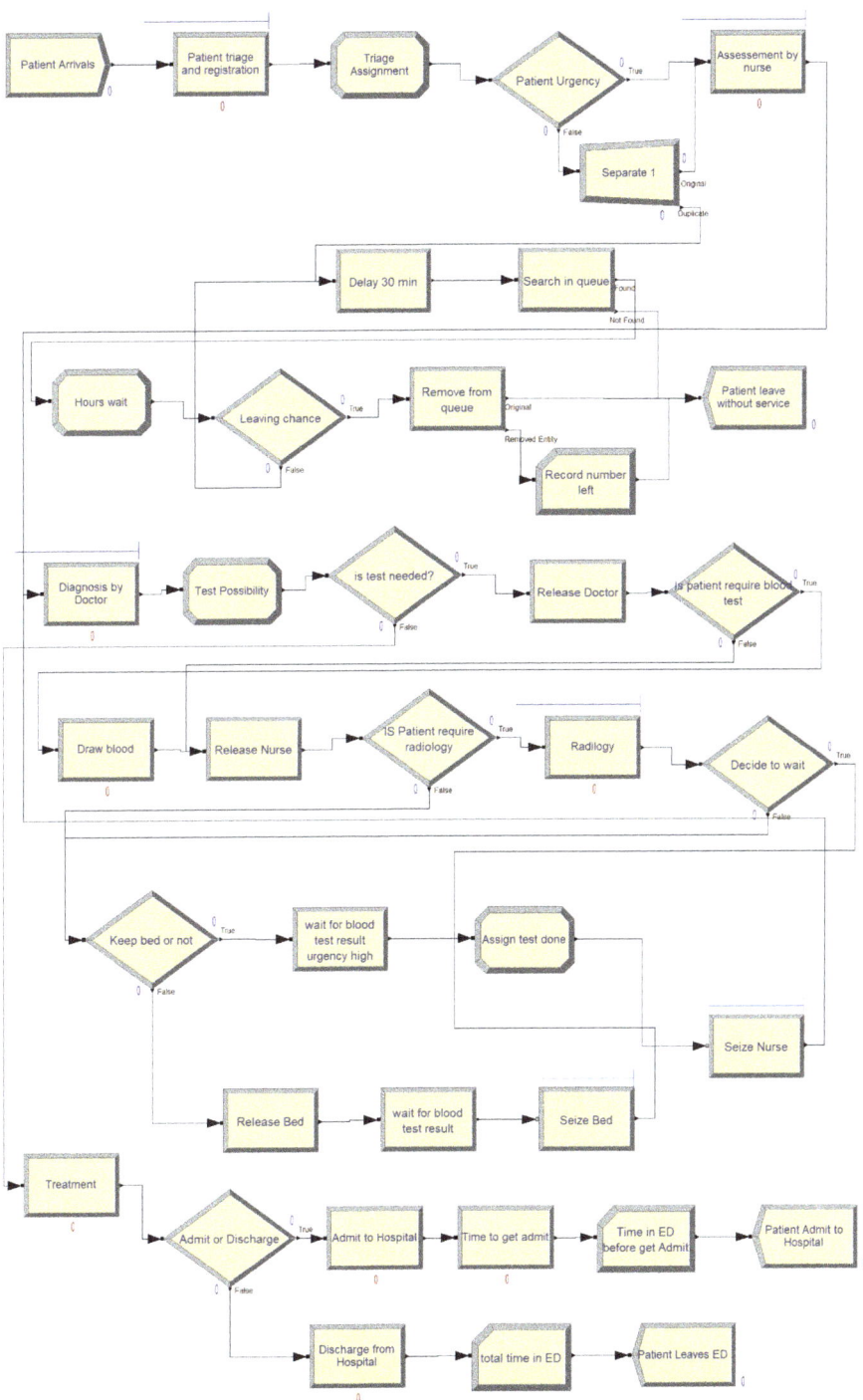

Figure 2. Emergency department process flow model in Arena.

Table 1. Current resource allocation in emergency departments.

	First Shift	Second Shift	Third Shift	Total
Doctors	1	4	1	6
Triage nurses	1	3	1	5
Bedside nurses	2	8	2	12
Radiologists	1	1	1	3
Beds		16		

3.3. Data Collection

The first step is the collection of data that is used as input to the model. The data described in Figure 3 are collected from hospital administration as well as through time study. The data are collected between 1 June 2022 to 29 July 2022. The arrival time of about 7000 patients is gathered from hospital administration. Similarly, a member of the research team conducted a time study in the emergency department to determine the service time of about 100 patients. Time spent on triage and nurse assessments, doctor diagnoses, discharge procedures, registration, blood tests, radiology, etc., are all estimated using the time study.

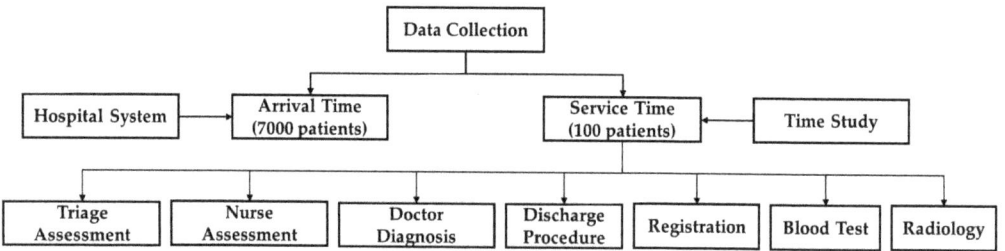

Figure 3. Data collection for the model.

3.4. Arrival Data

The hospital administrative database containing details related to visiting patients is utilized to generate the patients' arrival times and probabilities employed in the emergency department simulation model. The arrival of patients is based on a schedule, is updated hourly and daily considering peak and off-peak hours. Data are used from approximately 7000 patients, collected over a period of two months. The arrivals are spread out over each hour using a variety of distributions, as illustrated in Table 2.

Table 2. Hourly distribution of patient arrival.

Period	Distribution	Patient Arrival Expression	Squared Error
00:00–1:00	Exponential	EXPO (0.952)	0.015192
1:00–2:00	Exponential	EXPO (1.05)	0.003993
2:00–3:00	Exponential	EXPO (0.976)	0.001173
3:00–4:00	Exponential	EXPO (0.952)	0.000472
4:00–5:00	Lognormal	LOGN (0.66, 0.313)	0.000874
5:00–6:00	Exponential	EXPO (0.833)	0.009568
6:00–7:00	Lognormal	LOGN (0.742, 0.467)	0.025989
7:00–8:00	Lognormal	LOGN (0.557, 0.167)	0.001615
8:00–9:00	Exponential	EXPO (1.26)	0.006111
9:00–10:00	Normal	NORM (11.3, 5.77)	0.016496
10:00–11:00	Normal	NORM (20.6, 5.81)	0.023891
11:00–12:00	Normal	NORM (21.2, 5.89)	0.014977
12:00–13:00	Normal	NORM (22.6, 7.11)	0.020261

Table 2. Cont.

Period	Distribution	Patient Arrival Expression	Squared Error
13:00–14:00	Normal	NORM (18.1, 5.74)	0.026783
14:00–15:00	Normal	NORM (14.8, 4.87)	0.008851
15:00–16:00	Normal	NORM (18.8, 5.74)	0.018294
16:00–17:00	Uniform	UNIF (3.5, 26.5)	0.017746
17:00–18:00	Normal	NORM (6.57, 4.8)	0.023369
18:00–19:00	Exponential	EXPO (1.62)	0.003426
19:00–20:00	Exponential	EXPO (1.26)	0.01278
20:00–21:00	Exponential	EXPO (1.02)	0.001825
21:00–22:00	Exponential	EXPO (1.26)	0.013155
22:00–23:00	Exponential	EXPO (1.1)	0.002558
23:00–24:00	Exponential	EXPO (1.33)	0.006698

3.5. Triage Level and Percent Distribution

The nurse triages the patients as they enter the model. Patients are assigned a triaged score based on the nurse's initial evaluation. On a scale from 1 to 5, where 1 denotes the highest priority or most urgency and 5 denotes the lowest priority or least importance, the triaged score is established. Table 3 summarizes the percentage of arriving patients in each triage level and the Weibull expression for the triage time. This percentage is calculated using real data from the hospital.

Table 3. Number of patients for each triage level.

Triage Level	Number of Patients (%)	Cumulative (%)
1	1	1
2	15	16
3	56	72
4	25	97
5	3	100

Triage time distribution follows Weibull Expression as 1.5 + WEIB (4, 1.63), where error is 0.0024.

The same nurse performs patient registration once the patients are divided into categories according to their triage level. The triage and registration times are collected from a time and motion study ($n = 100$) undertaken in the emergency department for 24 h. The triage time and patient registration time, which are calculated for 100 patients, are distributed using the Weibull distribution. The distribution is satisfactory with a fitting error of 0.0024. This distribution os used as input data to the model in order to simulate the operation of the emergency department.

3.6. Probability of Patients Leaving Systems

The patient either waits in the queue or is examined by the nurse depending on the triage level. Patients with less urgent needs enter the queue. However, the number of patients leaving the system rises as waiting times increase. Table 4 summarizes the information about the number of patients leaving the system based on data gathered from the hospital. It is observed that during the first half hour, some patients are seen leaving the system after observing lengthy queues. Moreover, it is noticed that after 7 h, the number of patients leaving the system reaches saturation, with the cumulative percentage remaining at 33% through hours 8, 9, 10, and so on (refer to the following Table 4).

Table 4. Probability data of patients leaving the system.

Time (h)	Number of Patients Leaving per Hour	Percentage	Cumulative Percentage
0.5		Based on queue length	
1	2	2%	2%
2	2	2%	4%
3	4	4%	8%
4	2	3%	11%
5	6	6%	17%
6	9	9%	26%
7	7	7%	33%
8			
9		33% onwards	
10			

3.7. Probability of Laboratory Test Depend on the Triage Level

Following the doctor's diagnosis, the patient either undergoes the test or receives immediate treatment. If the patient has to take the test, the treatment begins only after the results are known. It is also observed that the number of patients undergoing tests or direct treatment depends on the triage level (refer to Table 5). In addition to the doctors, nurses, and test times, the model also incorporates the discharge procedure time as well as the admission time for in-patient treatment (in case the patient is asked to be admitted). The triage level has an impact on admission probability as well. For example, Triage level 1 patient would have an admission probability of 1, while the Triage level 5 would have an admission probability of 0 (refer to Table 5).

Table 5. The probabilities of the test and admission.

Triage Level	Probabilities		
	Blood Test	Radiology	Admission
1	0.85	0.80	1
2	0.75	0.10	0.54
3	0.50	0.50	0.20
4	0.20	0.30	0.15
5	0.01	0.20	0

3.8. Service Time Data

The patient is either admitted to or discharged from the hospital following their treatment. The patient's probability of being admitted to the hospital as estimated from administrative data is 0.27. The following Table 6 presents the distributions of various service time data used in the model.

Table 6. Characteristics of Inputs used in the model.

Input (Time in Minutes)		Distribution	Expression	Error
Assessment by the nurse		Triangular	TRIA (7.5, 9.73, 15.5)	0.001621
Diagnosis by the doctor		Normal	NORM (6.28, 0.873)	0.001433
Treatment	Triage levels 1 and 2	Triangular	TRIA (6.5, 8, 11.5)	0.006077
	Triage levels 3, 4, and 5	Normal	NORM (4.18, 1.13)	0.004335
Blood test		Normal	NORM (3.58, 0.681)	0.001122
Radiology		Triangular	TRIA (4.5, 9, 10.5)	0.013475
Discharge procedure		Normal	NORM (9.56, 1.26)	0.007743
Admission time to Inpatient		Exponential	5 + EXPO (102)	0.003841

3.9. Performance Measures

The model is established in order to reduce the waiting time, service time, and number of patients leaving the system. It also aims to optimize the number of doctors and nurses in the system with their maximum limit defined. The simulation run is conducted for a week in order to attain the desired results. Moreover, several scenarios are explored using the developed model, for example, a case of resource allocation being raised or optimized.

3.10. Model Initialization

A warm-up period of 24 h is used in the model to eliminate initialization bias. The warm-up period is acquired using Welch's approach [44] in this research. The number of runs is determined using the statistical method developed by Kelton [45]. After the model is run a predetermined number of times, the output data such as average, half width and standard deviation for all performance measures are collected in this step. Finally, the estimation of the number of simulation runs needed to achieve the 95% confidence level of accuracy is calculated using the statistical t-distribution approach. The estimated number of simulation runs for various performance measures are presented in the following Table 7. The results of statistical analysis indicate that a minimum number of 45 simulation runs for this model is required for meaningful results.

Table 7. Estimation for the number of runs in the model.

Item	Average	Half Width	STD	Required Half Width (Relative Error = 0.15)	No. of Runs Required	
					First Approximation (t)	Second Approximation (z) 95% Confidence Level
Patient triage 1 (wait time, h)	0.23	0.03	0.09	0.03	8.76	28.85
Patient triage 2 (wait time, h)	0.21	0.01	0.03	0.03	1.07	3.52
Patient triage 3 (wait time, h)	0.76	0.04	0.13	0.11	1.52	5.00
Patient triage 4 (wait time, h)	2.83	0.19	0.56	0.42	2.00	6.60
Patient triage 5 (wait time, h)	3.47	0.60	1.76	0.52	13.42	44.18
Patients leave without service	425.89	43.09	126.13	63.88	4.55	14.98

3.11. Model Validation and Verification

To validate and verify the number of hospital visits per week produced from the simulation model with those estimated using hospital data, the results were compared to ensure that the simulation model is accurate and validated. The outcome of the simulation model indicated that there are 1001.4 patients on average every week, with a half width of 34.52 and an SD of 114.93. Simulation results showed a 95% confidence interval that covers the calculated database average of 1016.2 patients each week. The overall flow, the analytical characterization of the arrival pattern, and the other processes in the model were all therefore confirmed by this experiment. Due to a lack of information in the hospital database, the simulation model's results for various performance measures were presented to professionals on the medical staff. Documentation of the model's structure, assumptions, and limitations were clearly explained to management and staff. The hospital management deemed all of the results to be reliable.

4. Goal Programming (GP) Model

The quality of care provided to patients can be ensured by having enough resources available in the department and ensuring that they are efficiently utilized. Goal programming is a linear programming technique that can be utilized to resolve multiple objectives by treating them as goals with target values and weight. It has, in fact, been widely utilized to simulate and solve scheduling-related issues in the healthcare system. For instance, Mohammadian et al. [46] used goal programming to address the issue of nurse scheduling in a large medical facility in Tehran. Similarly, Anna et al. [47] used the goal programming technique to establish the monthly work shift schedules of nurses, leading to more evenly distributed workloads. Additionally, Jerbi and Kamoun [48] implemented simulation and goal programming to reschedule the shifts of emergency department doctors in a Tunisian hospital. The goal programming model was designed to optimize and choose the most appropriate measures.

In this study, the objectives are to optimize the department resources levels in order to improve the overall efficiency and effectiveness. Therefore, goal programming is used to minimize the number of patients leaving the system without service, patient waiting time, as well as positive deviations from the number of doctors, number of nurses, and number of beds. This, in turn, minimizes the cost of operations in the emergency department of the hospital under consideration. Accordingly, an objective function is set (refer to Equation (1)), and corresponding constraints are defined (refer to Equations (2)–(7)). Weights w_1, w_2, w_3, w_4, w_5, and w_6 are varied to analyze their impact on the objective function. Percentage normalization of the weights is applied to normalize the OptQuest model.

$$\text{Minimize } Z = w_1 \frac{TL}{TTL} + w_2 \frac{\sum_{j=1}^{5} \frac{TW_j}{TTW_j}}{5} + w_3 \frac{d_3^+}{b_3} + w_4 \frac{d_4^+}{b_4} + w_5 \frac{d_5^+}{b_5} + w_6 \frac{d_6^+}{b_6}, \quad (1)$$

subject to

$$\sum_{k=1}^{3} D_k - d_3^+ + d_3^- = b_3, \quad (2)$$

$$\sum_{k=1}^{3} N_k - d_4^+ + d_4^- = b_4, \quad (3)$$

$$\sum_{k=1}^{3} TN_k - d_5^+ + d_5^- = b_5, \quad (4)$$

$$B - d_6^+ + d_6^- = b_6, \quad (5)$$

$$D_k, N_k, TN_k, B \geq 1, \quad (6)$$

$$d_3^+, d_3^-, d_4^+, d_4^-, d_5^+, d_6^+, d_6^- \geq 0. \quad (7)$$

In the above Equations (1)–(7),

w_i = weight or importance of goal i (i ∈ 1, 2...6);
TL = total number of patients that leave the hospital without service;
TTL = target total number of patients that leave the hospital without service;
TW_j = total waiting time in queue for Triage level j patients (j ∈ 1, 2...5);
TTW_j = target total waiting time in queue for Triage level j patients (j ∈ 1, 2...5);
b_i = target values for goal i (i ∈ 3, 4, ...6);
d_i^+ = positive deviation of goal i (i ∈ 3, 4, ...6);
d_i^- = negative deviation of goal i (i ∈ 3, 4, ...6);
k = number of shifts in the hospital emergency department (k ∈ 1, 2, 3);
D_k = number of doctors assigned in shift k (k ∈ 1, 2, 3);

N_k = number of bedside nurses assigned in shift k (k ϵ 1, 2, 3);
TN_k = number of triage assesment nurses assigned in shift k (k ϵ 1, 2, 3);
B = number of beds in hospital emergency department.

5. Results and Discussion

The simulation runs are performed for seven days and each run is replicated 45 times to eliminate any biases. The existing setting is treated as a base scenario (S0) to depict the current situation in the emergency department of KKUH. Subsequently, the base scenario simulation outcomes are assessed and reported to the hospital's emergency management. After a discussion with the management, as is customary, the hospital stuff suggested only increasing the amount of human resources, i.e., doctors and nurses to improve the set objectives. This option is treated as Scenario 1 (S1). It is evident that simply increasing the selective resources does not accomplish the set objectives. Thus, the only option ahead is to find the optimum level of all resources. The above-stated goal programming model is developed, and the OptQuest tool is used in combination with the simulation model. In Scenario 2 (S2), experiments utilizing OptQuest are conducted by assigning equal weights to all the set goals. Scenario 2 is implemented to ascertain how well the available resources or workforce level are being utilized. Scenario 2 also explores the trade-offs occurring between available resources, queues, waiting times, and the number of beds based on preferences. The most important management goals in the emergency department are reductions in waiting time and the number of patients leaving service. These goals are not completely met due to an equal weight strategy for all goals. Hence, after analyzing the outcome of Scenario 2 OptQuest simulation results, higher weights are applied to the most important objectives. This option of applying variable weights to a set of goals is treated as Scenario 3 (S3).

The simulation model is utilized to understand both the current scenario (or base scenario) and a number of potential improvements or scenarios. For the current scenario, as shown in Table 1, resources are assigned as follows. One doctor is allocated to the first shift, two doctors are assigned to the second shift, and three doctors are dedicated to the third shift. Similarly, there are two bedside nurses on duty on the first shift, eight on the second shift, and one on the third shift. Additionally, there is one triage nurse on the first shift, three on the second shift, and one on the third shift. The emergency department has a total of 16 beds. For the current scenario, an average performance evaluation of various measures across all replications is presented in the following Table 8.

Table 8. Performance evaluation of the current situation using the simulation model.

Performance Measure	Average Value	Half Width	Overall SD Across Replications
Patient waiting time to receive a bed	1.28 h	0.06 h	0.20 h
Total time spent in ED (in case patient is admitted)	4.07 h	0.07 h	0.22 h
Total time spent in ED (in case patient is discharged)	2.51 h	0.05 h	0.15 h
Patient waiting in queue:			
Total waiting time in queue based on triage level			
Triage level 1	0.23 h	0.03 h	0.10 h
Triage level 2	0.21 h	0.01 h	0.03 h
Triage level 3	0.75 h	0.04 h	0.12 h
Triage level 4	2.82 h	0.16 h	0.53 h
Triage level 5	3.36 h	0.53 h	1.76 h
Patient leaving queue:			
Total time spent in system before leave	2.02 h	0.08 h	0.28 h
Number of patients leaving	423	35	118

It is evident that for the base scenario, S0 (refer to Table 7), there is a significant scope for improvement if the resources can be allocated appropriately in different shifts. It can be seen that every performance metric exceeds the targets established in collaboration with hospital management. For example, the target number of patients leaving the system should be 200, but in the current situation, as indicated in the above Table 7, there are currently 423 patients departing the system without treatment. In a similar fashion, the target waiting time for all triage types of patients is set to less than 2 h, but in the current scenario, it is not satisfactory. Thus, improvements are recommended to address the current problem and each improvement is treated as a new scenario one by one. The outcomes of simulated scenarios are presented here, below.

The first improvement, as in Scenario 1, is the employment of additional doctors and nurses to the second shift when a greater number of patients are observed to be waiting in queue. In Figure 4, the number of patients waiting in queue at any given time can be observed. This is the recommendation given by the hospital administration, who believe that resolving the existing situation would require more resources, particularly more doctors and bedside nurses, during the second shift. Hospital management consistently believes that doctors and nurses are the most important people and focuses solely on the increase in the number of doctors and nurses, without considering all options and thoroughly assessing the system, which is never the right approach.

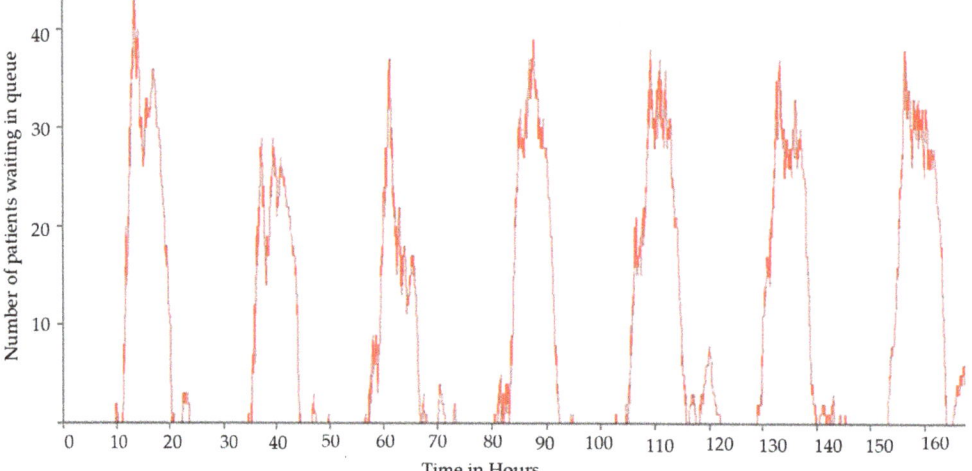

Figure 4. Number of patients waiting in queue for given time.

The hospital management recommends increasing the number of doctors and nurses working in the second shift by two and four, respectively. As indicated in the following Figure 5, the results are attained after the simulation model is run using the resource allocation plan suggested by hospital management. Figure 5 compares the base scenario, Scenario 0 and Scenario 1 for the two most important performance measures, i.e., the number of patients leaving the system and the total waiting time of the patients in the triages. Despite the fact that the number of patients leaving the queue drops from 423 to 380, it is still much more than the target value of 200. Similarly, no improvement is observed in patient waiting time in all triages. This shows that the amount of resources is increased, and, as a result, healthcare costs are also increased, yet no improvement is observed. This necessitates the deployment of an appropriate approach that can objectively produce the best results at a minimum cost. Thus, the only option ahead is to find the optimum level of all resources. As in Scenario 2, experiments utilizing OptQuest are conducted by assigning equal weights to all sets of goals.

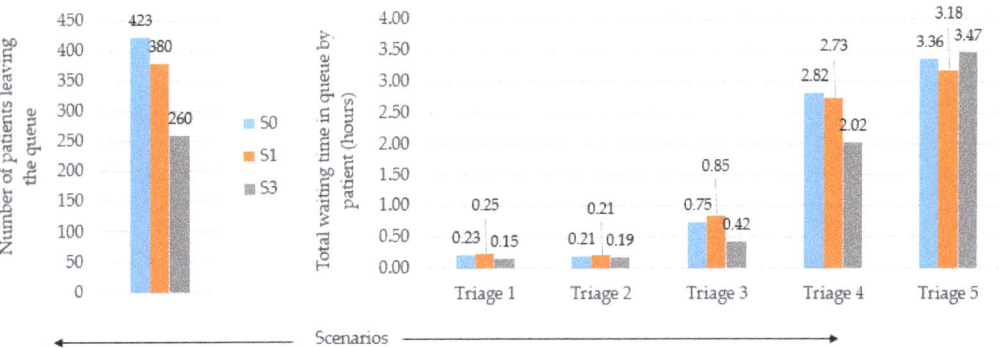

Figure 5. Performance measures for the base scenario, Scenarios 1 and 2.

In Scenario 2, OptQuest finds the best solution after nearly 700 different runs with various combinations of resource assignment, using equal weights for each goal. Table 9 below presents the OptQuest resource assignment for Scenario 2. It is observed that it recommends removing a doctor from the second shift and adding them to the third shift. It also suggests removing a bedside nurse from the first shift while proposing to add three bedside nurses and a triage nurse for total of four nurses to the third shift. It is evident from Figure 4 that a greater number of waiting patients becomes carried over to the third shift from the second shift, even though the arrival rate of patients in the third shift is very low compared to that of the patients in the second shift. Subsequently, comparative assessment of the base scenario and Scenario 2 is performed, and the obtained results are presented in Figure 5.

Table 9. Number of resources assigned for various scenarios.

Type of Resource	Shift Number	Assigned Number of Resources			
		Base Scenario, S0	Scenario 1	Scenario 2	Scenario 3
Doctors	1	1	1	1	1
	2	4	6	3	5
	3	1	1	2	4
Bedside nurses	1	2	2	1	1
	2	8	12	8	9
	3	2	2	5	4
Triage nurses	1	1	1	1	2
	2	3	3	3	3
	3	1	1	2	2
Beds		16	16	16	19

In Figure 5, it can also be noticed that the emergency department's performance in Scenario 2 is much better than it is in the base scenario. It is observed that both the number of patients leaving the queue and the average waiting time in triages for the patients are lowered by approximately 38% and 15%, respectively. In spite of this, Figure 5 also shows that the target for the number of patients leaving the system, which is set at 200, is not met. However, the target for waiting times in triages is met successfully in Scenario 2.

As these goals are not completely met due to an equal weight strategy for all goals, Scenario 3 is established in order to further enhance the emergency department's performance in order to meet the target for the number of patients leaving the queue. In Scenario 3, the total number of patients leaving the queue and the waiting times of the patients are given greater weight than other objectives. Table 9 displays the results and recommendations from Scenario 3. For instance, it is established that the emergency department needs to add three doctors for the third shift and one doctor for the second shift. Similarly, modifications in other resources from Scenario 2 to Scenario 3 can also be observed; refer to Table 9. It must be realized that Scenario 3 changes most of the resources instead of focusing on one or two resources, thereby allowing for effective and efficient resource allocation. The results shown in Table 10 re related to Scenario 3. It can be recognized that all of the performance indicators reduce noticeably. For instance, in comparison to the base scenario (refer to Table 8), the number of patients leaving the system falls by 61.70%, and the patient waiting time in the case of Triage 1 decreases significantly, by 86.95%. In addition, the desired targets of 200 patients leaving the queue and the patient waiting times in different triages are met. As a result, the need to consider all possible aspects is highlighted rather than presuming that a small number of them are accountable for inefficient operations.

Table 10. Scenario 3 simulation outcome with unequal weights.

Performance Measure	Average Value
Patient waiting time to receive a bed	0.48 h
Total time spent in ED (in case patient is admitted)	3.32 h
Total time spent in ED (in case patient is discharged)	1.83 h
Patient waiting in queue:	
Total waiting time in queue based on triage level:	
Triage level 1	0.03 h
Triage level 2	0.11 h
Triage level 3	0.28 h
Triage level 4	1.19 h
Triage level 5	2.12 h
Patient leaving queue	
Total time spent in system before leave	0.85 h
Number of patients leaving	162

Assessment of All Scenarios Using Process Analyzer

The objective is to perform comparative assessment of all of the four scenarios above. This process is conducted using the Arena process analyzer tool. For this, initially, the created model must be uploaded, inputs and outputs need to be added for examination, and the model needs to be rub in the process analyzer. In parallel, the experiment needs to be configured by defining the input parameter ranges, the number of simulation iterations, and other parameters. Thus, the process analyzer automatically runs numerous distinct scenarios and graphically compares the outcomes of various scenarios. It also helps to perform the assessment of the model modifications and their effects on system goals. The graph displayed in Figure 6 represents the outcome of the process analyzer in the form of box and whisker plots for each scenario, along with the minimum, maximum and median values.

From Figure 6, it is evident that for the performance measure of the 'number of patients leaving the emergency department without having service' reaches an average minimum level for Scenario 3 from that of the current scenario (or base scenario, S0). Similarly, the waiting time in hours for patients of all triage levels is gradually minimized from the current or base scenario to Scenario 3. Thus, it is proposed that there is a need to improve the current scenario to Scenario 3.

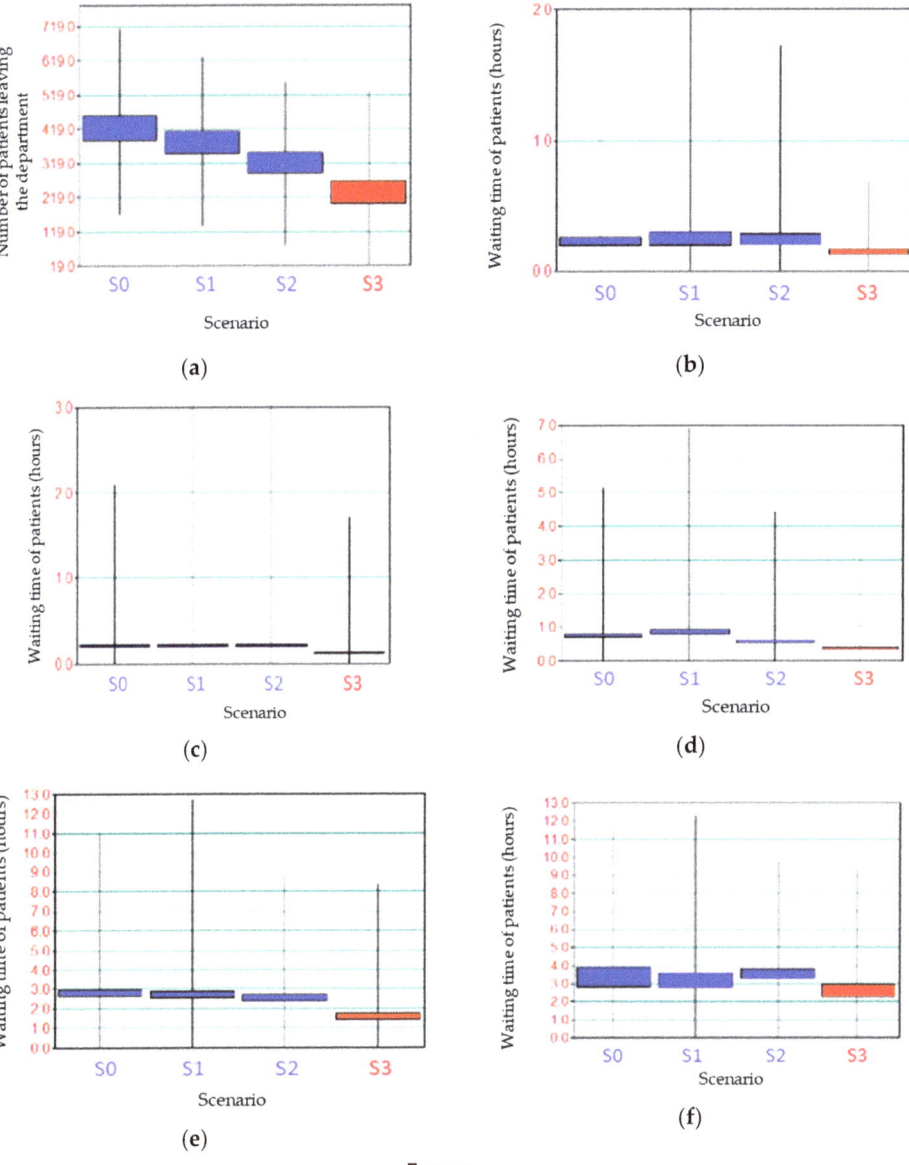

Figure 6. Performance of all scenarios. (**a**) Number of patients leaving the department without service; (**b**) waiting time of patients with Triage level 1; (**c**) waiting time of patients with Triage level 2; (**d**) waiting time of patients with Triage level 3; (**e**) waiting time of patients with Triage level 4; (**f**) waiting time of patients with Triage level 5.

6. Conclusions

The emergency department in any hospital has a vital role since it interacts with a number of patients every day. It performs numerous interactions between patients, employees, and other resources. Greater patient contentment and favorable hospital credibility depend on the emergency department operating responsibly and efficiently. Furthermore, its operational efficiency and performance depend on the number and allocation of the hospital's doctors, nurses, beds, and other resources. For example, any change in personnel (e.g., number of nurses or doctors, specific shift assignments) should be carefully considered based on system performance. As a result, it is crucial to provide or assign the proper number of resources to every shift. Prolonged waiting times driven by improper resource allocation have a significant negative impact on patient experience. Therefore, in this study, we explored the emergency department of a hospital in Saudi Arabia and offered recommendations in order to reduce patient wait times and the number of patients that leave the queue untreated. We built a detailed model in Arena and carried out goal programming. For this case, we observed that, if three additional doctors are assigned to the third shift and one to the second shift, the number of patients leaving the system without service decreases from 423 to 162. In a similar manner, for the current scenario, if two additional bedside nurses are added to the third shift and one additional bedside nurse is assigned to the second shift, as well as when an extra triage nurse is added to the first and third shifts each and the number of beds is increased from the 16 beds employed currently to 19 beds, a 61.7% drop in the number of patients leaving without service and a substantial drop in the waiting time for patients with all types of triage are observed. This highlights the fact that hospital management should focus on all available resources instead of emphasizing just one or two of them, because the developed model successfully portrayed the appropriate resource allocation required to improve customer/patient satisfaction levels.

Finally, it can be concluded that simulation and optimization could benefit the hospital by performing reallocation of the existing resources. The proposed model uses the simulation outcome as input to OptQuest and the goal programming model. The few research directions that the researchers can take into consideration for further advancement are as follows: incorporation of resource scheduling using genetic algorithms and/or simulated annealing and development of an artificial intelligence machine learning model to evaluate the performance of emergency departments at different dynamic staffing levels using the multiple simulation output from OptQuest. The authors aim to propose a more generalized model for emergency departments in future publications by incorporating more possibilities and specifics in the current model.

Author Contributions: Conceptualization, A.U.R., Y.S.U., S.H.M. and M.H.A.; methodology, A.U.R., Y.S.U., S.H.M. and H.A.; formal analysis, A.U.R., Y.S.U. and S.H.M.; investigation, Y.S.U. and S.H.M.; resources, A.U.R. and H.A.; data curation, A.U.R., Y.S.U., S.H.M. and M.H.A.; writing—original draft preparation, A.U.R., Y.S.U. and S.H.M.; writing—review and editing, A.U.R., Y.S.U., S.H.M., M.H.A. and H.A.; project administration, A.U.R. and M.H.A.; funding acquisition, A.U.R. All authors have read and agreed to the published version of the manuscript.

Funding: Deputyship for Research and Innovation, "Ministry of Education" in Saudi Arabia funded this research work through the project number (IFKSUDR_H105).

Institutional Review Board Statement: Not applicable.

Informed Consent Statement: Not applicable.

Data Availability Statement: All the data are available in the article.

Acknowledgments: The authors extend their appreciation to the Deputyship for Research and Innovation, "Ministry of Education" in Saudi Arabia for funding this research work through the project number (IFKSUDR_H105).

Conflicts of Interest: The authors declare no conflict of interest.

References

1. Rockwell Automation. Arena Simulation Software in Healthcare—Control Costs, Respond to New Regulations and Enhance Patient Experience. Available online: https://www.rockwellautomation.com/en-pl/products/software/arena-simulation/discrete-event-modeling/healthcare.html (accessed on 21 May 2023).
2. Vanbrabant, L.; Braekers, K.; Ramaekers, K.; Van Nieuwenhuyse, I. Simulation of Emergency Department Operations: A Comprehensive Review of KPIs and Operational Improvements. *Comput. Ind. Eng.* **2019**, *131*, 356–381. [CrossRef]

3. Lynn, S.G.; Kellermann, A.L. Critical Decision Making: Managing the Emergency Department in an Overcrowded Hospital. *Ann. Emerg. Med.* **1991**, *20*, 287–292. [CrossRef]
4. Lim, M.E.; Worster, A.; Goeree, R.; Tarride, J.-É. Simulating an Emergency Department: The Importance of Modeling the Interactions between Physicians and Delegates in a Discrete Event Simulation. *BMC Med. Inform. Decis. Mak.* **2013**, *13*, 59. [CrossRef] [PubMed]
5. Kozan, E.; Diefenbach, M. Hospital Emergency Department Simulation for Resource Analysis. *Ind. Eng. Manag. Syst.* **2008**, *7*, 133–142.
6. Sinreich, D.; Jabali, O.; Dellaert, N.P. Reducing Emergency Department Waiting Times by Adjusting Work Shifts Considering Patient Visits to Multiple Care Providers. *IIE Trans.* **2012**, *44*, 163–180. [CrossRef]
7. Ahmed, M.A.; Alkhamis, T.M. Simulation Optimization for an Emergency Department Healthcare Unit in Kuwait. *Eur. J. Oper. Res.* **2009**, *198*, 936–942. [CrossRef]
8. Chen, W.; Guo, H.; Tsui, K.-L. A New Medical Staff Allocation via Simulation Optimisation for an Emergency Department in Hong Kong. *Int. J. Prod. Res.* **2020**, *58*, 6004–6023. [CrossRef]
9. Zeltyn, S.; Marmor, Y.N.; Mandelbaum, A.; Carmeli, B.; Greenshpan, O.; Mesika, Y.; Wasserkrug, S.; Vortman, P.; Shtub, A.; Lauterman, T.; et al. Simulation-Based Models of Emergency Departments: Operational, Tactical, and Strategic Staffing. *ACM Trans. Model. Comput. Simul.* **2011**, *21*, 1–25. Available online: https://dl.acm.org/doi/10.1145/2000494.2000497 (accessed on 21 May 2023). [CrossRef]
10. Vanbrabant, L. Simulation and Optimisation of Emergency Department Operations. *4OR* **2021**, *19*, 469–470. [CrossRef]
11. Malik, M.; Šormaz, D. Data-Driven Simulation Model of Operating Rooms in Hospital. *Procedia Manuf.* **2019**, *39*, 371–380. [CrossRef]
12. Blake, J.T.; Carter, M.W. A Goal Programming Approach to Strategic Resource Allocation in Acute Care Hospitals. *Eur. J. Oper. Res.* **2002**, *140*, 541–561. [CrossRef]
13. Arenas, M.; Bilbao, A.; Caballero, R.; Gómez, T.; Rodríguez, M.V.; Ruiz, F. Analysis Via Goal Programming of the Minimum Achievable Stay in Surgical Waiting Lists. *J. Oper. Res. Soc.* **2002**, *53*, 387–396. [CrossRef]
14. Chouba, I.; Yalaoui, F.; Amodeo, L.; Arbaoui, T.; Blua, P.; Laplanche, D.; Sanchez, S. An Efficient Simulation-Based Optimization Approach for Improving Emergency Department Performance. In *Studies in Health Technology and Informatics*; IOS Press: Amsterdam, The Netherlands, 2019; Volume 264, pp. 1939–1940. [CrossRef]
15. Feng, Y.-Y.; Wu, I.-C.; Chen, T.-L. Stochastic Resource Allocation in Emergency Departments with a Multi-Objective Simulation Optimization Algorithm. *Health Care Manag. Sci.* **2017**, *20*, 55–75. [CrossRef] [PubMed]
16. Storrow, A.B.; Zhou, C.; Gaddis, G.; Han, J.H.; Miller, K.; Klubert, D.; Laidig, A.; Aronsky, D. Decreasing Lab Turnaround Time Improves Emergency Department Throughput and Decreases Emergency Medical Services Diversion: A Simulation Model. *Acad. Emerg. Med.* **2008**, *15*, 1130–1135. [CrossRef] [PubMed]
17. Moslehi, S.; Masoumi, G.; Barghi-Shirazi, F. Benefits of Simulation-Based Education in Hospital Emergency Departments: A Systematic Review. *J. Educ. Health Promot.* **2022**, *11*, 40. [CrossRef]
18. Bahari, A.; Asadi, F. A Simulation Optimization Approach for Resource Allocation in an Emergency Department Healthcare Unit. *Glob. Heart* **2020**, *15*, 14. [CrossRef]
19. Yeh, J.-Y.; Lin, W.-S. Using Simulation Technique and Genetic Algorithm to Improve the Quality Care of a Hospital Emergency Department. *Expert Syst. Appl.* **2007**, *32*, 1073–1083. [CrossRef]
20. Oddoye, J.P.; Jones, D.F.; Tamiz, M.; Schmidt, P. Combining Simulation and Goal Programming for Healthcare Planning in a Medical Assessment Unit. *Eur. J. Oper. Res.* **2009**, *193*, 250–261. [CrossRef]
21. Silva, E.; Pereira, M.F.; Vieira, J.T.; Ferreira-Coimbra, J.; Henriques, M.; Rodrigues, N.F. Predicting Hospital Emergency Department Visits Accurately: A Systematic Review. *Int. J. Health Plan. Manag.* **2023**, *38*, 904–917. [CrossRef]
22. Rostami-Tabar, B.; Ziel, F. Anticipating Special Events in Emergency Department Forecasting. *Int. J. Forecast.* **2022**, *38*, 1197–1213. [CrossRef]
23. Cabrera, E.; Taboada, M.; Iglesias, M.L.; Epelde, F.; Luque, E. Simulation Optimization for Healthcare Emergency Departments. *Procedia Comput. Sci.* **2012**, *9*, 1464–1473. [CrossRef]
24. Rerkjirattikal, P.; Huynh, V.-N.; Olapiriyakul, S.; Supnithi, T. A Goal Programming Approach to Nurse Scheduling with Individual Preference Satisfaction. *Math. Probl. Eng.* **2020**, *2020*, e2379091. [CrossRef]
25. Castanheira-Pinto, A.; Gonçalves, B.S.; Lima, R.M.; Dinis-Carvalho, J. Modeling, Assessment and Design of an Emergency Department of a Public Hospital through Discrete-Event Simulation. *Appl. Sci.* **2021**, *11*, 805. [CrossRef]
26. Roh, T.; Quinones-Avila, V.; Campbell, R.L.; Melin, G.; Pasupathy, K.S. Evaluation of interventions for psychiatric care: A simulation study of the effect on emergency departments. In Proceedings of the 2018 Winter Simulation Conference (WSC), Gothenburg, Sweden, 9–12 December 2018; pp. 2507–2517.
27. Zhang, L.; Kill, C.; Jerrentrup, A.; Baer, F.; Amberg, B.; Nickel, S. Improving quality of care in a multidisciplinary emergency department by the use of simulation optimization: Preliminary results. In Proceedings of the 2018 Winter Simulation Conference (WSC), Gothenburg, Sweden, 9–12 December 2018; pp. 2518–2529.
28. Moustaid, E.; Meijer, S. A System Approach to Study Waiting Times at Emergency Departments in Metropolitan Environments. In Proceedings of the 2019 Winter Simulation Conference (WSC), National Harbor, MD, USA, 8–11 December 2019; pp. 996–1007.

29. Swan, B.; Ozaltin, O.; Hilburn, S.; Gignac, E.; McCammon, G. Evaluating an Emergency Department Care Redesign: A Simulation Approach. In Proceedings of the 2019 Winter Simulation Conference (WSC), National Harbor, MD, USA, 8–11 December 2019; pp. 1137–1147.
30. Harper, A.; Mustafee, N.; Yearworth, M. The Issue of Trust and Implementation of Results in Healthcare Modeling and Simulation Studies. In Proceedings of the 2022 Winter Simulation Conference (WSC), Singapore, 11–14 December 2022; pp. 1104–1115.
31. Kar, E.; Eldabi, T.; Fakhimi, M. Hybrid Simulation in Healthcare: A Review of the Literature. In Proceedings of the 2022 Winter Simulation Conference (WSC), Singapore, 11–14 December 2022; pp. 1211–1222.
32. Philip, A.M.; Prasannavenkatesan, S.; Mustafee, N. Simulation Modelling of Hospital Outpatient Department: A Review of the Literature and Bibliometric Analysis. *Simulation* **2023**, *99*, 573–597. [CrossRef]
33. Laker, L.F.; Torabi, E.; France, D.J.; Froehle, C.M.; Goldlust, E.J.; Hoot, N.R.; Kasaie, P.; Lyons, M.S.; Barg-Walkow, L.H.; Ward, M.J.; et al. Understanding Emergency Care Delivery through Computer Simulation Modeling. *Acad. Emerg. Med.* **2018**, *25*, 116–127. [CrossRef]
34. Harper, A.; Mustafee, N. A Hybrid Modelling Approach Using Forecasting and Real-Time Simulation to Prevent Emergency Department Overcrowding. In Proceedings of the 2019 Winter Simulation Conference (WSC), National Harbor, MD, USA, 8–11 December 2019; pp. 1208–1219.
35. Tang, S.; McDonald, S.; Furmaga, J.; Piel, C.; Courtney, M.; Diercks, D.; Cordova, A.R. 185 Data-Driven Staffing Decision-Making at an Emergency Department in Response to COVID-19. *Ann. Emerg. Med.* **2020**, *76*, S71–S72. [CrossRef]
36. Prabhu, V.G.; Taaffe, K.; Pirrallo, R.; Jackson, W.; Ramsay, M. Physician Shift Scheduling to Improve Patient Safety and Patient Flow in the Emergency Department. In Proceedings of the 2021 Winter Simulation Conference (WSC), Phoenix, AZ, USA, 12–15 December 2021; pp. 1–12.
37. Doudareva, E.; Carter, M. Using Discrete Event Simulation to Improve Performance At Two Canadian Emergency Departments. In Proceedings of the 2021 Winter Simulation Conference (WSC), Phoenix, AZ, USA, 12–15 December 2021; pp. 1–12.
38. Mustafee, N.; Powell, J.H.; Martin, S.; Fordyce, A.; Harper, A. *Investigating the Use of Real-Time Data in Nudging Patients' Emergency Department (ED) Attendance Behaviour*; Society for Modeling and Simulation International: San Diego, CA, USA, 2017.
39. Harper, A.; Mustafee, N. Participatory Design Research for the Development of Real-Time Simulation Models in Healthcare. *Health Syst.* **2023**, 1–12. [CrossRef]
40. Prabhu, V.G.; Taaffe, K.; Shehan, M.; Pirrallo, R.; Jackson, W.; Ramsay, M.; Hobbs, J. How Does Imaging Impact Patient Flow in Emergency Departments? In Proceedings of the 2022 Winter Simulation Conference (WSC), Singapore, 11–14 December 2022; pp. 961–972.
41. Su, B.; Kwak, J.; Pourghaderi, A.R.; Lees, M.H.; Tan, K.B.K.; Loo, S.Y.; Chua, I.S.Y.; Quah, J.L.J.; Cai, W.; Ong, M.E.H. Simulation-Based Analysis of Evacuation Elevator Allocation for a Multi-Level Hospital Emergency Department. In Proceedings of the 2022 Winter Simulation Conference (WSC), Singapore, 11–14 December 2022; pp. 358–369.
42. Abourraja, M.N.; Marzano, L.; Raghothama, J.; Asl, A.B.; Darwich, A.S.; Meijer, S.; Lethvall, S.; Falk, N. A Data-Driven Discrete Event Simulation Model to Improve Emergency Department Logistics. In Proceedings of the 2022 Winter Simulation Conference (WSC), Singapore, 11–14 December 2022; pp. 748–759.
43. Su, B.; Kwak, J.; Pourghaderi, A.R.; Lees, M.H.; Tan, K.B.K.; Loo, S.Y.; Chua, I.S.Y.; Quah, J.L.J.; Cai, W.; Ong, M.E.H. A Model-Based Analysis of Evacuation Strategies in Hospital Emergency Departments. In Proceedings of the 2021 Winter Simulation Conference (WSC), Phoenix, AZ, USA, 12–15 December 2021; pp. 1–12.
44. Heidelberger, P.; Welch, P.D. Simulation Run Length Control in the Presence of an Initial Transient. *Oper. Res.* **1983**, *31*, 1109–1144. [CrossRef]
45. Kelton, D.V. *Simulation with Arena*, 5th ed.; International Economy Edition; Mc Graw Hill: New York, NY, USA, 2010. Available online: https://www.amazon.com/Simulation-Arena-Kelton-International-Economy/dp/1259098605 (accessed on 12 March 2023).
46. Mohammadian, M.; Babaei, M.; Amin Jarrahi, M.; Anjomrouz, E. Scheduling Nurse Shifts Using Goal Programming Based on Nurse Preferences: A Case Study in an Emergency Department. *Int. J. Eng.* **2019**, *32*, 954–963. [CrossRef]
47. Anna, I.D.; Cahyadi, I.; Sandiayani, F. Scheduling of Nurse's Work Shift of Emergency Room Unit Using Goal Programming. In Proceedings of the 2021 IEEE 7th Information Technology International Seminar (ITIS), Surabaya, Indonesia, 6–8 October 2021; pp. 1–6.
48. Jerbi, B.; Kamoun, H. Using Simulation and Goal Programming to Reschedule Emergency Department Doctors' Shifts: Case of a Tunisian Hospital. *J. Simul.* **2009**, *3*, 211–219. [CrossRef]

Disclaimer/Publisher's Note: The statements, opinions and data contained in all publications are solely those of the individual author(s) and contributor(s) and not of MDPI and/or the editor(s). MDPI and/or the editor(s) disclaim responsibility for any injury to people or property resulting from any ideas, methods, instructions or products referred to in the content.

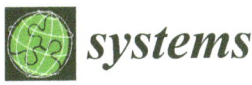

Article

Evaluating the Impact of Increased Dispensing of Opioid Agonist Therapy Take-Home Doses on Treatment Retention and Opioid-Related Harm among Opioid Agonist Therapy Recipients: A Simulation Study

Narjes Shojaati and Nathaniel D. Osgood *

Department of Computer Science, University of Saskatchewan, Saskatoon, SK S7N 5C9, Canada; narjes.shojaati@usask.ca
* Correspondence: nathaniel.osgood@usask.ca

Abstract: Modified opioid agonist therapy (OAT) guidelines that were initially introduced during the COVID-19 pandemic allow prescribers to increase the number of take-home doses to fulfill their need for physical distancing and prevent treatment discontinuation. It is crucial to evaluate the consequence of administering higher take-home doses of OAT on treatment retention and opioid-related harms among OAT recipients to decide whether the new recommendations should be retained post-pandemic. This study used an agent-based model to simulate individuals dispensed daily or weekly OAT (methadone or buprenorphine/naloxone) with a prescription over a six-month treatment period. Within the model simulation, a subset of OAT recipients was deemed eligible for receiving increased take-home doses of OAT at varying points during their treatment time course. Model results demonstrated that the earlier dispensing of increased take-home doses of OAT were effective in achieving a slightly higher treatment retention among OAT recipients. Extended take-home doses also increased opioid-related harms among buprenorphine/naloxone-treated individuals. The model results also illustrated that expanding naloxone availability within OAT patients' networks could prevent these possible side effects. Therefore, policymakers may need to strike a balance between expanding access to OAT through longer-duration take-home doses and managing the potential risks associated with increased opioid-related harms.

Keywords: agent-based modelling; opioid agonist therapy; COVID-19-related public health order; methadone; buprenorphine/naloxone; retention in opioid agonist therapy; opioid-related harms

1. Introduction

Opioid agonist therapy (OAT) utilizes methadone or buprenorphine/naloxone to prevent withdrawal in individuals exhibiting opioid use disorder (OUD) [1–3] and elevate treatment retention, as achieving this goal is linked with a decreased risk of suffering from an overdose [3,4]. However, due to its low treatment retention rate, OAT is often underutilized [5–9]. OAT recipients are required to frequently visit their prescribing doctors until they qualify for an increased dispensing of opioid agonist therapy take-home doses. Under these circumstances, many patients either decline treatment or are not retained in the treatment for sufficiently long enough to secure approval for graduated numbers of their take-home doses [9,10].

In the context of COVID-19-related healthcare delivery modifications [11], in some jurisdictions, regular access to OAT and retention in treatment were further disrupted [12,13], raising the risk of overdose and death for individuals who discontinue OAT [3,13]. This pandemic experience calls for procedures and policies that guarantee constant access to OAT. New guidance for expanded access to OAT during the COVID-19 pandemic was approved across several countries, including in the US and Canada [14,15]. In Ontario, this guidance supported an increase in the number of take-home doses for individuals who may have been eligible under the existing treatment guidelines [15]. Expanded access to OAT during the COVID-19 pandemic may lead to a high treatment adherence [16,17]. However, it is not clear whether this new guideline for administering higher take-home doses of OAT will still be beneficial as the world moves beyond the unique circumstances of the COVID-19 pandemic.

Methadone and buprenorphine/naloxone are both opioid agonist medications used in the treatment of opioid addiction. Methadone, a synthetic opioid agonist medication, has a long-lasting effect and helps alleviate withdrawal symptoms and reduce cravings [18]. Buprenorphine/naloxone is an oral medication that combines buprenorphine and naloxone, with a higher concentration of buprenorphine compared to naloxone. Buprenorphine acts as a partial opioid agonist, helping to reduce withdrawal symptoms and cravings, while the naloxone in buprenorphine/naloxone serves as a deterrent against misuse. When taken orally as prescribed, naloxone has a limited impact due to poor absorption in the gastrointestinal tract. However, if buprenorphine/naloxone is misused via injections, naloxone becomes active and can block the effects of other opioids as a result [19]. In emergency situations that require the rapid reversal of an opioid overdose, naloxone, as a potent opioid antagonist on its own, is typically administered via routes such as intranasal, intramuscular, intravenous, or subcutaneous means. These routes facilitate faster absorption rates and immediate effects, allowing for a more rapid response to the medication and effectively reversing the overdose. Hence, considering the differences in the concentrations of buprenorphine and naloxone within this combination and administration method, the naloxone present in buprenorphine/naloxone is insufficient to effectively reverse an overdose on its own [20].

Computational simulation models [21] are efficient tools for evaluating the possible effects of different intervention strategies and are used for better understanding the mechanisms underlying the observed trends. Agent-based modelling [22] is one of the primary types of computational simulation methods employed in the field of public health, with that choice being generally being dependent on the research question and the scope of the respective study. Agent-based models can highlight heterogeneous properties with ease, reflect individual-level behaviours, and generate potential health consequences and histories as a result of such behaviours. Although there are several simulation models that exist for studying OAT [23–29], the current study is the first agent-based model simulation to assess the impact of increased dispensing of take-home doses of OAT utilizing data sources from Canadian OAT recipients. In the present study, an agent-based model can capture a clear understanding of the trajectory of patients using methadone or buprenorphine/naloxone for OAT and investigate the potential effects of administering higher take-home doses of OAT on treatment retention and opioid-related harms among OAT recipients.

The primary objectives of this study were to evaluate the impact of increased dispensing of take-home doses of methadone and buprenorphine/naloxone on treatment retention and opioid-related harm among OAT recipients, and to examine the health consequences of whether the new guidelines for administering higher take-home doses of OAT should be continued in the future. Furthermore, this study aimed to investigate the effect of fostering a supportive environment within OAT communities. While previous research has documented varying effects of peers on individuals undergoing opioid agonist treatment, such as deterring prescription refills [30,31] or, conversely, providing assistance during overdose events to reduce opioid-related harm [32,33], the secondary objective of this study was to explore the effects of promoting a peer support network within OAT communities, with a specific focus on the involvement of naloxone-equipped peers during opioid overdose emergencies [34,35]. The remainder of this paper is organized as follows: Section 2 describes the model, including agent-based modelling, and the experimental design. Section 3 elucidates the results. Section 4 includes the corresponding discussion and concludes the paper.

2. Materials and Methods

The impact of the clinical decision to increase the number of take-home doses of OAT and patient outcomes among OAT recipients was investigated using an agent-based model. This study presents the dynamics of individuals' behaviors actively treated with OAT (methadone or buprenorphine/naloxone). Data for the agent-based model presented in this work was obtained from a detailed study from the Institute for Clinical Evaluative Sciences (ICES) [36], which captured many relevant health variables for Ontario residents [17]. The simulation software AnyLogic Version 8.8.0 [37] was used to create the model.

2.1. Agent-Based Modelling

The use of agent-based modelling in this study supports scenario-based assessments of the impact of the increase in the dispensing of OAT take-home doses on treatment retention and opioid-related harms among individuals receiving daily or weekly dispensed OAT. The model used in this study featured a single type of agent, representing an individual experiencing an opioid use disorder (OUD).

Within the model, individuals experiencing opioid use disorder were endowed with sociodemographic characteristics that influence their possible peer network, including the location of residence (urban or suburb) and neighborhood income quintile. OUD behaviour is governed using two state charts which are depicted in Figure 1. These state charts characterize the possible state space for individuals experiencing OUD whether they are undergoing treatment or not.

The treatment state chart represents the dynamics of the treatment options available for each individual experiencing an OUD. Individuals experiencing an OUD are out of treatment if they never choose a treatment or have discontinued the previous one. An individual who has never previously entered treatment can choose either methadone or buprenorphine/naloxone treatment. Further, patients are dispensed OAT in a daily or weekly manner, which is equivalent to a one-day supply or 5–6 days supply for all prescriptions, respectively. Individuals are classified among these four groups based on historical distributions [17]. During each visit to a physician for OAT, individuals who do not possess naloxone have the opportunity to obtain a naloxone kit, which can be used to assist their peers in the event of an opioid overdose.

Every patient in these four subsets of treatment have the potential to experience treatment disruption. The model treats such disruptions as being of two types: gaps in therapy from 5 to 14 days, respectively, are classed as interruptions, while those of more than 14 days are termed as treatment discontinuations and lead the patient to enter the out-of-treatment state. There are specific hazard rates governing individuals in each treatment type and leading to occurrence of an opioid overdose, opioid-related death, and all-cause death based on historical data [17]. Treatment retention is viewed as having been successfully achieved when the patient enters the post-treatment state after 6 months of therapy without any interruptions.

The illicit opioid use status state chart reflects the various illicit opioid use stages determined by treatment through which each OAT recipient progresses, including uncontrolled illicit opioid use, restricted opioid use while under treatment, and stopping illicit opioid use while in a post-treatment stage. While an OAT recipient is in an in-treatment restriction state, they have a probability of being deemed eligible for dispensing of increased take-home doses of OAT, based on historical distributions [17].

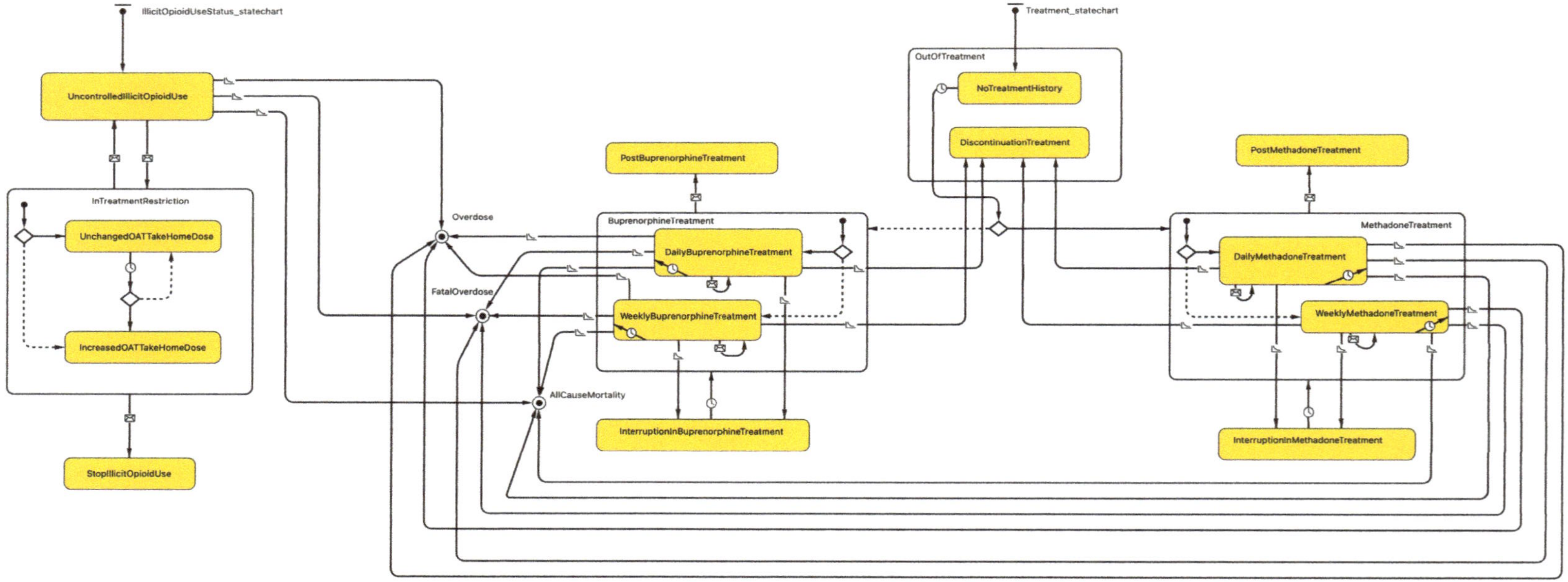

Figure 1. Patient receiving OAT state chart structure. When viewed in a landscape mode, the treatment state chart is positioned to the **right** while the illicit opioid use status state chart is to the **left**.

Among the daily buprenorphine/naloxone recipients without any change in their dose status, they are required to make daily visits to the clinic to receive their dispensed take-home doses. Additionally, for those with a change in their take-home dose status, their visits are scheduled every 14 days. Similarly, among the weekly buprenorphine/naloxone recipients with no change in their dose status, they are required to make weekly visits to the clinic to obtain their dispensed take-home doses. For individuals with a change in their take-home dose status, their visits are scheduled every 14 days. In a comparable manner, methadone daily recipients with no change in their dose status have daily visits to the clinic to receive their dispensed take-home doses. However, for those with a change in their take-home dose status, their visits occur every other day. Methadone weekly recipients without any change in their dose status make weekly visits to the clinic to receive their dispensed take-home doses. In contrast, for individuals with a change in their take-home dose status, their visits are scheduled every 14 days.

As policymakers may consider implementing targeted interventions or additional support measures for patients at a higher risk of opioid-related harms due to an increased dispensing of OAT, this study simulated the creation of a supportive peer network among patients to enhance the access to naloxone kits for overdose prevention. Therefore, considering agent heterogeneity and preferential attachment, a network was constructed with multiple disconnected components, wherein OAT recipients, regardless of changes in their take-home dose, have the potential to acquire a naloxone kit when attending to receive their dispensed OAT; that kit can then be used to reverse overdoses amongst other patients in their network.

2.2. Network

To simulate the possibility of a patient receiving naloxone administration from their peers in the case of an opioid overdose, a network exhibiting preferential attachment was implemented between patients. Within this network, it was assumed that an individual (ego) is always intended to connect with alters in the same location of residence, neighborhood income, and treatment type. In order to achieve this objective, the network construction process underwent two steps. First, an Erdos–Renyi network [38] was established connecting each ego with an average number of 15 candidate alters. Second, candidate alters that did not meet the desired criteria of having the same residence location, neighborhood income, and treatment type were then promptly removed, resulting in the formation of a network exhibiting a preferential attachment composed of multiple disconnected components. Figure 2 illustrates the distribution of the final network.

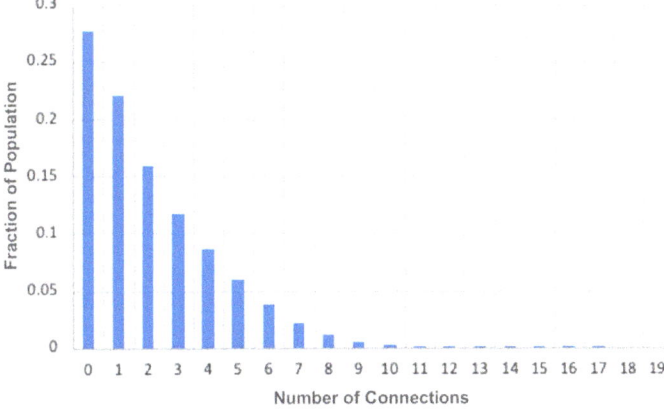

Figure 2. The degree distribution for each individual's social circle induced through the network construction process.

2.3. Outcome Measures

Primary model outcome measures were set as cumulative opioid overdoses, cumulative opioid-related deaths, and cumulative treatment retention among people treated with methadone or buprenorphine/naloxone over six months of treatment without any interruptions.

2.4. Parameterization and Validation

The model was parameterized with assumptions characteristic of the Ontario adult population experiencing OUDs and simulates a population of 50,000 individuals enrolled in OAT. The main source of data for parameterization was a published original investigation [17] which utilized the narcotics monitoring system database and the ICES repository to detect prescription claims for OAT in Ontario between March 2020 and October 2020, respectively.

Despite the uncertainties associated with the data values presented by the authors of [17], due to the restrictions in the study population, the potential influence of pandemic-related factors, and the possibility of changes in take-home dose dispensing patterns [17], these data deliver a significant level of value in informing for the current study. Table A1 presents a summary of the parameters for the patients receiving methadone or buprenorphine/naloxone treatment either on a daily or weekly basis and considers their eligibility for changes in take-home doses of OAT. The parameters were reported in terms of the rates per year and include opioid overdose, discontinuation and interruption of therapy, all-cause mortality, and opioid-related deaths that are based on the parameterizations postulated by the authors of [17]. Table A1 shows that—with the notable exception of weekly methadone patients eligible for increased take-home doses—methadone patients generally have higher opioid overdose rates compared to buprenorphine/naloxone patients. This suggests that buprenorphine/naloxone may have a lower risk of overdose compared to methadone, potentially due to its partial agonist properties. Table A1 also indicates that buprenorphine/naloxone patients exhibit higher rates of therapy discontinuation and interruption compared to methadone patients across different settings. This could be attributed to buprenorphine/naloxone being less effective for certain individuals in managing their opioid dependency along with the limited availability of buprenorphine/naloxone treatment providers and clinics. Additionally, within Table A1, in cases where the number of deaths among recipients was small (≤ 5), either all-cause mortality or opioid-related mortality was treated as 0.001. However, the all-cause mortality and opioid-related death rates generally appeared to be higher for methadone patients, particularly for those who were not eligible for increased take-home doses. The data presented in Table A1 was then utilized to specify the transition rates, such as the opioid overdose rate, discontinuation rate of therapy, interruption rate in therapy, all-cause mortality rate, and opioid-related death rate, for each of the two different methadone or buprenorphine/naloxone recipient sub-state charts depicted in Figure 1.

Table A2 provides insights into the socio-demographic factors related to the patients of interest, including their urban location of residence and neighborhood income quintile [17]. This table showcases the distribution of patients residing in urban areas across various treatment groups and their eligibility for increased take-home doses. The data presented in Table A2 reveals that the majority of patients, irrespective of the medication type, reside in urban areas. This may suggest a higher number of opioid users living under urban settings and potentially indicates that opioid treatment programs may be more accessible and concentrated in these areas. Further, in most cases (except for weekly methadone patients not eligible for increased take-home doses) methadone patients have a higher percentage of individuals from urban areas compared to buprenorphine/naloxone patients. This may reflect accessibility or availability advantages in securing methadone treatment across urban settings. Table A2 also highlights the distribution of patients based on their eligibility for increased take-home doses. In general, patients who are eligible for increased take-home doses tend to exhibit higher levels of urban dwelling compared to those who are not eligible. This finding suggests that increased take-home doses may be more commonly provided to patients living in urban settings, potentially indicating a higher likelihood of meeting the criteria for extending take-home doses among patients in urban areas. Additionally, Table A2 presents the distribution of patients based on neighborhood income levels. The declining percentage of patients as one moves from the lowest to the highest income category implies a potential lower prevalence of extensive opioid use and/or individuals seeking opioid agonist treatment in higher-income neighborhoods. When interpreting this result, it is important to consider the difference between the total population residing in the urban areas and rural areas. Additionally, the distribution of individuals across the different neighborhood income levels should also be considered. The data presented in Table A2 was utilized to define the custom distributions for the residence location and neighborhood income of the diverse agents in the model.

Table A3 provides an overview of the remaining parameters, which involve different treatment types, varying disposal timings, and the potential for changes in the disposal time [17]. The parameters listed in Table A3 were utilized as custom distributions to initialize the model and as parameters for implementing the interventions during model simulation. Furthermore, Table A3 includes parameters that are specifically relevant to opioid users outside OAT settings, for which the assumptions have been grounded in the relevant literature. These parameters, such as the opioid overdose rate per year, all-cause mortality rate per year, and opioid-related death rate per year, have been utilized to determine the transition rates in the illicit opioid use state chart, depicted as a sub-state chart in Figure 1.

Finally, the model underwent a thorough verification and validation process to assess its accuracy. Firstly, the assumptions made within the model were visually represented using state charts and possible transitions. This visual representation allowed for a clearer understanding of the assumptions and facilitated their evaluation for accuracy and coherence. The model's assumptions were then carefully articulated and validated against its code logic, ensuring that there were no discrepancies or errors between the assumptions and the code. Secondly, the model's emergent behavior was compared to real-world data to assess its accuracy. This step ensured that the model's outcomes closely matched the observed outcomes in the real world [17], increasing confidence in its validity. Thirdly, the coefficient of variation for treatment retention was found to be less than 0.05 for both treatment types, indicating a relatively low level of variation. Similarly, the coefficient of variation for opioid overdose in both treatment types and opioid-related deaths in the methadone treatment group was less than 0.20. However, due to the limited number of opioid-related deaths amongst the buprenorphine recipients (≤ 5), the coefficient of variation did not provide informative insights for this outcome in the buprenorphine group. By fulfilling these requirements, this model successfully passed our tests by demonstrating the clarity of its assumptions provided by the state charts and its alignment with real-world data [17].

2.5. Scenarios

Alongside the baseline scenario that examined the no extended take-home doses for OAT recipients across the 6-month treatment horizon, three scenarios were defined to explore the differential results of providing extended take-home doses for OAT recipients starting at various times of treatment. The number of eligible OAT recipients for extended take-home doses remained constant within these three scenarios, while the time of implementation of the extended take-home doses policy varied to begin with after the second, third, and fourth month of treatment, respectively. Furthermore, these three scenarios were combined with varying probabilities of OAT patients obtaining a naloxone kit during a physician visit (i.e., 5%, 10%, and 15%, respectively) to assess the impact of naloxone disposal within OAT patients' networks. For each scenario, an ensemble of 100 realizations was run, each with varying random seeds. Finally, percentage changes from the baseline for all three outcomes of interest were reported over the six-month treatment horizon.

3. Results

The baseline scenario posits approximately 10,500 individuals, which represents 20.8% of the OAT population receiving the six-month buprenorphine/naloxone treatment, while approximately 39,700 individuals comprising 79.1% of the OAT population receive the six-month methadone treatment, respectively.

Among the people treated with buprenorphine/naloxone, 1600 individuals representing 15.2% of this population received daily dispensed buprenorphine/naloxone while others received weekly dispensed buprenorphine/naloxone. Among people treated with methadone, 13,900 individuals representing 35.0% of this population received daily dispensed methadone, and the rest of the individuals received weekly dispensed methadone. With no additional interventions applied, the baseline scenario yielded approximately 80 opioid overdoses and 10 opioid-related deaths with the six-month buprenorphine/naloxone treatment, accounting for 0.7% and 0.09% of this population, respectively; in contrast, methadone treatment gave rise to a higher burden, with approximately 750 opioid overdoses and 70 opioid-related deaths having occurred during the six-month treatment period, accounting for 1.8% and 0.1% of this population, respectively. Finally, out of the population receiving the six-month buprenorphine/naloxone treatment, 7900 individuals, representing 75.4%, continued treatment without interruption and discontinuation for six months, thereby achieving a six-month retention with buprenorphine/naloxone treatment; in contrast, 30,800 individuals, which was equivalent to 77.5%, achieved six-month retention with methadone treatment. These results demonstrate the baseline distribution of OAT recipients across distinct types of treatment and disposal methods based on empirical data [17].

3.1. Individuals Receiving Methadone Treatment

Among the methadone-treated individuals receiving daily dispensed OAT, 8200 individuals, equivalent to 58.8% of this population, were eligible to transition to take-home doses, and among the methadone-treated individuals receiving weekly dispensed OAT, 18,700 individuals, representing 72.5%, were eligible to extend to 13 take-home doses.

3.1.1. Providing Extended Take-Home Doses among the People Treated with Methadone

Table 1 shows the six-month outcomes of interest for providing extended take-home doses among people treated with methadone within the successive time frames. Earlier permission for the provision of extended methadone take-home doses to eligible patients was found to exhibit a beneficial impact on all three outcomes of interest. Providing extended take-home doses among people treated with methadone increased treatment retention (by 2.8%, 2.0%, and 1.4% when permission for extended take-home doses was granted within the second month of treatment, the third month of treatment, and the fourth month of treatment, respectively). Furthermore, providing extended take-home doses among people treated with methadone decreased both the total number of opioid overdoses by 7.3%, 6.1%, and 3.5%, and the total number opioid-related deaths by 13.0%, 10.7%, and 6.9%, when permission for extended take-home doses was granted within the second month of treatment, the third month of treatment, and the fourth month of treatment, respectively. These results suggest that ensuring a guaranteed access to take-home doses of methadone as early as the second month of treatment can lead to higher treatment retention rates and reduce the harms related to opioids. This positive outcome may be attributed to reducing the barriers to accessing suitable methadone doses, providing relief from withdrawal symptoms and reducing cravings for methadone recipients.

Table 1. Results of providing extended take-home doses among people treated with methadone: six-month outcome percentage change from the baseline.

Policy	Change in Opioid Overdose (%)	Change in Opioid-Related Deaths (%)	Change in Treatment Retention (%)
Providing Extended Take-Home Doses after the			
Second month	−7.3%	−13.0%	+2.8%
Third month	−6.1%	−10.7%	+2.0%
Fourth month	−3.5%	−6.9%	+1.4%

3.1.2. Providing Extended Take-Home Doses and Expanding Naloxone Availability among People Treated with Methadone

Table 2 characterizes the six-month outcomes of interest arising from providing extended take-home doses and expanding naloxone availability among the people treated with methadone. Across all outcomes, the greatest impact was achieved with a 15% naloxone expansion combined with permission for the provision of extended methadone take-home doses granted within the second month of treatment. These results highlight the significant reduction in opioid-related harms when methadone recipients within the peer support network were empowered with readily available naloxone. By having naloxone readily available, methadone recipients can promptly intervene during an opioid overdose emergency for their peers, potentially saving lives and reducing the severity of harm.

Table 2. Results of providing extended take-home doses and expanding naloxone availability among the people treated with methadone: six-month outcome percentage change from the baseline.

Policy		Change in Opioid Overdose (%)	Change in Opioid-Related Deaths (%)	Change in Treatment Retention (%)
Providing Extended Take-Home Doses after the	Expanding Naloxone Availability by			
Second month	5%	−46.8%	−47.5%	+2.8%
Second month	10%	−58.5%	−61.4%	+2.7%
Second month	15%	−65.4%	−66.4%	+2.8%
Third month	5%	−46.8%	−47.8%	+2.0%
Third month	10%	−58.4%	−60.9%	+2.0%
Third month	15%	−65.3%	−66.2%	+2.0%
Fourth month	5%	−46.2%	−48.3%	+1.4%
Fourth month	10%	−58.3%	−59.9%	+1.2%
Fourth month	15%	−64.9%	−66.1%	+1.3%

3.2. Individuals Receiving Buprenorphine/Naloxone Treatment

Among the buprenorphine/naloxone-treated individuals receiving daily dispensed OAT, 700 individuals, representing 43.8% of this population, were eligible to transition to take-home doses, and among the buprenorphine/naloxone-treated individuals receiving weekly dispensed OAT, 6600 individuals, representing 74.3% of this population, were eligible to extend to 13 take-home doses.

3.2.1. Providing Extended Take-Home Doses among the People Treated with Buprenorphine/Naloxone

Table 3 shows the six-month outcomes of interest for providing extended take-home doses among the people treated with buprenorphine/naloxone within the successive time frames. Earlier granting of permission for the provision to extend buprenorphine/naloxone take-home doses to eligible patients has a small beneficial impact on treatment retention and a large undesirable impact on opioid overdose and opioid-related deaths. Providing extended take-home doses among people treated with buprenorphine/naloxone increases treatment retention (by 1.5%, 1.0%, and 0.7% when permission for extended take-home doses was applied within the second month of treatment, the third month of treatment and the fourth month of treatment, respectively). However, providing extended take-home doses among people treated with buprenorphine/naloxone also increased both the total number of opioid overdoses by 8.9%, 7.7%, and 3.9%, and the total number of opioid-related deaths by 3.4%, 7.2%, and 6.3%, when permission to use extended take-home doses was granted within the second month of treatment, the third month of treatment and the fourth month of treatment, respectively. These results suggest that ensuring a guaranteed access to take-home doses of buprenorphine/naloxone as early as the second month of treatment can lead to higher treatment retention rates. This finding suggests that when patients have the opportunity to receive take-home doses, they are more likely to remain engaged in their treatment program. However, this greater flexibility and convenience in managing their medication comes with some drawbacks for buprenorphine/naloxone recipients. The opioid-related harms tend to increase among this group, which may be attributed to the lack of direct monitoring of patients receiving buprenorphine/naloxone in OAT. Unlike methadone, buprenorphine/naloxone may be less effective in providing a long-term stability due to its pharmacological properties [39]; while not directly represented in the model, such factors may contribute to patterns reflected in the empirical data that are used to parameterize the model. Furthermore, individuals receiving buprenorphine/naloxone treatment who are experiencing a change in their take-home dose status are scheduled for visits every 14 days. This extended interval between visits may result in a loss of contact with healthcare providers, which could potentially contribute to an increase in opioid-related harms.

Table 3. Results of providing extended take-home doses among people treated with buprenorphine/naloxone: six-month outcome percentage change from the baseline.

Policy	Change in Opioid Overdose (%)	Change in Opioid-Related Deaths (%)	Change in Treatment Retention (%)
Providing Extended Take-Home Doses after			
Second month	+8.9%	+3.4%	+1.5%
Third month	+7.7%	+7.2%	+1.0%
Fourth month	+3.9%	+6.3%	+0.7%

3.2.2. Providing Extended Take-Home Doses and Expanding Naloxone Availability among People Treated with Buprenorphine/Naloxone

Table 4 shows the six-month outcomes of interest for providing extended take-home doses and expanding naloxone availability among the people treated with buprenorphine/naloxone. Even with a 5% naloxone expansion, a beneficial impact relative to the baseline would be achieved over all three different time frames of providing extended take-home doses. Achieving the best treatment retention and reducing both opioid overdose and opioid-related deaths has been made by a 15% naloxone expansion combined with an early (second treatment month) grant of permission for the provision of extended buprenorphine/naloxone take-home doses. When naloxone is easily accessible within the peer support network, it can be promptly administered during an overdose emergency. The timely administration of naloxone effectively counteracts the effects of opioids and restores normal respiration, thus reducing the risk of fatal outcomes associated with overdose incidents. Therefore, through empowering buprenorphine/naloxone recipients within the peer support network with readily available naloxone, the potential for reducing opioid-related harms is enhanced.

Table 4. Results of providing extended take-home doses and expanding naloxone availability among people treated with buprenorphine/naloxone: six-month outcome percentage change from the baseline.

Policy		Change in Opioid Overdose (%)	Change in Opioid-Related Deaths (%)	Change in Treatment Retention (%)
Providing Extended Take-Home Doses after the	Expanding Naloxone Availability by			
Second month	5%	−10.2%	−10.2%	+1.4%
Second month	10%	−19.9%	−21.7%	+1.6%
Second month	15%	−23.3%	−22.6%	+1.4%
Third month	5%	−13.6%	−15.8%	+1.4%
Third month	10%	−21.5%	−26.5%	+1.1%
Third month	15%	−25.9%	−32.8%	+1.2%
Fourth month	5%	−15.9%	−17.2%	+0.8%
Fourth month	10%	−24.4%	−21.9%	+1.1%
Fourth month	15%	−28.5%	−20.8%	+0.8%

4. Discussion

This simulation study of individuals receiving OAT in a context inspired by data from Ontario, Canada, suggests that facilitating methadone or buprenorphine/naloxone recipients' transition to take-home doses or receiving extended take-home doses would result in a higher treatment retention compared with the status quo. A crucial finding of this study was that expanding the access to take-home doses earlier during the subsequent six-month treatment period among OAT recipients is likely to elevate treatment retention. Th results further suggest that the use of these extended take-home doses would decrease the occurrence of opioid overdose and opioid-related deaths among methadone recipients. Meanwhile, among those prescribed buprenorphine/naloxone, the results suggest that extended take-home doses might increase the risk of opioid overdose and opioid-related deaths. Furthermore, these results suggest that expanding naloxone availability can mitigate the adverse effect of increased take-home doses guidance on opioid overdose and opioid-related deaths among buprenorphine/naloxone recipients.

The differences in the pharmacological properties of methadone and buprenorphine/naloxone may contribute to variations in the treatment outcomes that were seen in the empirical data used for model parameterization. Factors such as the duration of action, receptor binding affinity, and pharmacokinetic profiles could impact the treatment response and the risk of adverse events [39]. For example, the longer duration of action and higher receptor binding affinity of methadone [18] may result in a greater stability and decreased risk of overdose among those receiving extended take-home doses.

Alternatively, buprenorphine/naloxone has a shorter duration of action and a lower receptor binding affinity compared to methadone, which could reduce its effectiveness in providing a long-term stability. As potential contributors to relevant patterns in the empirical data used to evidence the model, these factors may contribute to the current observation in that an increased availability of the buprenorphine/naloxone outside of the clinic without close supervision may lead to a higher risk of opioid misuse, overdose, and their related deaths. Additionally, it is important to note that individual patient characteristics, such as tolerance levels, treatment history, and support systems, can influence these outcomes. The stability of patients in their treatment can also impact their response to the take-home doses.

Moreover, it is important to emphasize that individuals undergoing buprenorphine/naloxone treatment and undergoing a change in their take-home dose status are only required to attend clinic visits every 14 days. This prolonged gap between visits for all individuals undergoing buprenorphine/naloxone treatment with a change in their take-home dose poses a concern, as it may reduce the frequency of contact with their healthcare providers. The potential consequences of limited contact include a diminished opportunity to address any emerging challenges or concerns promptly, such as adjusting their medication dosage or addressing new risk factors.

The creation of supportive peer networks and the availability of naloxone have demonstrated promising results in preventing opioid overdose incidents due to several reasons. Firstly, supportive peer networks provide individuals in OAT with a sense of belonging and mutual support, which may enhance their treatment engagement and reduce the risk of relapse. Secondly—and in an effect captured in the model presented here—the availability of naloxone, a medication used to reverse opioid overdose, plays a critical role in harm reduction. When naloxone is readily accessible—including through such peer networks—it can be promptly administered during an overdose emergency, reducing the risk of fatal outcomes. By having naloxone readily available, one can act quickly to intervene and potentially save lives. The combination of supportive peer networks and naloxone availability creates a complementary approach to preventing opioid overdose incidents.

Patient-centered care for OAT recipients involves adapting the treatment and support services to meet the unique needs and preferences of each individual [12]. This study examined various aspects of patient-centered care, including the implementation of flexible take-home doses and the establishment of supportive peer networks. Reflecting the ability of patients to exercise a greater level of control over their treatment through flexible take-home doses and reduced challenges in weaving their dose administration into daily scheduling, this model captured a resulting increase in the treatment retention. Moreover, the creation of supportive peer networks, coupled with the availability of naloxone, demonstrated the potential to prevent opioid overdose incidents. In this context, concern has been raised in that the storage of a large quantity of OAT medication at home, particularly methadone, might place other family members or other co-domiciliaries at risk of opioid overdoses—a consideration that suggests the importance of promoting safe storage. Furthermore, there are specific criteria that must be met before providing patients with new or higher take-home doses, which adds to the complexity of these clinical decisions.

Several limitations of this study need to be noted. First, while the implemented agent-based model monitors the behavior of OAT recipients over a six-month treatment period informed using reported data and investigates the patterns of changes between the baseline and subsequent scenarios, it is essential to recognize that it does not employ a conceptual framework with distinct evidence-based rules for the full diversity of the causal mechanisms involved; indeed, the current state of evidence falls well short of what would be required to support such a representation. It is therefore particularly important to acknowledge that the main data source used in this model may still be subject to residual confounding, which can impact the reported results. Thus, it is advisable to interpret these findings with caution. Partly to support the incorporation of evolving evidence, the implemented model is accessible online. Beyond incorporating the updated parameter estimates, the availability of the model can further aid in refining the model structural assumptions with a refined theory. Second, it is important to note that the model simplifies the complexity of implementing and maintaining a peer support network among OAT patients in real-world settings. Establishing and maintaining a successful peer support network in practice requires a significant amount of effort and consideration of the diversity within the OAT population. Third, while the literature [3,40] suggests a potential for an elevated risk of overdose and mortality during the initial stages of methadone treatment, it bears emphasis that this model has not been parameterized to reflect this aspect of the context and does not report the timing of the events within the six-month treatment time frame. This limitation is primarily attributed to the constraints imposed by the currently utilized data sources. Finally, additional evaluations may be required to validate the findings thoroughly. For instance, in accordance with the empirical data, opioid-related rates, including overdose and deaths, were not excluded from the all-cause death rate for OAT recipients. Moreover, due to the potential changes in the levels of tolerance among OAT recipients over time, there are uncertainties regarding opioid-related harm rates outside of OAT. However, since these rates remained constant across all scenarios and that the amounts of opioid-related harm outside of OAT were not among the outcomes of interest for the current study, these limitations are expected to have only a minimal impact on the overall results. Moreover, the model was simplified by greatly limiting its representation of agent heterogeneity by virtue of employing overall empirical data, and the model does not account for disparities in the access to treatment services.

The findings of this study are in accordance with that of several other previous case studies [41–46] in suggesting that benefits can be secured if the modified guidance for administering higher take-home doses of OAT continues beyond the COVID-19 pandemic. Through implementing longer-duration take-home doses in methadone treatment programs, there is a potential to decrease the occurrence of opioid overdose and opioid-related deaths. To further address overdose incidents and prevent fatalities among OAT recipients, while also enhancing treatment retention, promoting the usage of naloxone among peers [34,35], and facilitating its accessibility without a prescription [47] may be effective.

Based on these results, policymakers may need to consider several factors when formulating or revising policies related to OAT. Policymakers may need to strike a balance between expanding access to OAT through longer-duration take-home doses and managing the potential risks associated with increased opioid-related harms, suggesting the value of conducting a thorough risk assessment and considering additional safety measures to ensure the well-being of patients. Moreover, policymakers may acknowledge that the benefits of longer-duration take-home doses vary among patients. They may underscore the significance of modifying treatment plans to tailor to individual needs and consider factors such as gender, income level, residential location, and treatment history when assessing a patient's stability and risk profile. This information might aid in determining the most suitable treatment duration and level of supervision for each patient. To achieve this aim, policymakers might place an emphasis on establishing robust monitoring and surveillance systems to closely monitor the outcomes and safety of OAT patients receiving longer-duration take-home doses. This could involve regular check-ins, adherence monitoring, and systems to promptly identify and respond to any concerning trends or adverse events. Finally, this study highlights that policymakers may benefit from collaboration among systems scientists, healthcare providers, and data custodians to further investigate the impact of longer-duration take-home doses on treatment outcomes and opioid-related harms. Such collaborations facilitate research and studies that aim to identify context-specific policy recommendations that are highly dependent on patient populations, local regulations, and existing guidelines.

Author Contributions: Conceptualization, N.S. and N.D.O.; methodology, N.S. and N.D.O.; software, N.S.; validation, N.S. and N.D.O.; formal analysis, N.S.; writing—original draft preparation, N.S.; writing—review and editing, N.S. and N.D.O.; visualization, N.S.; supervision, N.D.O. All authors have read and agreed to the published version of the manuscript.

Funding: This research received no external funding.

Data Availability Statement: The implemented model can be found at https://doi.org/10.5281/zenodo.8201137 (accessed on 31 July 2023).

Conflicts of Interest: The authors declare no conflict of interest.

Appendix A

Table A1. Summary of the opioid-related parameters for methadone and buprenorphine/naloxone treatment based on the study published by the authors of [17] used in the model parametrization: daily and weekly dispensing of OAT and eligibility for changes in take-home doses.

Parameter	Opioid Overdose rate (1/Year)	Discontinuation Rate of Therapy (1/Year)	Interruption Rate in Therapy (1/Year)	All-Cause Mortality Rate (1/Year)	Opioid-Related Death Rate (1/Year)
Daily methadone patients not eligible for increased take-home doses	0.095	0.636	0.239	0.013	0.005
Weekly methadone patients not eligible for increased take home doses	0.018	0.196	0.074	0.011	0.003
Daily methadone patients eligible for increased take-home doses	0.069	0.510	0.190	0.015	0.006
Weekly methadone patients eligible for increased take-home doses	0.014	0.141	0.051	0.008	0.001 *
Daily buprenorphine/naloxone patients not eligible for increased take-home doses	0.035	0.932	0.293	0.001 *	0.001 *
Weekly buprenorphine/naloxone patients not eligible for increased take-home doses	0.014	0.308	0.129	0.008	0.001 *
Daily buprenorphine/naloxone patients eligible for increased take-home doses	0.065	0.851	0.253	0.001 *	0.001 *
Weekly buprenorphine/naloxone patients eligible for increased take-home doses	0.017	0.260	0.095	0.008	0.001 *

* To deal with the statistical variability associated with small sample counts, a value of 0.001 is used when the reported number of deaths among recipients is less than or equal to 5.

Table A2. Summary of the socio-demographic parameters for methadone and buprenorphine/naloxone Treatment based on the study published by the authors of [17] used in the model parametrization: daily and weekly dispensing of OAT and eligibility for changes in take-home doses.

Parameter	Location of Residence	Neighborhood Income				
	Urban	One (Lowest)	Two	Three	Four	Five (Highest)
Daily methadone patients not eligible for increased take-home doses	88.7%	48.2%	21.5%	13.4%	10.2%	6.8%
Weekly methadone patients not eligible for increased take home doses	85.5%	41.3%	22.1%	16.0%	11.6%	9.1%
Daily methadone patients eligible for increased take-home doses	89.9%	39.4%	23.8%	16.0%	13.0%	7.8%
Weekly methadone patients eligible for increased take-home doses	88.1%	38.0%	24.4%	17.3%	12.3%	8.0%
Daily buprenorphine/naloxone patients not eligible for increased take-home doses	80.9%	48.8%	16.3%	15.6%	11.9%	7.4%

Table A2. Cont.

Parameter	Location of Residence	Neighborhood Income				
	Urban	One (Lowest)	Two	Three	Four	Five (Highest)
Weekly buprenorphine/naloxone patients not eligible for increased take-home doses	86.5%	34.0%	22.9%	18.6%	14.3%	10.2%
Daily buprenorphine/naloxone patients eligible for increased take-home doses	88.2%	39.5%	24.1%	14.9%	11.8%	9.6%
Weekly buprenorphine/naloxone patients eligible for increased take-home doses	86.5%	34.8%	24.4%	17.9%	12.6%	10.3%

Table A3. Summary of Remaining Parameters in the Model Parametrization.

Parameter	Values	Reference
OAT recipients' population size	50,000	Assumed
The number of OAT recipients in each treatment type (methadone and buprenorphine/naloxone)	Custom distribution	Parametrized [17]
The number of OAT recipients in each disposal timing (daily or weekly) across different treatment types	Custom distribution	Parametrized [17]
The number of OAT recipients considering their eligibility for changes in take-home doses across different treatment types and disposal timings	Custom distribution	Parametrized [17]
Rate of the opioid overdose per year for opioid users outside the OAT	Uniform distribution between 0.009 and 0.048, respectively	Assumed [17]
Rate of opioid-related death per year for opioid users outside the OAT	Uniform distribution between 0.0179 and 0.0562, respectively	Assumed [48]
Rate of non-opioid-related death per year for opioid users outside the OAT	0.001	Assumed [49]

References

1. Proctor, S.L.; Copeland, A.L.; Kopak, A.M.; Herschman, P.L.; Polukhina, N. A Naturalistic Comparison of the Effectiveness of Methadone and Two Sublingual Formulations of Buprenorphine on Maintenance Treatment Outcomes: Findings from a Retrospective Multisite Study. *Exp. Clin. Psychopharmacol.* **2014**, *22*, 424. [CrossRef] [PubMed]
2. Bruneau, J.; Ahamad, K.; Goyer, M.-È.; Poulin, G.; Selby, P.; Fischer, B.; Wild, T.C.; Wood, E. Management of Opioid Use Disorders: A National Clinical Practice Guideline. *CMAJ* **2018**, *190*, E247–E257. [CrossRef]
3. Sordo, L.; Barrio, G.; Bravo, M.J.; Indave, B.I.; Degenhardt, L.; Wiessing, L.; Ferri, M.; Pastor-Barriuso, R. Mortality Risk during and after Opioid Substitution Treatment: Systematic Review and Meta-Analysis of Cohort Studies. *BMJ* **2017**, *357*, j1550. [CrossRef] [PubMed]
4. Stone, A.C.; Carroll, J.J.; Rich, J.D.; Green, T.C. One Year of Methadone Maintenance Treatment in a Fentanyl Endemic Area: Safety, Repeated Exposure, Retention, and Remission. *J. Subst. Abus. Treat.* **2020**, *115*, 108031. [CrossRef] [PubMed]
5. Bell, J.; Strang, J. Medication Treatment of Opioid Use Disorder. *Biol. Psychiatry* **2020**, *87*, 82–88. [CrossRef] [PubMed]
6. Yarborough, B.J.H.; Stumbo, S.P.; McCarty, D.; Mertens, J.; Weisner, C.; Green, C.A. Methadone, Buprenorphine and Preferences for Opioid Agonist Treatment: A Qualitative Analysis. *Drug Alcohol Depend.* **2016**, *160*, 112–118. [CrossRef]
7. Williams, A.R.; Nunes, E.V.; Bisaga, A.; Pincus, H.A.; Johnson, K.A.; Campbell, A.N.; Remien, R.H.; Crystal, S.; Friedmann, P.D.; Levin, F.R. Developing an Opioid Use Disorder Treatment Cascade: A Review of Quality Measures. *J. Subst. Abus. Treat.* **2018**, *91*, 57–68. [CrossRef]
8. Timko, C.; Schultz, N.R.; Cucciare, M.A.; Vittorio, L.; Garrison-Diehn, C. Retention in Medication-Assisted Treatment for Opiate Dependence: A Systematic Review. *J. Addict. Dis.* **2016**, *35*, 22–35. [CrossRef]
9. Volkow, N.D.; Frieden, T.R.; Hyde, P.S.; Cha, S.S. Medication-Assisted Therapies—Tackling the Opioid-Overdose Epidemic. *N. Engl. J. Med.* **2014**, *370*, 2063–2066. [CrossRef]
10. Mancino, M.; Curran, G.; Han, X.; Allee, E.; Humphreys, K.; Booth, B.M. Predictors of Attrition from a National Sample of Methadone Maintenance Patients. *Am. J. Drug Alcohol Abus.* **2010**, *36*, 155–160. [CrossRef]

11. Canadian Institute for Health Information. *Overview: COVID-19's Impact on Health Care Systems [Story]*; Canadian Institute for Health Information: Ottawa, ON, Canada, 2023.
12. Corace, K.; Suschinsky, K.; Wyman, J.; Leece, P.; Cragg, S.; Konefal, S.; Pana, P.; Barrass, S.; Porath, A.; Hutton, B. Evaluating How Has Care Been Affected by the Ontario COVID-19 Opioid Agonist Treatment Guidance: Patients' and Prescribers' Experiences with Changes in Unsupervised Dosing. *Int. J. Drug Policy* **2022**, *102*, 103573. [CrossRef] [PubMed]
13. Ahamad, K.; Bach, P.; Brar, R.; Chow, N.; Coll, N.; Compton, M.; Hering, R. *Risk Mitigation in the Context of Dual Public Health Emergencies: Interim Clinical Guidance*; British Columbia Centre on Substance Use: Vancouver, BC, Canada, 2020.
14. Welsh, C.; Doyon, S.; Hart, K. Methadone Exposures Reported to Poison Control Centers in the United States Following the COVID-19-Related Loosening of Federal Methadone Regulations. *Int. J. Drug Policy* **2022**, *102*, 103591. [CrossRef] [PubMed]
15. Centre for Addiction and Mental Health. COVID-19 Opioid Agonist Treatment Guidance. Published 2020. Updated August 2021. Available online: https://Www.Camh.Ca/-/Media/Files/Covid-19-Modifications-to-Opioid-Agonist-Treatment-Delivery-Pdf.Pdf (accessed on 20 October 2022).
16. Kitchen, S.A.; Campbell, T.J.; Men, S.; Bozinoff, N.; Tadrous, M.; Antoniou, T.; Wyman, J.; Werb, D.; Munro, C.; Gomes, T. Impact of the COVID-19 Pandemic on the Provision of Take-Home Doses of Opioid Agonist Therapy in Ontario, Canada: A Population-Based Time-Series Analysis. *Int. J. Drug Policy* **2022**, *103*, 103644. [CrossRef] [PubMed]
17. Gomes, T.; Campbell, T.J.; Kitchen, S.A.; Garg, R.; Bozinoff, N.; Men, S.; Tadrous, M.; Munro, C.; Antoniou, T.; Werb, D. Association between Increased Dispensing of Opioid Agonist Therapy Take-Home Doses and Opioid Overdose and Treatment Interruption and Discontinuation. *JAMA* **2022**, *327*, 846–855. [CrossRef]
18. Kreek, M.J.; Borg, L.; Ducat, E.; Ray, B. Pharmacotherapy in the Treatment of Addiction: Methadone. In *Women, Children and Addiction*; Routledge: Oxfordshire, UK, 2014; pp. 88–104. ISBN 1-315-87382-6.
19. A Yokell, M.; D Zaller, N.; C Green, T.; D Rich, J. Buprenorphine and Buprenorphine/Naloxone Diversion, Misuse, and Illicit Use: An International Review. *Curr. Drug Abus. Rev.* **2011**, *4*, 28–41. [CrossRef]
20. Rzasa Lynn, R.; Galinkin, J.L. Naloxone Dosage for Opioid Reversal: Current Evidence and Clinical Implications. *Ther. Adv. Drug Saf.* **2018**, *9*, 63–88. [CrossRef]
21. Almagooshi, S. Simulation Modelling in Healthcare: Challenges and Trends. *Procedia Manuf.* **2015**, *3*, 301–307. [CrossRef]
22. Tracy, M.; Cerdá, M.; Keyes, K.M. Agent-Based Modeling in Public Health: Current Applications and Future Directions. *Annu. Rev. Public Health* **2018**, *39*, 77–94. [CrossRef]
23. Altice, F.L.; Azbel, L.; Stone, J.; Brooks-Pollock, E.; Smyrnov, P.; Dvoriak, S.; Taxman, F.S.; El-Bassel, N.; Martin, N.K.; Booth, R. The Perfect Storm: Incarceration and the High-Risk Environment Perpetuating Transmission of HIV, Hepatitis C Virus, and Tuberculosis in Eastern Europe and Central Asia. *Lancet* **2016**, *388*, 1228–1248. [CrossRef]
24. Nielsen, A.E. *Quantifying Spatial Potential Access Equity in an Agent Based Simulation Model of Buprenorphine Treatment Policy in the United States*; Portland State University: Portland, OR, USA, 2018.
25. Wakeland, W.; Nielsen, A. *Modeling Opioid Addiction Treatment Policies Using System Dynamics*; Portland State University: Portland, OR, USA, 2013.
26. Chetty, M.; Kenworthy, J.J.; Langham, S.; Walker, A.; Dunlop, W.C. A Systematic Review of Health Economic Models of Opioid Agonist Therapies in Maintenance Treatment of Non-Prescription Opioid Dependence. *Addict. Sci. Clin. Pract.* **2017**, *12*, 6. [CrossRef]
27. Stringfellow, E.J.; Lim, T.Y.; Humphreys, K.; DiGennaro, C.; Stafford, C.; Beaulieu, E.; Homer, J.; Wakeland, W.; Bearnot, B.; McHugh, R.K. Reducing Opioid Use Disorder and Overdose Deaths in the United States: A Dynamic Modeling Analysis. *Sci. Adv.* **2022**, *8*, eabm8147. [CrossRef] [PubMed]
28. Homer, J.; Wakeland, W. A Dynamic Model of the Opioid Drug Epidemic with Implications for Policy. *Am. J. Drug Alcohol Abus.* **2021**, *47*, 5–15. [CrossRef] [PubMed]
29. Pitt, A.L.; Humphreys, K.; Brandeau, M.L. Modeling Health Benefits and Harms of Public Policy Responses to the US Opioid Epidemic. *Am. J. Public Health* **2018**, *108*, 1394–1400. [CrossRef]
30. Brands, B.; Leslie, K.; Catz-Biro, L.; Li, S. Heroin Use and Barriers to Treatment in Street-Involved Youth. *Addict. Res. Theory* **2005**, *13*, 477–487. [CrossRef]
31. Russell, C.; Neufeld, M.; Sabioni, P.; Varatharajan, T.; Ali, F.; Miles, S.; Henderson, J.; Fischer, B.; Rehm, J. Assessing Service and Treatment Needs and Barriers of Youth Who Use Illicit and Non-Medical Prescription Drugs in Northern Ontario, Canada. *PLoS ONE* **2019**, *14*, e0225548. [CrossRef] [PubMed]
32. Mackesy-Amiti, M.E.; Finnegan, L.; Ouellet, L.J.; Golub, E.T.; Hagan, H.; Hudson, S.M.; Latka, M.H.; Garfein, R.S. Peer-Education Intervention to Reduce Injection Risk Behaviors Benefits High-Risk Young Injection Drug Users: A Latent Transition Analysis of the CIDUS 3/DUIT Study. *AIDS Behav.* **2013**, *17*, 2075–2083. [CrossRef]
33. Pilarinos, A.; Kwa, Y.; Joe, R.; Thulien, M.; Buxton, J.A.; DeBeck, K.; Fast, D. Navigating Opioid Agonist Therapy among Young People Who Use Illicit Opioids in Vancouver, Canada. *Int. J. Drug Policy* **2022**, *107*, 103773. [CrossRef]
34. Lagu, T.; Anderson, B.J.; Stein, M. Overdoses among Friends: Drug Users Are Willing to Administer Naloxone to Others. *J. Subst. Abus. Treat.* **2006**, *30*, 129–133. [CrossRef]
35. Marshall, C.; Perreault, M.; Archambault, L.; Milton, D. Experiences of Peer-Trainers in a Take-Home Naloxone Program: Results from a Qualitative Study. *Int. J. Drug Policy* **2017**, *41*, 19–28. [CrossRef]

36. Schull, M.J.; Azimaee, M.; Marra, M.; Cartagena, R.G.; Vermeulen, M.J.; Ho, M.; Guttmann, A. ICES: Data, Discovery, Better Health. *Int. J. Popul. Data Sci.* **2019**, *4*, 1135. [CrossRef]
37. Borshchev, A. Multi-method Modelling: AnyLogic. In *Discrete-Event Simulation and System Dynamics for Management Decision Making*; Wiley: Hoboken, NJ, USA, 2014; pp. 248–279.
38. Erdős, P.; Rényi, A. On the Evolution of Random Graphs. *Publ. Math. Inst. Hung. Acad. Sci.* **1960**, *5*, 17–60.
39. Whelan, P.J.; Remski, K. Buprenorphine vs. Methadone Treatment: A Review of Evidence in Both Developed and Developing Worlds. *J. Neurosci. Rural Pract.* **2012**, *3*, 45–50. [CrossRef] [PubMed]
40. Hickman, M.; Steer, C.; Tilling, K.; Lim, A.G.; Marsden, J.; Millar, T.; Strang, J.; Telfer, M.; Vickerman, P.; Macleod, J. The Impact of Buprenorphine and Methadone on Mortality: A Primary Care Cohort Study in the United Kingdom. *Addiction* **2018**, *113*, 1461–1476. [CrossRef]
41. Bennett, A.S.; Elliott, L. Naloxone's Role in the National Opioid Crisis—Past Struggles, Current Efforts, and Future Opportunities. *Transl. Res.* **2021**, *234*, 43–57. [CrossRef] [PubMed]
42. Bennett, A.S.; Townsend, T.; Elliott, L. The COVID-19 Pandemic and the Health of People Who Use Illicit Opioids in New York City, the First 12 Months. *Int. J. Drug Policy* **2022**, *101*, 103554. [CrossRef] [PubMed]
43. Brothers, S.; Viera, A.; Heimer, R. Changes in Methadone Program Practices and Fatal Methadone Overdose Rates in Connecticut during COVID-19. *J. Subst. Abus. Treat.* **2021**, *131*, 108449. [CrossRef] [PubMed]
44. Krawczyk, N.; Fawole, A.; Yang, J.; Tofighi, B. Early Innovations in Opioid Use Disorder Treatment and Harm Reduction during the COVID-19 Pandemic: A Scoping Review. *Addict. Sci. Clin. Pract.* **2021**, *16*, 68. [CrossRef]
45. O'Carroll, A.; Duffin, T.; Collins, J. Harm Reduction in the Time of COVID-19: Case Study of Homelessness and Drug Use in Dublin, Ireland. *Int. J. Drug Policy* **2021**, *87*, 102966. [CrossRef]
46. Durand, L.; Keenan, E.; Boland, F.; Harnedy, N.; Delargy, Í.; Scully, M.; Mayock, P.; Ebbitt, W.; Vázquez, M.O.; Corrigan, N. Consensus Recommendations for Opioid Agonist Treatment Following the Introduction of Emergency Clinical Guidelines in Ireland during the COVID-19 Pandemic: A National Delphi Study. *Int. J. Drug Policy* **2022**, *106*, 103768. [CrossRef]
47. Tanne, J.H. *FDA Approves over the Counter Sale of Naloxone to Reverse Drug Overdoses*; British Medical Journal Publishing Group: London, UK, 2023; ISBN 1756-1833.
48. Linas, B.P.; Savinkina, A.; Madushani, R.; Wang, J.; Yazdi, G.E.; Chatterjee, A.; Walley, A.Y.; Morgan, J.R.; Epstein, R.L.; Assoumou, S.A. Projected Estimates of Opioid Mortality after Community-Level Interventions. *JAMA Netw. Open* **2021**, *4*, e2037259. [CrossRef]
49. de Villa, E. Toronto Overdose Action Plan: Status Report 2020. Available online: https://www.toronto.ca/legdocs/mmis/2020/hl/bgrd/backgroundfile-147549.pdf (accessed on 10 June 2023).

Disclaimer/Publisher's Note: The statements, opinions and data contained in all publications are solely those of the individual author(s) and contributor(s) and not of MDPI and/or the editor(s). MDPI and/or the editor(s) disclaim responsibility for any injury to people or property resulting from any ideas, methods, instructions or products referred to in the content.

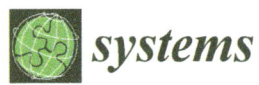

Article

Participatory Modeling with Discrete-Event Simulation: A Hybrid Approach to Inform Policy Development to Reduce Emergency Department Wait Times

Yuan Tian [1,*], Jenny Basran [2,3], James Stempien [2,3], Adrienne Danyliw [3], Graham Fast [3], Patrick Falastein [4] and Nathaniel D. Osgood [1]

1. Department of Computer Science, University of Saskatchewan, Saskatoon, SK S7N 5C9, Canada; osgood@cs.usask.ca
2. College of Medicine, University of Saskatchewan, Saskatoon, SK S7N 5E5, Canada; jenny.basran@saskhealthauthority.ca (J.B.); jas510@mail.usask.ca (J.S.)
3. Saskatchewan Health Authority, Saskatoon, SK S7K 0M7, Canada; adrienne.danyliw@saskhealthauthority.ca (A.D.); graham.fast@saskhealthauthority.ca (G.F.)
4. Saskatchewan Health Quality Council, Saskatoon, SK S7N 3R2, Canada; pfalastein@hqc.sk.ca
* Correspondence: yut473@mail.usask.ca

Abstract: We detail a case study using a participatory modeling approach in the development and use of discrete-event simulations to identify intervention strategies aimed at reducing emergency department (ED) wait times in a Canadian health policy setting. A four-stage participatory modeling approach specifically adapted to the local policy environment was developed to engage stakeholders throughout the modeling processes. The participatory approach enabled a provincial team to engage a broad range of stakeholders to examine and identify the causes and solutions to lengthy ED wait times in the studied hospitals from a whole-system perspective. Each stage of the approach was demonstrated through its application in the case study. A novel and key feature of the participatory modeling approach was the development and use of a multi-criteria framework to identify and prioritize interventions to reduce ED wait times. We conclude with a discussion on lessons learned, which provide insights into future development and applications of participatory modeling methods to facilitate policy development and build multi-stakeholder consensus.

Keywords: participatory modeling; discrete-event simulation; emergency department; patient flow

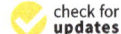

Citation: Tian, Y.; Basran, J.; Stempien, J.; Danyliw, A.; Fast, G.; Falastein, P.; Osgood, N.D. Participatory Modeling with Discrete-Event Simulation: A Hybrid Approach to Inform Policy Development to Reduce Emergency Department Wait Times. *Systems* 2023, 11, 362. https://doi.org/10.3390/systems11070362

Academic Editor: Wayne Wakeland

Received: 1 May 2023
Revised: 6 July 2023
Accepted: 8 July 2023
Published: 17 July 2023

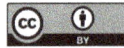

Copyright: © 2023 by the authors. Licensee MDPI, Basel, Switzerland. This article is an open access article distributed under the terms and conditions of the Creative Commons Attribution (CC BY) license (https://creativecommons.org/licenses/by/4.0/).

1. Introduction

Evidence-based decision making is the foundation for health policymaking and health service planning. There remain many practical challenges to integrating the results of research to identify evidence-based interventions to implement in a given context, especially in the face of the uncertainty and complexity that characterize many healthcare delivery systems. Although research presents a multitude of acceptable evidence-based options, it is difficult to determine which interventions will have the greatest impact given the heterogeneity in the population and the health-service delivery system. Complex or uncertain disease epidemiology, including multimorbidity, can introduce additional challenges to decision making. In addition, a large number of stakeholders with differing perspectives and competing priorities are typically involved in the decision-making processes. Failure to achieve consensus among these stakeholders can hinder the effective implementation of interventions [1–3].

As a result of these challenges and the increasing availability of advanced computer technology, there has been a growing interest in using modeling and simulation techniques to assist in the decision-making process in the health sector [4,5]. The design and development of health services would benefit from using these techniques to systematically integrate diverse evidence sources into a computer model and validate the underlying causal mechanisms that drive complex healthcare problems. More importantly, these models allow assessment and comparison of the effects of proposed changes or resource configurations in service design through "what-if" scenarios, providing insights on potential impacts in a cost-effective and timely manner compared to real-world trials. A number of simulation studies have successfully applied computer modeling methods to inform strategic planning and health policy-making for stroke care improvement, alcohol-related harm reduction, cardiovascular disease interventions, and managing diabetes in pregnancy [6–9].

Despite this growing interest and an increasing number of simulation studies in health-related fields, serious and widespread application of systems modeling and simulation remains lacking in informing health-policy development [5,10–14]. Low stakeholder engagement is a major factor that hinders the translation of model findings into evidence-based policy and practice [13,15,16]. Recent studies in the context of healthcare found that relatively few simulation models addressed the needs of policymakers, and models were often constructed without the involvement of health-system managers or policymakers (who are considered the 'end users') in the research process [4,5,15,17]. Many factors contributed to the "implementation gap" between model findings and serious application in the health field; for instance, the communication gap between research and stakeholder groups [15], the lack of involvement of researchers when important policy decisions are made [18], and the trust issues throughout different modeling stages that involve interactions between the model, the modeler, and the stakeholders [19]. Harper et al. proposed a trust model and discussed different aspects of trust building in the life cycle of a simulation study [20].

Successful development of health interventions or policies depends on stakeholder support for the proposed improvements or actions. There is a growing recognition of the value of using a participatory modeling approach in simulation studies to bridge the communication gap and enable collaboration between stakeholders and modelers in building the simulation models [3,7,21]. The participatory modeling (also referred to as collaborative modeling, participative modeling, or facilitated modeling) approaches involve the joint creation of a computer model that reproduces a shared representation of the system in silico with the end users, stakeholders, and experts to facilitate collaborative learning, build consensus, and inform the group's decision making [22]. In these approaches, expert modelers directly collaborate with a team of end users or stakeholders throughout the whole simulation study life cycle, as opposed to the traditional approaches where the modelers conduct the simulation studies independently and only present the findings to the stakeholders [4]. A participatory approach to simulation modeling helps strengthen relationships and improve knowledge translation when designing health services and policies for complex problems [23].

This case study describes modeling ED and acute care patient flow using a four-stage participatory modeling approach with discrete-event simulation (DES) in a Canadian health-policy setting. The paper complements the literature by reporting on the use of a participatory approach in developing DES models of patient flow in the emergency department (ED) to inform the design and planning of effective wait time reduction strategies from a whole-system perspective. The DES models, built in collaboration with a multidisciplinary group of stakeholders, served as a decision-support tool that integrated existing data, research evidence, expert knowledge, and local context to assess the potential impact of different intervention scenarios.

The modeling findings have been utilized to inform policy development and subsequent actions. We detailed our DES model's structure and major quantitative results in previous work [24]; discussions on major simulation findings can be found therein. In the current study, we provide methodological details of the participatory approach used in model development and model use with stakeholders. We focus here on describing the following key aspects of the participatory modeling process:

- building trust in the modeling approach and seeking buy-in from the project leads for further development during the project initialization;

- leveraging existing conceptual mapping tools used in the health system for conceptual modeling;
- using co-production methods to build trust in the model and its outputs;
- identify and prioritize intervention scenarios using a multi-criteria framework.

We then discuss lessons learned and implications for adopting the participatory modeling approach in the health-policy setting.

2. Brief Review of Participatory Modeling Approaches

2.1. Motivation

In the past two decades, there has been little improvement in translating simulation findings into policy and practice [12,25–31], with communication gaps and a lack of understanding of policymakers' needs contributing to the underutilization of model findings in healthcare decision making [15,31]. There is a rising awareness that more needs to be done to ensure that research results in better knowledge translation and improved health services and patient outcomes. Engaging stakeholders in research has been highlighted as a possible mechanism to increase the value, use, and relevance of research [32]. Scholars have called for collaborative engagement with health professionals, managers, decision makers, and patient representatives in simulation studies to increase the likelihood of successful implementation of simulation outputs [3,9,12,30]. In addition, a range of programs were established to support stakeholder engagement in health research, such as the development of the US Patient-Centered Outcomes Research Institute and knowledge translation activities in Canada [32].

Participatory modeling approaches have been proposed as one way for engaging stakeholders and improving stakeholders' knowledge and understanding of a system and its dynamics under a variety of conditions in order to support shared learning or the decision-making process [3,9,21,22,33,34]. It also increases trust in and use of scientific information in decision making [35]. It is a deliberate learning process that involves a diverse range of modeling activities that draw on stakeholders' knowledge to develop a shared and formalized understanding and representation of the reality or system [22,31]. In a participatory modeling process, stakeholders can be involved in one or more modeling stages with different levels of engagement, ranging from passive participation (e.g., being merely informed about model findings) to active participation where stakeholders might contribute to problem identification, data collection, model design, and model use [31,34].

2.2. Applied Fields and Purpose

Participatory approaches to modeling have gained recognition in a number of sectors, including natural resource management (e.g., water management) [31,36], environmental planning [34,37], and health research and policy [3,33,38–40]. Voinov et al. reviewed participatory modeling studies in resource management and environmental planning that involved multiple sectors and stakeholders [34]. There has been an increase in the popularity of participatory modeling in recent years, as evidenced by the rising number of papers published on the topic [34,41]. The authors presented different components for stakeholder participation within the development of specific environmental models and summarized tools and methods for participatory modeling in different modeling stages [34,41]. Participatory modeling approaches are also being used in public health and health services research. Freebairn et al. described the novel use of participatory simulation modeling combined with system science methodology in informing health policies through three case studies aimed at reducing alcohol-related harms, childhood obesity, and diabetes in pregnancy in real-world policy settings in Australia [3,42]. The authors published a series of papers on these case studies that provided valuable lessons, detailed procedures, and concrete guidance in using participatory dynamic simulation modeling methods in health policy settings, such as integrating knowledge translation and mobilization into participatory processes, converting conceptual system maps into a dynamic simulation, and building consensus with stakeholders for policy actions [3,7,9,43]. Frerichs et al.

and Gerritsen et al. discussed and showcased the potential of using community-based participatory modeling approaches in public health and health equity research [44,45].

Depending on the form of participatory modeling approach used, participatory modeling processes may serve somewhat different purposes. Most participatory modeling projects focused on developing a collective understanding of the issues among the participants, and the model was viewed as a tool to support shared learning or community-based learning; while others engaged stakeholders to inform policy-making or mobilize actions [3,31,33,40,42,44,46,47]. Using the participatory modeling approach was found to have several benefits, including providing a better evidence base for policy decisions, improving the quality of the research, and increasing the dissemination and implementation of interventions [40,48,49]. A number of tools and methods can be employed to facilitate stakeholder engagement in participatory modeling processes. Voinov et al. provided a systematic overview and assessment of various participatory modeling methods and discussed their strengths and weaknesses [22]. The authors proposed a typology of methods used in participatory modeling with illustrated workflows and provided practical guidance for method selection. Depending on the modeling stage, either qualitative (e.g., rich pictures or causal loop diagrams) or quantitative methods (e.g., agent-based modeling or system dynamics) could be utilized.

2.3. Specific Participatory Modeling Approaches and Tools

2.3.1. Soft Operation Research Methodology

Soft Systems Methodology (SSM) is a broader participatory modeling methodology that emphasizes the use of rich picture tools to learn about a problem situation and start exploratory discussions with people [50]. It also embraces the systems perspective to explore problematic situations with relevant stakeholders. SSM used a sequence of steps from problem finding and rich picture building to solution identification and action mobilization [22,50]. It has been used as a problem structuring approach in a number of sectors (e.g., strategic planning and policy development concerning agriculture) [51], but its application in the healthcare setting is limited [46]. There are other "soft" problem structuring methods used for studying complex and unstructured problems involving multiple stakeholders with diverse perspectives, such as strategic options development and analysis, and hierarchical process modeling [52,53].

2.3.2. Group Model Building

Group model building (GMB) refers to a set of techniques used to engage client groups directly in the process of problem finding, model construction, and use through facilitated workshops or sessions [39,54,55]. Group model building has matured as a field, specifically as a community-based participatory approach for social learning or the development of system dynamics (SD) models [39,45,47,54–56]. Depending on the type of problem, the end product often results in either qualitative models (causal loop diagrams) or quantitative models (such as SD models).

2.3.3. PartiSim Framework for DES

Tako and Kotiadis developed a facilitated modeling approach named PartiSim [21,57–59]. PartiSim (short for participative simulation) is a multi-methodology framework that integrates DES with SSM. The PartiSim framework integrates stakeholder input and facilitation as part of the process of conducting DES studies. The framework is divided into six primary stages in the simulation study life cycle, each with its own set of activities, deliverables, and tools to help the modeling team engage stakeholder participation in the study. The authors employed the PartiSim framework while collaborating with healthcare organizations on a variety of operational issues in healthcare settings [60]. The authors reflected on practical challenges encountered in facilitating the conceptual modeling process, particularly panel composition and team roles in handling conflicts and promoting involvement among stakeholder teams and modeling teams [57]. The authors also discussed and reported on the post-model coding step, specifically scenario development and experiments [59]. The authors achieved success in implementing model findings in an obesity service to improve patient waiting times [60].

2.3.4. Other Participatory Modeling Approaches Used in Case Studies

Unlike the formal frameworks or methodologies introduced above, several studies reported the use of participatory modeling through case studies [3,7,9,42,43]. These studies elaborated on the rationale and procedure of the participatory modeling approach used [7], integration of rapid review with participatory modeling processes for knowledge mobilization [3], the conversion of conceptual mapping into a quantitative simulation model [9], and decision makers' experience in the participatory modeling processes [42].

2.3.5. Participatory Modeling Tools

Participatory modeling can be used in either qualitative or quantitative modeling. For qualitative modeling, a number of tools can be used at different modeling stages or combined with more general frameworks or methodologies such as SSM, GMB, or PartiSim. Diagramming or graphical tools, such as rich pictures (as a part of the SSM), causal loop diagrams, and cognitive (or conceptual) mapping, were often used in participatory modeling to generate visual representations of the components of the problems [9,22]. These qualitative maps or diagrams are utilized for collaborative exploration and group understanding of a complex issue by representing diverse relationships among many interacting components, illustrating how changes in one area affect other factors, and drawing the feedback loops that are assumed to explain the dynamic behaviors [9,22]. Unlike participatory modeling approaches for qualitative modeling, which are primarily concerned with fostering trust and understanding among stakeholders, participatory modeling approaches in quantitative modeling are more focused on "solving" a specific problem and frequently produce forecasts or quantitative estimates [22]. Participatory modeling can be embedded in the development and use of SD, DES [21], and agent-based models (ABM) [22].

2.4. Hybrid Modeling and Simulation

With new developments in the simulation tools and the rising complexity of the studied systems and decision-making needs, a growing number of studies in the field of modeling and simulation (M&S) have embraced a hybrid approach [61–63]. This involves combining multiple simulation techniques (e.g., in the form of mixing SD, DES, and ABM) or integrating hard or soft operation research (OR) methods in one or more stages of a simulation study (e.g., combining SSM with DES) [61–63]. The adoption of hybrid approaches becomes increasingly appealing, especially from a practical standpoint, as hybrid approaches can overcome some limitations of using any single M&S technique and complement each other [61,62]. This approach can further facilitate the nimble evolution of model scope and formulation in light of the growing understanding of the system and changing policy evaluation needs and context. One of the main areas of application of hybrid M&S was found to be healthcare [61]. A combination of multiple simulation techniques (e.g., SD, ABM, DES, and social network analysis) has been employed to investigate a range of complex health-related issues and systems, such as disease prevention and care management [43,64–66], projection of disease burden [67], health workforce dynamics [68], and immunoepidemiology of infectious diseases [69]. Reflecting the diversity in the mixing of different methods in simulation studies, Mustafee et al. presented a conceptual classification of hybrid M&S and discussed innovation in the M&S field by highlighting *hybrid modeling* [70–72]. Unlike *hybrid simulation*, which combines two or more simulation techniques (e.g., SD, DES, or ABM) primarily in the model implementation stage of a simulation study, *hybrid modeling* extends *hybrid simulation* by emphasizing the combined application of simulation techniques together with theories, frameworks, methods, or tools in the broader OR domain or from other disciplines in stages of the modeling process of a simulation study beyond implementation [70–72]. *Hybrid modeling* can involve the synthesis of a qualitative soft OR technique (such as SSM or a participatory approach) with a simulation technique [62]. For instance, McDonald et al. used a community-engaged collaborative modeling approach to co-create an ABM with the indigenous community to better understand the water services [73]. Jiang et al. combined the use of causal loop diagrams in the conceptual modeling stage with ABM to study breastfeeding interventions [74]. Other forms of *hybrid modeling* include the co-application of simulation techniques with cross-disciplinary methods from other fields or domains [70]. Tian et al. proposed a hybrid approach by linking multiple techniques with an SD model to investigate stroke prevention and care [75]. Kreuger et al. discussed the combined use of agile design in software engineering with hybrid simulation design and use [76]. *Hybrid modeling* stands at the forefront of fostering innovations in both the theoretical and practical aspects of M&S, especially in light of new developments in conceptual modeling to better understand and depict studied systems [62], and in stakeholder engagement to capture domain knowledge from diverse stakeholders and build trust in simulation models [70,71].

3. Case Study Context
3.1. The Problem of Emergency Department Crowding and Wait Times

ED crowding, often reflected in lengthy wait times for emergency care, is a worldwide healthcare delivery issue that negatively affects patient safety, experience, and clinical outcomes, such as increased mortality rates and worse patient satisfaction [77–81]. The causes of ED crowding and lengthy ED wait times are multi-factorial and complex [77,82]. Among 11 developed nations, Canadians reported the longest ED waits [83,84]. Lengthy ED wait times are a major concern for Canadians [85], and several Canadian provinces have launched initiatives to address the ED crowding and patient wait times [78]. The government of Saskatchewan challenged the health system to tackle the waiting time problem in EDs [86]. In response to the challenges of improving timely access to emergency care, the Saskatchewan ED Waits and Patient Flow Initiative was launched to address ED wait times. The provincial initiative was charged with developing and implementing ED wait time reduction strategies provincially [86]. Given the complex nature of the issue, limited resources for allocation, and an extensive set of evidence-based options from both the literature and expert opinions, it is challenging to quantify the impact of each plausible contributing factor. It is also costly to pilot each evidence-based intervention individually or collectively for the studied EDs. Ideally, we would desire a safe and cost-effective approach to understand the causes and examine the likely consequences of proposed changes in advance. With the dual objectives of identifying the causes of lengthy ED wait times and comparing potential solutions to allocate limited resources, this study investigated the ED patient flow in six Saskatchewan hospitals. At the time of the research, the six hospitals were located in three health regions, which collectively served 63% of the Saskatchewan population.

3.2. Whole-System ED Patient Flow Modeling

There is a significant amount of literature on using simulation, particularly DES, to study ED crowding, streamline ED patient flow, and reduce wait times [12,28,30,87–89]. However, most of these ED simulation studies have high unit specificity with a focus only on care processes in a single ED [25,28,30]. Only a few studies investigated ED crowding or wait times as part of a larger system, such as a whole hospital or complete acute care system [90–92]. There has been limited improvement in multi-facility and whole-system modeling in the area of ED simulation studies that utilize DES [25,28,30,89].

Despite the broad agreement that the ED problem largely requires system-wide solutions and that solutions within the ED alone are insufficient, there remains a lack of whole-system multifacility modeling, as documented in the ED literature. Empirical evidence suggests that ED performance depends on adjoining systems, such as acute care, primary care, and sub-acute care to function efficiently [28,30,56,88,93]. Jun et al. concluded that future simulation results on ED crowding or wait times need to depict the interaction of major service departments and support services in a hospital to gain insights from analyzing the system as a whole, rather than in a unit-specific piecemeal fashion [25]. Gunal et al. argued that unit-specific and facility-specific ED simulation studies, which ignore the subtle linkages between the ED and other units or services within the hospital, might oversimplify the complexity of hospital activities within a simulation model and overlook side effects and unintended consequences [28]. Zhang echoed that healthcare management would benefit from DES models, which capture the intricate interactions of healthcare services rather than just limiting them to single units [89]. Salmon et al. also found high unit specificity among ED simulation studies, thus calling for the examination of system influences beyond the ED itself to better understand emergency department operations from a whole-system perspective [30].

This paper complements the literature by demonstrating how multi-facility whole-system DES models of patient flow can be used to design policies to improve ED patient flow and reduce wait times. Notably, the study embraced the systems view and studied ED wait times as a part of a larger integrated acute care system with multiple interacting subsystems or units.

4. Materials and Methods

4.1. Overview

This study described a participatory modeling approach for embedding stakeholder engagement in the development and use of DES models to support effective and coordinated policy development to reduce ED wait times. The participatory modeling approach used in this study drew on several existing frameworks for working with groups [21,56,94] and was adapted to the local context. The approach was applied through collaboration between the Saskatchewan ED Waits and Patient Flow Initiative, Saskatchewan Ministry of Health, regional health authorities, Saskatchewan Health Quality Council, clinicians, health professionals, researchers, and health policy planners. The study was exempted by the University of Saskatchewan Research Ethics Board.

The participatory modeling approach used in this study can be broken down into four major stages: (1) project initialization; (2) conceptual modeling; (3) model implementation; and (4) model use and policy co-development. Figure 1 illustrates the overall participatory modeling process with a detailed visualization of the model use and policy co-development stage.

4.2. Stage 1: Project Initialization

The initialization phase assembled the project team, defined the purpose and scope, and assessed the feasibility of using computational modeling to understand ED patient flow and inform the policy development process. The primary objective of this phase was to seek initial buy-in from the project lead (GF) and physician leads (JB and JS) of the ED Waits and Patient Flow Initiative. The goal was to help them recognize the value of computer simulation models as decision-support tools for addressing the ED patient flow challenges with a broader group of regional and provincial stakeholders. To achieve this, a proof-of-concept analysis was carried out to demonstrate the ability of computational models to simulate ED patient flow, synthesize evidence, data, and expert opinions, and allow for the evaluation and comparison of alternative wait time reduction strategies via virtual experiments.

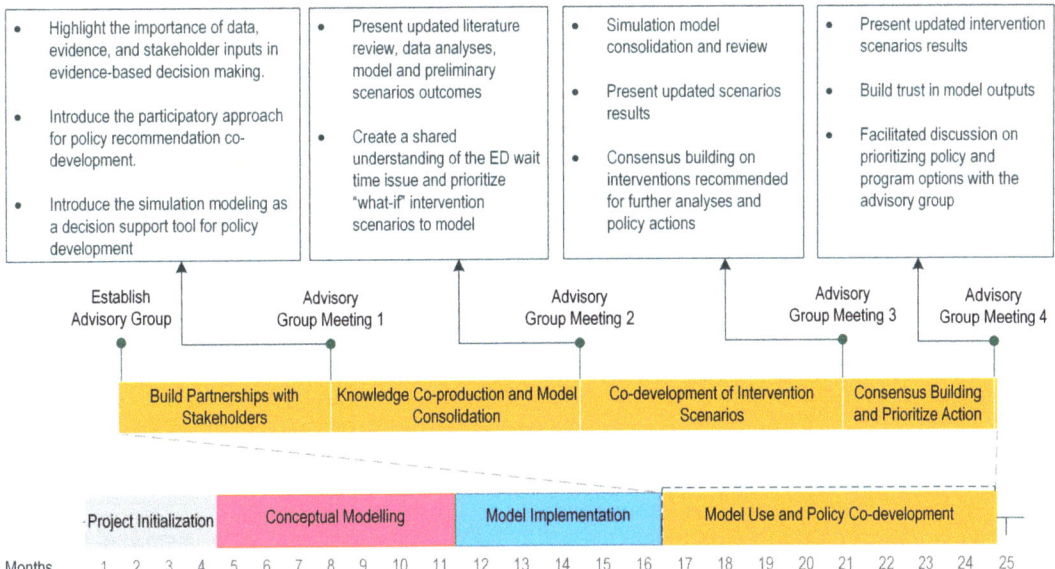

Figure 1. Participatory modeling process.

Team Composition

The modeling project team was led by a project lead (GF) who was primarily responsible for managing the project, overseeing model development, and communicating with important stakeholders, including regional leaders and policy partners. The domain experts on the team included ED physicians, a geriatrician, family physicians, clinical experts, patient flow managers, and quality improvement consultants. These experts provided information about the current patient flow situation in the studied EDs and hospitals and offered clinical guidance for model development and use. Two key physician leads (JB and JS) shared duties with the project lead and jointly facilitated modeling meetings and stakeholder communication. One of the domain experts (JB), who was a geriatrician, also served as the project champion. Two technical advisors (NO) oversaw high-level model conceptualization and development to ensure that the model was suitably scoped, rigorously validated, and could be delivered within a policy-friendly time frame. The lead modeler and researcher (YT) was responsible for designing the participatory modeling process with the project leads and technical advisors, managing data requirements, synthesizing evidence for model conceptualization, building and validating simulation models, developing intervention scenarios with stakeholders, and conducting simulation runs. Another modeler served as an intern for five months during the project's initialization phase to assess the feasibility of using computational modeling to inform decision making through proof-of-concept analysis. Two quality improvement consultants (AD and PF) helped facilitate meetings with stakeholders.

4.3. Stage 2: Conceptual Modeling

The first step of the study was to understand the existing ED waits situation by getting an overview of the entire ED patient flow and care processes in the studied EDs and hospitals. Conceptual modeling refers to a series of activities for abstracting a qualitative model from the problem situation and the real system with relevant domain experts and stakeholders [2,95]. The conceptual modeling process in the present study was inspired by elements from existing conceptual modeling frameworks [2,95] and comprised three key activities for knowledge discovery and information elicitation: (1) conceptualizing the problem, specifically the causes of ED wait times, and identifying a preliminary set of experimental factors (model inputs that can be changed); (2) understanding the data and care processes in the studied EDs and hospitals; and (3) defining the scope and boundaries of the model. The sequence of these activities was not linear, and they were pursued in a highly iterative fashion. We used tools that were borrowed or adapted from qualitative improvement toolkits [96] and lean management techniques [97]. Prior to the formation of the modeling team, the provincial initiative's working groups had conducted initial conceptual mapping of the ED wait time issue. Rather than introducing new conceptual mapping tools, the modeling team opted to review and enhance the previous work to generate new insights and foster a more comprehensive understanding of the problem situation.

Problem conceptualization started with a qualitative representation of the factors contributing to the ED wait times. A comprehensive literature review was conducted at this stage to identify important contributing factors to ED wait times. The modeling team also consulted with a wide range of domain experts and regional stakeholders through informal meetings and onsite visits to acquire knowledge about the studied sites. The perspectives of stakeholders and relevant domain experts were both crucial at this stage, as they assisted the modeler in better understanding the contextual factors in the studied EDs. A driver diagram was developed to depict the causes that could influence ED wait times from multiple perspectives. A driver diagram is a quality improvement tool used to illustrate a project team's understanding of the factors that contribute to the project objective [96]. It displays key areas (primary and secondary drivers) to influence in order to achieve the aim of an improvement project when tackling a complex problem.

To understand the data and care processes in the studied EDs and hospitals, the modeling team worked with process improvement consultants, patient flow managers, regional stakeholders, and patients and family advisors through rapid process improvement workshops to develop value stream maps (VSMs) of the current state of ED patient flow. VSM is a lean management technique that uses a flowchart to draw the current (and future) state of a specific process (or service), with the goal of identifying waste, reducing process time, and improving the flow [98]. At the time of this research, many lean tools were already in use as part of the lean implementation in the province's healthcare system [99]. Rather than re-inventing the wheel, the modeling team leveraged these existing conceptual mapping tools and instead focused on understanding and refining the VSMs. The modeling team met with process improvement consultants and individuals who have expertise in patient flow management in the studied hospitals and conducted onsite visits. The VSMs of ED and acute patient flow illustrated the major steps in the patient's journey from registration to discharge. They also mapped the ED activities (both necessary and non-value-added activities), current care processes, and lead times from the whole-system perspective. Additionally, input data for the model was analyzed using administrative databases based on the driver diagram and VSMs.

In the subsequent stage of the process, the model scope and level of detail were discussed and defined. The primary outcome of the study was the wait time in EDs, which made DES an appropriate choice for the modeling approach as it is well-suited for modeling queuing systems with constraints. The modeler, technical advisors, and project champion collaboratively defined major components (entities, attributes, activities, and resources) to be included in the DES models. Furthermore, assumptions and simplifications were made with input from domain experts and technical advisors.

4.4. Stage 3: Model Implementation

4.4.1. Turning Conceptual Modeling into DES Models

To operationalize the conceptual model as a computational model, the modeler worked with patient flow managers, clinical experts, and quality improvement consultants to identify critical components (e.g., units), interactions, and patient cohorts to be captured in the first iteration of the development of DES models. This was an iterative process throughout the project cycle that involved reviewing evidence and the conceptual models, analyzing administrative databases, and ongoing consultation with clinical experts to determine important processes and agents to be represented in the DES models.

In the early phase of the model development, to communicate and consult with clinical and domain experts on model logic, we added 3D visualization of the floor plan of the studied EDs to showcase the patient movement in the simulation. We conducted face validation and external validation to maintain the credibility of the model. Multiple patient cohorts (e.g., ED visits for family practice sensitive conditions, hospitalization for ambulatory care sensitive conditions, etc.) were identified in the conceptual modeling stage. We extracted these patients cohorts from administrative databases, analyzed their use of ED and acute care services, and characterized them in the DES models.

4.4.2. Capacity Building and Health System Modeling Workshop

Most project stakeholders knew very little about computational modeling and its use in healthcare. Their participation and involvement in the project were largely driven by the priority of the issue and their trusted relationship with the lead domain experts and the provincial initiative. However, many stakeholders were curious about modeling methods. A 4-day health system modeling workshop, led by the modeling team, was hosted by the Saskatchewan Health Quality Council and the provincial initiative. Thirty-five participants (including several provincial leaders) from Saskatchewan health regions, health organizations, and the Ministry of Health participated in this modeling workshop on computational modeling and system thinking in healthcare [100]. Several participants were data content experts and had worked with the modeling team on parameterizing the simulation models of patient flow for the hospitals studied. The modeling team also presented the initial DES models of patient flow to the participants.

4.5. Stage 4: Model Use and Policy Co-Development

After completing the initial model development and validation, the project moved to the model use and policy co-development stage. We formed an advisory group that included stakeholders from three health regions and ministry departments within the healthcare system. To work towards shared goals and aligned actions to reduce ED wait times, we invited the advisory group to participate in four facilitated advisory group meetings to co-develop intervention solutions for implementation to reduce ED wait times in the studied EDs. We highlighted the use of simulation models for integrating data, evidence, and stakeholder inputs to support evidence-informed policy development.

The advisory group was formed by the provincial initiative. The advisory group included all relevant senior stakeholders from the Ministry of Health branches, executive leaders from three regional health authorities, physician leads and clinical experts, researchers, and patient advisors. Figure 1 illustrates the major activities that involve interaction and engagement with stakeholders in the model use and policy co-development process. It also highlights four major advisory group meetings with the engagement of the full panel of the advisory group during this process. The first meeting introduced the use of simulation models for policy co-development with stakeholders. The second meeting reviewed the preliminary scenario results and discussed creating additional intervention scenarios based on stakeholders' assessments of their regional priorities, readiness, and drivers for lengthy

ED wait times in the studied EDs. The last two meetings were centered around discussing the model results and reaching an agreement on recommended interventions for further analyses and the eventual development of a business case for implementation.

4.5.1. The First Meeting

The first advisory group meeting introduced the use of simulation models for policy co-development. The meeting emphasized the participatory approach being undertaken to support evidence-informed policy development with the active engagement of the advisory group. We presented our data analyses on a number of patient groups that were identified as potentially contributing to the problem of lengthy ED wait times. Then we summarized our literature review and environmental scan on two topics: (1) what interventions had been tried, what worked, and what did not work; and (2) promising practices from other jurisdictions and lessons learned from other organizations experiencing similar ED crowding or flow issues. Finally, we proposed the use of simulation models as a decision-support tool to synthesize data, evidence, and input from the advisor group to explore and compare the impact of proposed interventions. The modeling team also described the collaborative model development and model validation activities with patient flow managers, physicians, and data analysts. The advisory group agreed with using the participatory modeling approach to develop policy recommendations for the budgeting cycle.

After the first meeting, the modeling team started to conduct simulation runs of interventions that emerged from evidence and data. In addition, key contacts were identified for the three health regions where the six studied hospitals were situated. Engagement with regional and smaller stakeholder groups also occurred after the first meeting. We held multiple regional advisory group meetings with leaders of specific regional health authorities to gather information about hospitals studied in their region, their local contexts, data sources, interventions of interest, readiness, and priorities. Specifically, a multi-criteria prioritization framework for scenario development was designed and used with the regional leads (seen in Figure 2 and Table 1). The modeling team distributed this framework to key contacts in each health region before the second meeting. The key contact (a senior regional leader) discussed with managers and directors in their region about what interventions they would like to explore via simulation modeling to reduce ED wait times given their current state and local challenges. We also instructed them to review and assess each proposed intervention using the criteria in the framework. We then gathered an initial list of intervention scenarios that each region would like to explore using the models.

4.5.2. The Second Meeting

The second meeting began by presenting the early findings of five model intervention scenarios for five hospitals. For each intervention scenario, we presented the reduction in ED waits over three years and the supporting evidence for the proposed models of care or interventions. These intervention scenarios were identified by the modeling team through literature review, data analyses, and consultation with domain experts. These initial scenario runs were undertaken for demonstration purposes and exploration of "what-if" interventions, rather than for necessarily selecting the most desired scenario. The results of the scenario exploration stimulated discussions with the stakeholders.

In the wake of the above, we focused on discussing the development of additional modeling scenarios according to regional priorities and readiness. In the second meeting, we reviewed the list of interventions proposed by each health region. The regional leads explained the rationale behind each proposed scenario and reflected their regional priorities and alignments with the initiative's goals. Ideally, it would be desirable to include all proposed scenarios from the regions in the simulation model; however, given the large number of scenarios that we received, the advisory group agreed on incorporating the top-ranked scenarios for each region based on the multi-criteria framework described in Figure 2 and Table 1. The modeling team took on the task of finalizing the list of scenarios for each health region and discussing data requirements and relevant evidence after the second meeting.

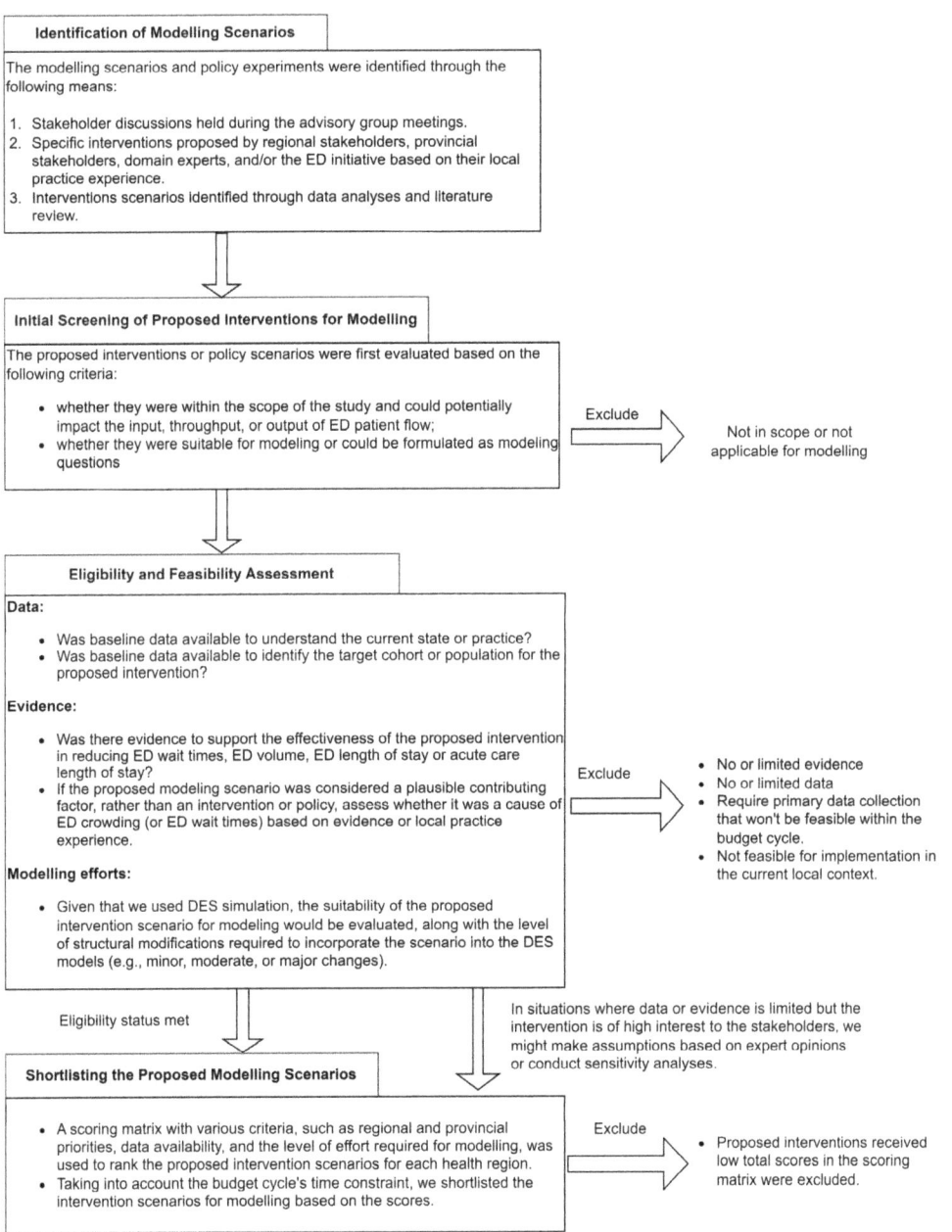

Figure 2. The intake process for modeling scenarios.

Table 1. Scoring Matrix. Criteria used for prioritizing requested modeling scenarios.

Component	Criteria	Description	Scoring (in the Range of 0 to 5)
Data	Regional Data Availability	Degree to which regional data is collected or available for understanding the current state or the targeted cohort for the intervention scenario	0 = no data; 1 = limited data with poor quality; 2 = partial data with poor quality; 3 = partial data with good quality; 4 = almost complete data; 5 = we have everything we need
	Administrative Data Availability	Degree to which data are readily available in administrative databases for modeling or understanding the current state or target cohort.	
Evidence	Literature Support for Modeling	Degree to which evidence (e.g., meta-analysis and systematic reviews) provides relevant outcome metrics for modeling	0 = very low; 1 = low; 2 = low to moderate; 3 = moderate; 4 = moderate to high; 5 = high
Modeling	Modeling Effort	The amount of effort and time it will take for the modeler to incorporate and simulate the scenario using the DES model.	0 = extreme effort; 1 = significant effort; 2 = moderate effort; 3 = moderate to low effort; 4 = low effort; 5 = almost no effort at all
Stakeholders Inputs	Organizational Readiness	Degree to which the organization is ready and committed to implementing the idea	0 = not ready at all; 1 = not ready; 2 = neural or uncertain; 3 = moderately ready; 4 = mostly ready; 5 = ready to go immediately
	Regional Priority	Degree to which the health region agrees that this will address their ED wait times or patient flow issues	0 = not at all; 1 = unlikely; 2 = somewhat unlikely; 3 = neutral or uncertain; 4 = somewhat likely; 5 = very likely
	Provincial Priority	Degree to which the provincial stakeholders and ED waits initiative agrees that this will address ED wait times or patient flow issues	
	Length of Time to Impact Drivers	The length of time it would take to see an effect on ED waits, volume, ED LOS or acute LOS.	0 = >7 years; 1 = 5–7 years; 2 = 3–5 years; 3 = 1–3 years; 4 = within 1 year; 5 = immediate
	Length of Time to Get Service Ready	The length of time required to alter or design service.	

4.5.3. The Third and Fourth Meetings

The modeling team worked with each health region to refine and clarify the requested intervention scenarios using the multi-criteria prioritization framework. The third and fourth meetings consisted of an extensive review and discussion of the scenario results requested by each region, respectively. The modeling team presented the impact of each intervention scenario on ED wait times for the hospitals studied in the corresponding health region. For each scenario, we reviewed data input, supporting evidence (if any), evidence used in the model, key assumptions, and implementation ideas (e.g., how to achieve the expected wait reductions and what needs to be done in terms of implementation). To ensure a comprehensive exploration of intervention options to reduce wait times, additional intervention scenarios were requested during this time and incorporated into the simulation model.

To build trust in the modeling tool and continuously validate the model given the new changes made to incorporate different patient groups, we held a model challenge session between the third and fourth meetings. We invited clinical and data experts as well as interested parties to review the model structure, parameter values, and assumptions. Specific questions on the components being evaluated included: (1) how well the model component reflected the reality considered important by the clinical or domain experts; (2) whether the model output generated outputs that matched the real data; and (3) model assumptions, data sources, and data quality. We were able to gather feedback, suggestions, and critiques on (1) model input and data sources; (2) methodologies used; and (3) assumptions and ideas for future developments. This helped to further improve the DES models.

4.6. A Multi-Criteria Framework for Identifying and Prioritizing Policy Options with Stakeholders

It was challenging to select the most effective strategies to reduce ED wait times, given the large number of evidence-based options available that addressed different aspects of clinical practice and processes in the patient journey through the ED. Factors contributing to ED wait times might also differ between EDs due to variations in local context and organizational factors. Additionally, diverse opinions existed regarding the causes and solutions for the ED wait time issue in the studied hospitals. To address this, a multi-criteria framework was developed for the co-development of interventions with the stakeholders and the advisory group. The purpose of the framework is to promote transparent collaboration and communication with stakeholders during the policy development stage to identify feasible solution space. It is important to note that this framework is distinct from a multi-objective optimization framework and is not programmed into the DES models.

At the stage of co-development of intervention scenarios, we gathered and generated a large inventory of possible intervention scenarios from various sources, including (1) those supported by evidence; (2) those proposed by diverse stakeholder groups and domain experts; (3) those identified as likely to be promising through data analyses; (4) those currently considered for implementation; and (5) existing programs under consideration for expansion. Rather than accepting all scenarios for modeling without questioning, we screened and decided on the sets of interventions to be tested with the simulation models. The multi-criteria framework was used for identifying and prioritizing interventions or policies for modeling. The framework was developed following several knowledge translation principles and criteria to improve evidence-based decision making [101]. The multi-criteria framework has two components: (1) a modeling scenario intake process (seen in Figure 2) and (2) a scoring matrix (seen in Table 1). The framework took into account a number of criteria for managing scope, synthesizing evidence through a literature review, adapting knowledge to the local context, identifying gaps in practice, assessing feasibility, time to impact, and alignment with regional or provincial priorities.

4.6.1. The Intake Process for Modeling Scenario

To prevent "scope creep" and ensure that proposed intervention scenarios from stakeholders were appropriate and within scope [102], we created and used an intake process to screen the proposed interventions or recommended policies. The intake process is presented in Figure 2. The screening process involved evaluating each proposed modeling scenario against several criteria, including its suitability for modeling, availability of data, and supporting evidence about its potential impact on ED wait times or patient flow. It was important to note that local knowledge could not be unquestionably accepted and required assessment together with evidence and data. In addition, for each proposed intervention scenario, we identified a key contact (usually a stakeholder). We clarified the proposed intervention and data requirements with key contacts as needed. We also communicated to the stakeholders about our screening process to manage expectations.

The modeling team conducted the Initial screening and made a first decision on whether we would accept the proposed intervention scenarios for modeling. The proposed intervention scenarios for modeling were declined if one or more of the following conditions were met:

1. The proposed intervention scenario is not within the scope of the project;
2. Data are not available or the proposed intervention requires primary data collection that cannot be completed within the current timeline and budget cycle;
3. There is a lack of evidence regarding the efficacy of the proposed intervention in reducing ED wait times or improving ED patient flow;
4. If the intervention scenario is unsuitable for modeling, as determined by the modeling team, it will not be pursued;
5. If the intervention is not feasible for implementation in the current local context.

Although the modeling team conducted a literature review on the causes of and solutions to ED wait times during the conceptual modeling phase, the proposed intervention scenario might not have been included in the initial review. The second phase of screening involved a rapid review of the effectiveness of the requested intervention scenarios that were not captured in the initial literature review. If the evidence base was found to be thin but the intervention was of high interest to the stakeholders, the modeling team would work with the advisory group and domain experts to determine whether assumptions should be made about program efficacy based on expert opinions and whether sensitivity analyses should be conducted.

4.6.2. The Scoring Matrix

To facilitate policy recommendations at the third and fourth advisor meetings, the modeling team evaluated a list of proposed interventions aimed at reducing ED wait times for each health region using the intake process (Figure 2). Due to the high number of intervention scenarios received from various sources, a scoring matrix was used to further shortlist the interventions for modeling, as shown in Table 1. The modeling team, along with regional leaders and stakeholders in the advisory group, collaborated in filling out the scoring matrix, which evaluated each proposed intervention scenario based on the criteria outlined in Table 1. Each scenario—whether derived from data or evidence or requested by stakeholders—received a score. The scenarios were then sorted accordingly. The scoring matrices for each health region were developed and discussed during the third and fourth advisory meetings.

5. Application of the Participatory Modeling Approach

5.1. Stage 1: Project Initialization

Planning meetings were held to define the project scope and boundaries. It was agreed that the main goal of the project was to validate current assumptions about the causes of ED waits and examine a portfolio of possible intervention options to improve patient flow in the studied EDs, with a focus on ED wait times. Interventions or activities that solely focused on improving primary care, home care, mental health, or chronic disease management, but were unrelated to emergency care or wait times, were deemed out of scope. Two primary outcomes of interest were identified for the project: (1) time waiting for physician initial assessment: time between registration (or triage) and initial physician assessment; and (2) time waiting for an inpatient bed: time between the decision to admit the patient to an inpatient bed and the patient's departure from the ED for the inpatient unit.

Initially, the project leads were not convinced of the value of using a simulation approach to explore policy options related to ED patient flow due to their unfamiliarity with the modeling methods. To address this, a proof-of-concept analysis was conducted. The modeler consulted with several health experts, quality improvement consultants, and the provincial initiative to gather insights on the patient flow within the ED and acute care settings. Two preliminary ED patient flow simulation models were built under the guidance of the project champion and technical advisors. Figure 3 provides a flow chart of the simulated patient flow in the proof-of-concept DES model. The proof-of-concept models demonstrated how patient flow could be represented and how qualitative insights and high-level quantitative predictions on patient flow metrics could be generated. The analyses showed that computational models in principle had the potential to advance the evaluation of policy scenarios and improve the decision-making process. It is worth noting that the project champion played the role of an advocate for the simulating modeling approach in this stage and assisted in building trust and confidence with the project leads by articulating the proof-of-concept models in language familiar to the project leads. As a result, the project was sponsored, and a modeling team was formed as one of the working groups within the provincial initiative.

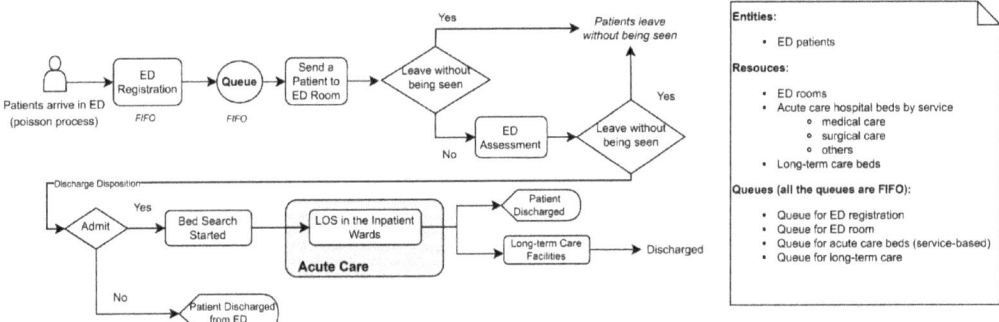

Figure 3. Flow chart showing the modeled ED and acute care patient flow in the proof-of-concept DES Model. LOS: length of stay; FIFO: first in, first out.

5.2. Stage 2: Conceptual Modeling

The initial conceptual modeling provided a theoretical basis for communicating with the domain experts, stakeholders, and the modeler. This was instrumental in guiding the modeler to develop DES models that captured the system problems with ED wait times while maintaining a reasonable scope and a moderate level of complexity.

5.2.1. Problem Conceptualization

The causes of ED crowding and lengthy ED wait times are complex [77,82]. ED crowding and long waiting times originate mainly from three interdependent components: the high volume of patients demanding ED care (input), the inability to assess and treat patients in a timely manner in the ED (throughput), and the boarding of inpatients in the ED after disposition decisions (output) [103]. Many potential contributing factors have been identified. They are present within each component of the input–throughput–output conceptual model of ED crowding [77,82,104–106]. Previous studies have investigated multiple input factors, such as the high volume of low-complexity patients in the ED, increased presentation with urgent and complex needs, and access to primary care [77,82,107]. Many throughput and output causes were also reported, such as ED staff shortages, limited availability of timely specialty consultation, delays in disposition decisions, and access block to inpatient units due to inadequate acute care beds or delayed discharge of inpatients [85,103,108]. Many input, throughput, and output solutions to ED crowding and wait times were trialed, modeled, and suggested with varying levels of success in different local contexts [77,109–111].

The modeling team jointly developed the driver diagram to depict five key areas to influence to reduce ED wait times. Figure 4 presents five primary drivers that are larger key topic areas related to the input, throughput, and output components of ED patient flow. Each primary driver was then linked with several secondary and tertiary drivers, which are less important or smaller in scale. The driver diagram was developed by incorporating diverse viewpoints from domain experts and stakeholders about the current state of the studied hospitals as well as evidence from the literature review. Domain experts and stakeholders were represented by physicians, nurse managers, operational leaders, and other health professionals from different health regions.

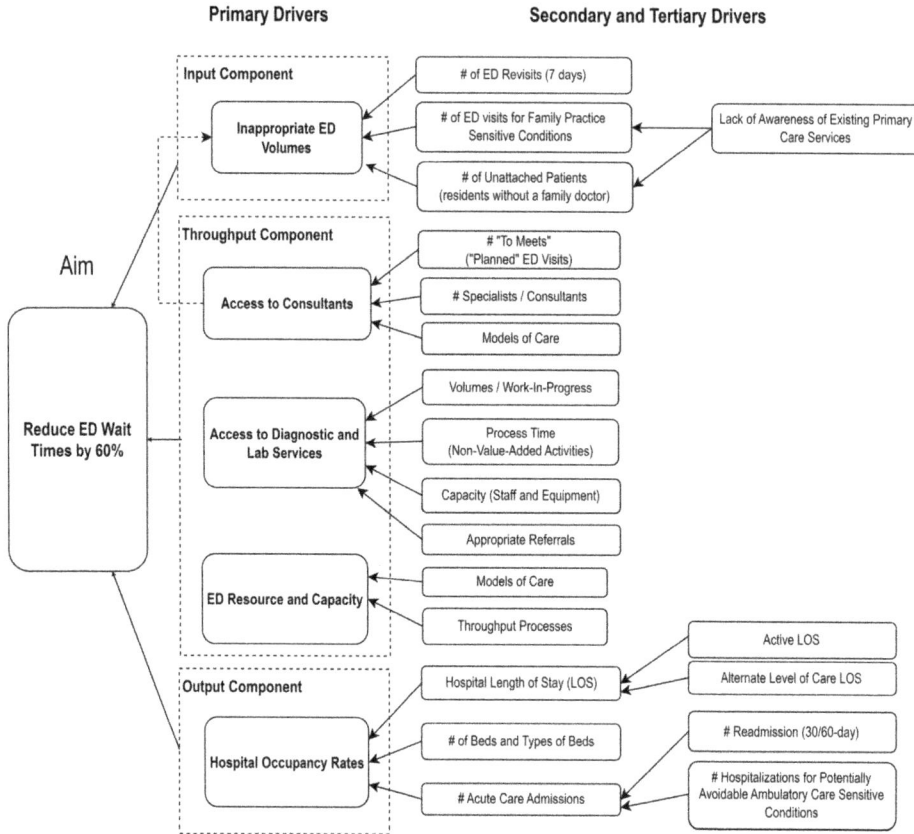

Figure 4. Driver diagram for lengthy ED wait times. LOS: length of stay.

5.2.2. Core Patient Flow Processes Emerging from the Value Stream Mapping

To gain insights into the flow of ED patients in the studied hospitals, the modeling team made use of VSMs that were created by healthcare professionals and improvement consultants during rapid process improvement workshops. Figure 5 illustrates the core care processes that emerged from the VSMs that were developed by regional teams that worked in the studied hospitals. It is worth noting that the regional teams took a whole-hospital perspective when mapping out the current state rather than just focusing solely on ED activities. Community and primary care services were also mapped out and connected to ED inputs and hospital discharges.

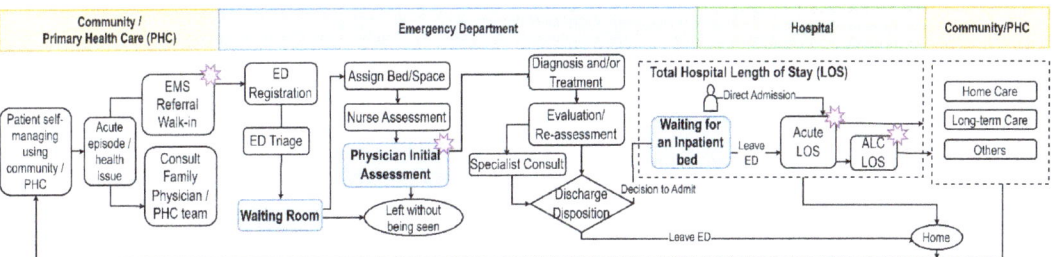

Figure 5. Core care processes emerging from the value stream maps. The stars indicate areas that require improvement, which were marked on value stream maps created during the rapid process improvement workshops. EMS: emergency medical services.

5.2.3. Model Scope and Level of Details

Figure 5 further helped to determine the scope of the simulation models and identify the boundaries of the model. The need to explore the inputs to the ED (e.g., ED volumes) was an obvious entry point into the simulation model. The requirement to study the cause of prolonged waits for inpatient beds suggested that the flow of acute care patients should be included in the model in order to capture the intricate interactions between the ED and other acute care services in the hospital. Although community and primary care services were also mapped out in Figure 5, they were excluded from the model based on guidance from the initiative leads and domain experts. Activities aimed solely at improving primary care, home care, or mental health care were also deemed beyond the intended scope of the study.

We then identified entities, activities, queues, and resources that fell within the model boundary. We focused on identifying components that were connected with secondary and tertiary drivers and areas requiring improvements in Figure 4. Knowledge of the domain experts and technical advisors was vital at this stage to help decide the level of detail that required modeling.

5.3. Stage 3: Model Implementation

During the conceptual modeling stage, the identification of key components, care processes, and model scope facilitated the selection of appropriate data sources and model inputs for the DES models. Patient-related model inputs were obtained from various administrative databases, including the National Ambulatory Care Reporting System, Discharge Abstract Database, Physician Billing Data Repository, and Person Health Registration System. These databases contain individual-level data on ED visits, hospitalizations, physician billing, and covered population demographics. Staff-related model inputs include ED-specific physician shifts, ED physician assessment time, registration time, and ED triage time. Resource-related model inputs include ED beds and acute care beds. The DES models were created using AnyLogic 8.7.2 (professional version; AnyLogic North America, Chicago, IL, USA) with the Java-based Process Modeling Library on an Intel® Core™ i7-9700 T CPU at 2.00 GHz, operating on Windows 10 Pro. Figure 6 shows the simulated patient flow from ED to acute care in the DES models.

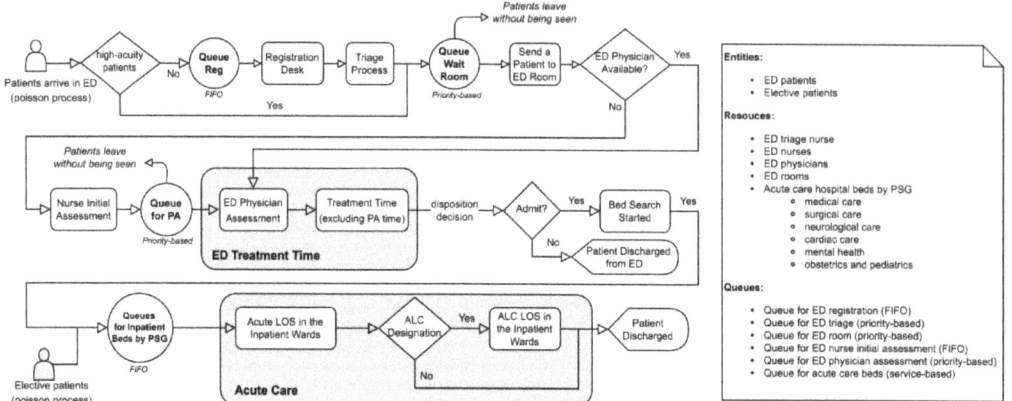

Figure 6. Flow chart showing the patient flow from ED to acute care [24]. Reg: registration; PA: physician assessment; ALC, alternate level of care; LOS, length of stay; PSG, patient service group; FIFO: first in, first out. Licensed material reproduced with permission from Springer Nature.

As ED patient flow was the central focus of the model, it needed to be explicitly modeled to ensure that the core ED care processes were captured. In addition, knowing that ED wait times could be the result of delays that occurred in other parts of the healthcare system—in particular acute care—made it essential to capture inpatient flow in acute care settings. The resulting model captured patients from ED presentation to discharge from the ED or an inpatient ward (for admitted patients), as illustrated in Figure 6. The model further incorporated the volume of patients admitted via elective admissions to an inpatient ward. The model allowed for adjustment of the volume of the ED, the arrival rate by hour and day of the week, the acuity, and the volume of the ED of a specific cohort (e.g., ED visits for family practice sensitive conditions). Clinical experts also proposed reasonable assumptions to be used in the models. For instance, high-acuity patients often receive immediate treatment and interventions upon arrival; therefore, registration or triage might occur concurrently with the treatment rather than before the treatment. For parameters that were unknown due to a lack of data in the administrative database, clinical experts (e.g., nurse managers and ED physicians) provided estimates for the studied EDs, including the duration of nurse initial assessment and the duration of physician assessment.

We developed 3D visualizations of the studied EDs in the early phase of model development to aid domain experts' understanding of the model logic and structure. Figure 7 illustrates examples of the visual representation of the studied EDs. Such visualization proved to be an effective approach in facilitating model interpretation and enabling effective communication with stakeholders without overwhelming them with detailed model logic and coding. The visualization allowed domain experts to provide valuable input and help refine model structure based on their clinical expertise and knowledge of the local contexts. For instance, this led to the incorporation of representations of chair spaces and surge stretchers in the EDs. Overall, incorporating visualization into the models improved model transparency and allowed for effective face validation of the models with domain experts.

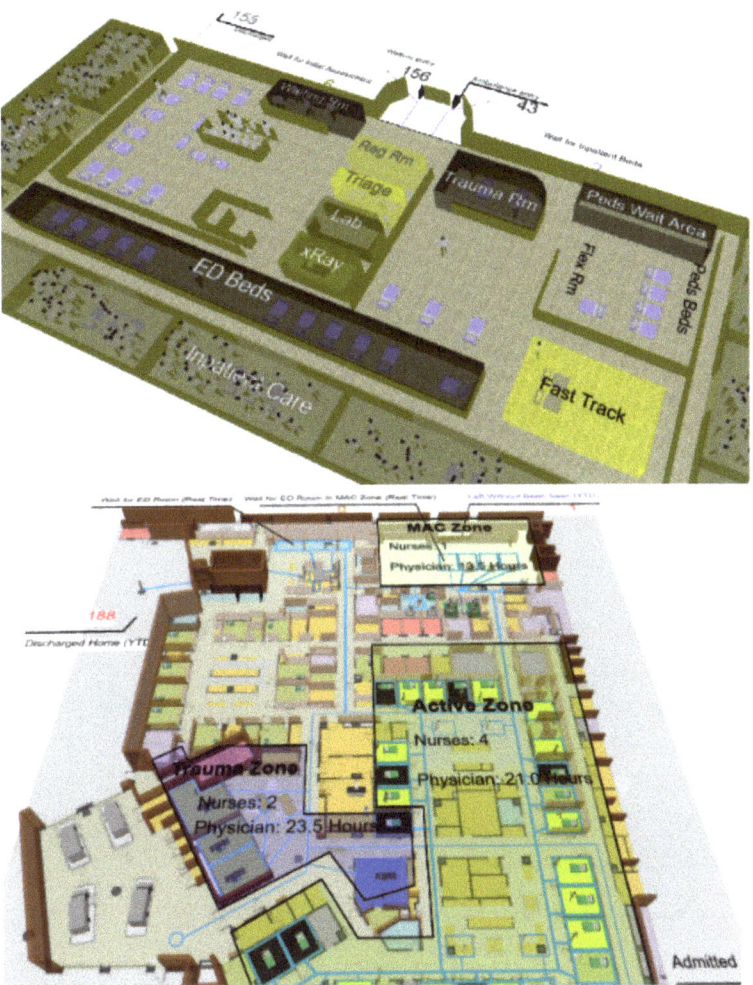

Figure 7. Examples of visual representation of the studied EDs.

The DES models were configured with a warm-up period of 5 months, followed by a 2-year run. Each scenario was replicated 40 times. The details on the model structure, inputs, assumptions, and experiment setup were reported in the previous study [24]. We focused on studying two ED wait time outcome measures: time waiting for physician initial assessment and time waiting for an inpatient bed. External model validation was performed by comparing the quantitative outputs of the simulation models in the baseline scenario (no intervention) with empirical data on the two outcome measures for the six studied EDs located in three health regions. Table 2 displays the validation results. It is important to highlight that we performed multiple validations at various stages of model development, particularly when structural modifications were incorporated or new model inputs or data were used in the DES models.

Table 2. Model validation [24].

Site	Mean Time Waiting for Physician Initial Assessment, Hours			Mean Time Waiting for Inpatient Bed, Hours		
	Simulated	Actual	Δ	Simulated	Actual	Δ
Site 1	1.99	2.04	−0.05	10.17	10.18	−0.01
Site 2	1.18	1.27	−0.09	7.81	7.88	−0.07
Site 3	1.26	1.26	0.00	11.13	11.01	0.12
Site 4	2.29	2.35	−0.06	4.65	4.61	0.04
Site 5	1.36	1.43	−0.07	1.38	1.29	0.09
Site 6	0.95	0.94	0.01	0.68	0.69	−0.01

Δ: difference (Simulated—Actual). Sites 2, 3, and 6 are in region A; site 5 is in region B; sites 1 and 4 are in region C. Licensed material reproduced with permission from Springer Nature.

5.4. Stage 4: Model Use and Policy Co-Development

The use of the multi-criteria framework allowed for a systematic approach to identify, screen, and shortlist the intervention scenarios to reduce ED wait times in each health region. This approach was critical in achieving the goal of co-developing effective interventions for reducing ED wait times. The use of the scoring matrix, as illustrated in Table 1, enabled the modeling team, regional leaders, and stakeholders in the advisory group to collaboratively assess each proposed intervention scenario based on a set of predefined criteria. This allowed for a transparent evaluation of the proposed interventions. The resulting shortlist of interventions, as shown in Table 3, reflected the varying priorities and readiness of each health region, as well as the unique contexts and varying perspectives of the stakeholders involved. After the third advisory group meeting, we incorporated several additional intervention scenarios for modeling based on discussions with stakeholders. These additional scenarios included combinations of individual interventions presented in Table 3 and expansion of existing programs in the healthcare system.

Table 3. Shortlisted intervention scenarios per health region in the third advisory group meeting.

Region	Scenario Name	Organizational Readiness	Regional Data Availability	Administrative Data Availability	Literature Support for Modeling	Regional Priority	Provincial Priority	Modeling Effort	Length of Time to Impact Drivers	Length of Time to Get Service Ready	Total Score
A	Attachment to primary care provider	3	3	5	5	5	4	4	3	3	35
	Reducing admissions for ACSCs	3	3	4	3	5	4	4	3	3	32
	Reducing ED visits for family practice sensitive conditions	3	3	4	1	5	4	4	3	3	30
	Alternate level of care reduction strategy	3	2	1	3	5	5	2	3	3	27
	High-quality care transitions (discharge planning and coordination)	3	3	4	4	4	4	1	4	3	30
	Hospital at home (early supported discharge) for surgical and neuro patients	4	4	4	5	4	4	5	3	3	36

Table 3. Cont.

Region	Scenario Name	Organizational Readiness	Regional Data Availability	Administrative Data Availability	Literature Support for Modeling	Regional Priority	Provincial Priority	Modeling Effort	Length of Time to Impact Drivers	Length of Time to Get Service Ready	Total Score
B	Expansion of community nurse practitioner services for COPD patients	5	5	3	2	5	4	3	5	4	36
	Hospitalist model for medical and surgical units	5	3	3	3	4	4	3	3	2	30
	Additional ED physician coverage	5	5	2	1	3	2	4	4	4	30
	Reducing ED visits for family practice sensitive conditions	4	4	4	1	4	3	4	3	3	30
C	ALC reduction strategy	-	1	3	3	-	5	2	3	3	20
	COPD clinical pathway	4	2	2	3	4	3	2	3	3	26
	High-quality care transitions (discharge planning and coordination)	-	3	4	4	3	4	1	3	4	26
	Hospital at home (early supported discharge) for surgical and neuro patients	4	4	4	4	4	3	5	3	5	36

ACSCs, ambulatory care sensitive conditions; COPD, chronic obstructive pulmonary disease; ALC, alternate level of care.

Considering the diverse range of proposed interventions aimed at specific patient groups, we systematically identified and extracted the corresponding target patient groups for each intervention in each studied ED or hospital and represented them in the DES models. Table 4 presents the effects of three selected scenarios on ED wait times, with one targeting the input component of the ED patient flow, and the other two targeting the output component. The quantitative simulation results of other proposed intervention scenarios have been described and discussed in detail elsewhere [24,112]. The three scenarios in Table 4 studied two patient groups: (1) patients aged under 75 who were hospitalized for ambulatory care sensitive conditions (ACSCs), and (2) inpatients who no longer need acute care but experienced delayed hospital discharge, also termed as alternate-level-of-care (ALC) patients.

Hospitalizations for ACSCs are considered largely preventable through improved primary care on an outpatient basis [113]. These conditions have been well documented in the literature. We analyzed the hospitalizations for five ACSCs: asthma, heart failure and pulmonary edema, chronic obstructive pulmonary disease (COPD), diabetes, and angina. We extracted the patient group using the most responsible diagnosis codes and cases with certain cardiac procedures were excluded for certain ACSC conditions [113,114]. Individuals aged 75 years and older were also excluded. It is worth noting that COPD is one of the ACSCs, and many health regions were interested in COPD prevention and care. Hospitalizations for these potentially avoidable ACSCs account for 1.9% to 4.4% of the hospitalizations in the five studied sites in Table 4.

Table 4. Effects of selected scenarios on ED wait times.

Scenario	Simulated Mean Time Waiting for Physician Initial Assessment, Hours			Simulated Mean Time Waiting for Inpatient Bed, Hours		
	Pre	Post	Δ	Pre	Post	Δ
Reduce ACSC-related hospitalizations by 10% (input)						
Site 1	1.99	1.95	−0.04	10.17	9.38	−0.79
Site 2	1.18	1.16	−0.02	7.81	7.43	−0.38
Site 3	1.26	1.22	−0.04	11.13	10.62	−0.51
Site 4	2.29	2.28	−0.01	4.65	4.47	−0.18
Site 5	1.36	1.36	0	1.38	1.22	−0.16
Reduce LTC-related ALC hospital days by 30% (output)						
Site 1	1.99	1.94	−0.05	10.17	7.83	−2.34
Site 2	1.18	1.12	−0.06	7.81	7.08	−0.73
Site 3	1.26	1.26	0	11.13	10.99	−0.14
Site 4	2.29	2.25	−0.04	4.65	3.95	−0.7
Site 5	1.36	1.36	0	1.38	1.23	−0.15
Reduce Non-LTC-related ALC hospital days by 30% (output)						
Site 1	1.99	1.93	−0.06	10.17	7.66	−2.51
Site 2	1.18	1.07	−0.11	7.81	6.21	−1.6
Site 3	1.26	1.26	0	11.13	10.91	−0.22
Site 4	2.29	2.25	−0.04	4.65	4.10	−0.55
Site 5	1.36	1.36	0	1.38	1.28	−0.1

Δ: simulated outcome postintervention minus that from the preintervention (baseline scenario). LTC: long-term care; ALC: alternate level of care; ACSC: ambulatory care sensitive conditions. Per scenario, 40 replications. We eliminated site 6 for these three selected scenarios because the ED in site 6 does not provide 24/7 service and has low ED admission rates; thus, the presented scenarios are not expected to have an impact on its ED patient flow and wait times. Sites 2 and 3 are in region A; site 5 is in region B; sites 1 and 4 are in region C.

We used ALC hospital days to measure the delays in hospital discharge experienced by ALC patients. The reasons for these delays can differ. They can occur when ALC patients are waiting for transfer to long-term care (LTC) facilities, resulting in LTC-related ALC hospital days. Alternatively, delays can occur before patients are discharged home but are awaiting post-acute care or home care, resulting in non-LTC-related ALC hospital days. The effect sizes of these three scenarios, such as 10% and 30%, were obtained from the advisory group and domain experts based on their assessments of achievable targets.

Reducing ACSC-related hospitalizations led to a slight decrease in the mean time spent waiting for an inpatient bed across EDs. The reduction in mean time waiting for an inpatient bed was greater in site 1 (Δ 0.79 h) owing to the higher proportion of ACSC-related hospitalizations in this hospital (4.1%). Reducing either LTC-related ALC days or non-LTC-related ALC days resulted in a larger reduction in mean time waiting for an inpatient bed for sites 1 and 2. The three selected scenarios had limited impact on the mean time waiting for physician initial assessment; therefore, they will not be able to solve the ED waits associated with physician assessment.

6. Discussion

The study presented a case study that aimed to support the identification of interventions to address the complex problem of lengthy ED wait times from a whole-system perspective in a Canadian policy development setting using a participatory modeling approach. We presented and discussed the quantitative results of the model findings in a previous contribution [24]. This paper focused on describing the formulation of the participatory modeling approach used and demonstrating its application in the process of developing DES models of EDs and acute care patient flow for six studied hospitals located in three Saskatchewan health regions. The participatory modeling approach involved engaging with key stakeholders in various modeling stages and co-developing interventions with stakeholders using a multi-criteria framework to identify, screen, and shortlist modeling scenarios to support effective policy development. The participatory modeling approach enabled the provincial initiative to effectively engage a broad range of stakeholders to examine and identify the causes and solutions to the ED wait time in the studied hospitals. Our methodology also contributed to the M&S field by introducing an innovative multiparadigm hybrid modeling approach that integrates qualitative and quantitative paradigms in different modeling stages [71].

To assess the impact of experts' and stakeholders' involvement in improving the model, we compared the proof-of-concept DES model (Figure 3) with the DES models developed using a participatory approach (Figure 6). While both models aimed to capture ED and acute care patient flow, significant differences were observed in their structures and development processes. The proof-of-concept DES model was constructed in an ad hoc manner, with the modeler taking the lead and consulting individual experts and stakeholders for information on the ED problem. The modeler represented the ED patient flow based on the obtained knowledge with very limited and ad hoc involvement of domain experts and stakeholders in the model development process. In contrast, the subsequent DES models were developed using a multistage participatory approach through iterative deliberation with stakeholders. Using the proposed participatory approach, domain experts and stakeholders collectively discussed evidence and shared knowledge about the causal mechanisms of the ED wait problem, identifying key drivers and areas requiring improvement through value stream mapping in the conceptual modeling stage. As a result of the different model building processes, notable differences emerged in the model structures. The proof-of-concept DES model primarily focused on ED patients, considering only ED-admitted patients for the acute care component, and featured simplified ED activities. In contrast, the later DES models incorporated detailed ED activities, included elective patients, stratified inpatients based on patient service groups, and accounted for separate alternate-level-of-care lengths of stay. The active and collaborative engagement of experts and stakeholders through the participatory approach contributed to these improvements in model structure and enhanced the modeler's understanding of the ED problem. The models were also better designed to evaluate proposed interventions by stakeholders. The use of qualitative tools and techniques in the conceptual modeling stage not only improved our shared understanding of the ED problem situation in the studied hospitals but also complemented the development of the DES models [62]. It is important to note that the ways in which the stakeholders and domain experts are engaged, either collaboratively or consultatively, also exert a significant impact on the development and quality of the models. Furthermore, the participatory approach allowed for a comprehensive system perspective. Given that ED and acute care systems are complex systems, individual experts or stakeholders may possess deep knowledge of specific aspects while lacking a holistic understanding. Engaging them collectively through the participatory approach provided a platform for multiple perspectives to be shared and fostered a broader understanding of the ED problem. In contrast, individual engagement could risk losing the systemic perspective that is crucial for addressing the ED wait times in the face of the complexity associated with the ED and acute care systems [115]. The system perspective enabled by applying a participatory modeling approach allowed us to study ED wait times as a part of a larger integrated acute care system. Our study contributed to the literature on whole-system DES models of ED patient flow for policy development.

Our study contributes to the conceptual modeling literature by demonstrating the use of the quality improvement toolkit and lean techniques as a problem structuring method to support problem conceptualization in the health policy development context [72]. Unlike other problem structuring methods which were rooted in the OR domain [53,116], we explored and used a number of existing tools that had already been used in the healthcare system, such as lean techniques and quality improvement tools for conceptual modeling. During the conceptual modeling stage, it is common for the modeling team to take the lead and utilize mapping tools that are unfamiliar to the domain experts or stakeholders. Persuading domain experts and patient flow managers to use new tools can be challenging and may require additional training and resources. Moreover, such stakeholders may not feel ownership of the project if they are only being consulted for information. In this study, instead of introducing new conceptual mapping tools, the modeling team explored and learned about existing quality improvement and mapping tools that were already in use within the healthcare system for structuring the problem. For instance, we used VSMs of ED patient flow that had already been developed by domain experts to conceptualize the problem of ED wait times. The use of these existing tools also facilitated communication with domain experts and flow managers about the ED wait time problem in the studied hospitals, given their familiarity with the lean techniques through the implementation of the lean methodology across the province's healthcare system at the time of this research. Such findings are consistent with previous research demonstrating that combining lean techniques with discrete-event simulation is a promising approach for studying care processes in the healthcare setting [117–119].

Two important facets of trust that influence the implementation of simulation findings are the stakeholder–model relationship and the stakeholder–modeler relationship, as the decision to implement changes based on simulation results is held by the stakeholders [19,20]. In contrast to the existing participatory modeling approaches in quantitative modeling, which primarily focus on resolving specific problems and generating quantitative forecasts or estimates [22], the novelty of our participatory modeling approach also lies in dedicated processes and activities specifically aimed at building trust in the computer modeling approach with the stakeholders and improving stakeholders' modeling knowledge. We conducted proof-of-concept analyses during project initialization and provided simulation modeling workshop to help stakeholders become familiar with the computer simulation approach. This helped foster trust at the beginning of the study and build confidence in the modeling approach that we used. Furthermore, our approach empowered stakeholders to develop skills to apply the modeling approach on their own. This, in turn, strengthened the stakeholder–model relationship, as they perceived the modeling approach to be more useful and credible. The stakeholder–modeler relationship is primarily centered around the stakeholders' perceived trust in the modeler's modeling and communication competencies, particularly whether stakeholders perceive that the modeler has a good and shared understanding of the problem situation in the early phases of a study [19,20]. The conceptual modeling component in our participatory approach played a key role in building trust in this relationship, thereby further improving trust in the stakeholder–model relationship.

Another contribution of our participatory approach lies in the development and use of the multi-criteria framework for co-developing interventions to address ED wait times. The use of the framework helped stakeholders reach an agreement regarding the feasible solution space and allowed a transparent assessment of the proposed actions. We included both the assessment of evidence and the availability of data in the framework to promote evidence-based decision making. In previous simulation studies, modeling scenarios were typically not fully designed to address the needs of stakeholders or policymakers. While stakeholders may have been involved in the development of intervention scenarios, their involvement was often limited to providing information rather than having a sense of ownership or being held "accountable" for the proposed intervention scenarios. In our study, we worked closely with stakeholders by involving them in the identification and prioritization of intervention scenarios through advisory group meetings. Stakeholders were held "accountable" for their proposed intervention scenarios, as a contact person was identified for each proposed scenario. The stakeholders and the modeling team collaborated to fill in a scoring matrix to prioritize intervention options based on criteria such as data availability, local practice, regional priority, and time to impact. This approach conferred on stakeholders a high degree of ownership and trust in the process and allowed regional leaders to view the scoring matrix of other regions. This process further aided in breaking the silos between organizations and various departments.

This case study further supported some learning regarding the application of the participatory modeling approach. We agreed with previous research findings on the importance of engaging stakeholders early on in the participatory modeling approach [42,48]. We would also like to highlight the role of the project champion in the team composition, as the project champion served as a key linkage between the modeling team and the stakeholder group and played a crucial role in building trust in the modeling methodology. Previous studies have also emphasized the importance of having a project champion in participatory modeling projects, as they can greatly contribute to the successful completion of such projects [10,57]. Our core engagement with stakeholders was in the co-development of intervention solutions to reduce ED wait times. Although we have been transparent about the model assumptions and model validations, we experienced challenges in building trust in the model outputs when the model outputs contradicted the stakeholders' prior beliefs or expectations. This phenomenon was also discussed in previous research [3,15]. In such cases, we found that it was important to facilitate ongoing and open dialogue with stakeholders through facilitated meetings.

7. Limitation and Future Work

The study has several limitations. The participatory modeling approach was applied to the case study of modeling ED and acute care patient flow using DES in a Canadian health policy setting. Due to the context-specific nature of the case study, the participatory modeling approach may not be directly applicable in other health-policy settings due to differences in organizational structures and policymaking environments. Second, the modeling team completed the scenario runs outside of the advisory group meetings, which might have reduced model transparency with stakeholders. An ideal solution would be to build models with a visual interface that allows for real-time experimentation during the advisory group meetings. However, this would require the identification of input variables related to the scenarios prior to the meetings and it is not always feasible to explore all the possible intervention solutions. Lastly, while the advisory group meetings were facilitated, formal scripts (e.g., PartiSim scripts) were not utilized, leading to a less structured approach that lacked standardization and might have resulted in missed opportunities.

The use of participatory modeling approaches with DES is still in its early stages in healthcare [59] and future research is needed to explore and develop innovative tools and processes that encourage stakeholder participation in the DES modeling processes and improve the implementation of the model findings. This includes combining tools or processes from diverse participatory modeling approaches (e.g., combining elements of GMB with PartiSim) and drawing insights from these experiences, and enhancing model validation [120]. This study further suggests the value of investigating the adaptation of existing tools employed in the healthcare system for use in the participatory modeling processes.

8. Conclusions

This study has successfully employed a four-stage participatory modeling approach with discrete-event simulation to identify intervention strategies for reducing ED wait times in a real-world health policy setting. The use of a participatory approach has enabled a broad range of stakeholders to examine and identify the causes and solutions to ED wait times and co-develop interventions for implementation. This approach has shown to be an effective way of engaging stakeholders throughout the modeling process and building consensus. Additionally, the study embraced a system view by studying ED wait times as a part of a larger integrated acute care system with multiple interacting subsystems or units, contributing to the literature on whole-system DES models of ED patient flow for policy development.

Author Contributions: Conceptualization, J.B., G.F., N.D.O. and Y.T.; methodology, Y.T., N.D.O., A.D. and P.F; software, Y.T.; validation, Y.T., J.B., J.S. and N.D.O.; formal analysis, Y.T.; investigation, Y.T., J.B., J.S., A.D. and P.F.; resources, Y.T., A.D. and P.F.; data curation, Y.T.; writing—original draft preparation, Y.T.; writing—review and editing, N.D.O., J.S., J.B. and A.D.; visualization, Y.T., P.F. and A.D.; supervision, N.D.O.; project administration, G.F. All authors have read and agreed to the published version of the manuscript.

Funding: This research received no external funding.

Data Availability Statement: The simulation model are available from the corresponding author (YT) upon reasonable request.

Acknowledgments: We would like to express our gratitude to Geoff McDonnell and Kurt Kreuger for their support and assistance in this research.

Conflicts of Interest: The authors declare no conflict of interest. The interpretation and conclusions contained herein do not necessarily represent those of the Government of Saskatchewan, the Saskatchewan Ministry of Health, the Saskatchewan Health Authority, or eHealth Saskatchewan.

References

1. Concannon, T.W.; Fuster, M.; Saunders, T.; Patel, K.; Wong, J.B.; Leslie, L.K.; Lau, J. A Systematic Review of Stakeholder Engagement in Comparative Effectiveness and Patient-Centered Outcomes Research. *J. Gen. Intern. Med.* **2014**, *29*, 1692–1701. [CrossRef] [PubMed]
2. Kotiadis, K.; Tako, A.A.; Vasilakis, C. A Participative and Facilitative Conceptual Modelling Framework for Discrete Event Simulation Studies in Healthcare. *J. Oper. Res. Soc.* **2014**, *65*, 197–213. [CrossRef]
3. Freebairn, L.; Rychetnik, L.; Atkinson, J.-A.; Kelly, P.; McDonnell, G.; Roberts, N.; Whittall, C.; Redman, S. Knowledge Mobilisation for Policy Development: Implementing Systems Approaches through Participatory Dynamic Simulation Modelling. *Health Res. Policy Syst.* **2017**, *15*, 83. [CrossRef]
4. Lamé, G.; Simmons, R.K. From Behavioural Simulation to Computer Models: How Simulation Can Be Used to Improve Healthcare Management and Policy. *BMJ Simul. Technol. Enhanc. Learn.* **2020**, *6*, 95. [CrossRef] [PubMed]
5. Pitt, M.; Monks, T.; Crowe, S.; Vasilakis, C. Systems Modelling and Simulation in Health Service Design, Delivery and Decision Making. *BMJ Qual. Saf.* **2016**, *25*, 38–45. [CrossRef]
6. Lich, K.H.; Tian, Y.; Beadles, C.A.; Williams, L.S.; Bravata, D.M.; Cheng, E.M.; Bosworth, H.B.; Homer, J.B.; Matchar, D.B. Strategic Planning to Reduce the Burden of Stroke among Veterans: Using Simulation Modeling to Inform Decision Making. *Stroke* **2014**, *45*, 2078–2084. [CrossRef]
7. Atkinson, J.-A.; O'Donnell, E.; Wiggers, J.; McDonnell, G.; Mitchell, J.; Freebairn, L.; Indig, D.; Rychetnik, L. Dynamic Simulation Modelling of Policy Responses to Reduce Alcohol-Related Harms: Rationale and Procedure for a Participatory Approach. *Public Health Res. Pract.* **2017**, *27*, 2711707. [CrossRef]
8. Hirsch, G.; Homer, J.; Evans, E.; Zielinski, A. A System Dynamics Model for Planning Cardiovascular Disease Interventions. *Am. J. Public Health* **2010**, *100*, 616–622. [CrossRef]
9. Freebairn, L.; Atkinson, J.-A.; Osgood, N.D.; Kelly, P.M.; McDonnell, G.; Rychetnik, L. Turning Conceptual Systems Maps into Dynamic Simulation Models: An Australian Case Study for Diabetes in Pregnancy. *PLoS ONE* **2019**, *14*, e0218875. [CrossRef]
10. Brailsford, S.C.; Harper, P.R.; Patel, B.; Pitt, M. An Analysis of the Academic Literature on Simulation and Modelling in Health Care. *J. Simul.* **2009**, *3*, 130–140. [CrossRef]
11. Atkinson, J.A.; Wells, R.; Page, A.; Dominello, A.; Haines, M.; Wilson, A. Applications of System Dynamics Modelling to Support Health Policy. *Public Health Res. Pract.* **2015**, *25*, e2531531. [CrossRef]
12. Mohiuddin, S.; Busby, J.; Savović, J.; Richards, A.; Northstone, K.; Hollingworth, W.; Donovan, J.L.; Vasilakis, C. Patient Flow within UK Emergency Departments: A Systematic Review of the Use of Computer Simulation Modelling Methods. *BMJ Open* **2017**, *7*, e015007. [CrossRef]
13. Taylor, S.J.E.; Eldabi, T.; Riley, G.; Paul, R.J.; Pidd, M. Simulation Modelling Is 50! Do We Need a Reality Check? *J. Oper. Res. Soc.* **2009**, *60*, S69–S82. [CrossRef]
14. Rutter, H.; Savona, N.; Glonti, K.; Bibby, J.; Cummins, S.; Finegood, D.T.; Greaves, F.; Harper, L.; Hawe, P.; Moore, L.; et al. The Need for a Complex Systems Model of Evidence for Public Health. *Lancet* **2017**, *390*, 2602–2604. [CrossRef]
15. Jahangirian, M.; Borsci, S.; Shah, S.G.S.; Taylor, S.J.E. Causal Factors of Low Stakeholder Engagement: A Survey of Expert Opinions in the Context of Healthcare Simulation Projects. *Simulation* **2015**, *91*, 511–526. [CrossRef]
16. Vázquez-Serrano, J.I.; Peimbert-García, R.E.; Cárdenas-Barrón, L.E. Discrete-Event Simulation Modeling in Healthcare: A Comprehensive Review. *Int. J. Environ. Res. Public Health* **2021**, *18*, 12262. [CrossRef] [PubMed]
17. Sobolev, B.G.; Sanchez, V.; Vasilakis, C. Systematic Review of the Use of Computer Simulation Modeling of Patient Flow in Surgical Care. *J. Med. Syst.* **2011**, *35*, 1–16. [CrossRef]
18. Brownson, R.C.; Royer, C.; Ewing, R.; McBride, T.D. Researchers and Policymakers: Travelers in Parallel Universes. *Am. J. Prev. Med.* **2006**, *30*, 164–172. [CrossRef] [PubMed]

19. Harper, A.; Mustafee, N.; Yearworth, M. The Issue of Trust and Implementation of Results in Healthcare Modeling and Simulation Studies. In Proceedings of the 2022 Winter Simulation Conference (WSC), Singapore, 11–14 December 2022; pp. 1104–1115.
20. Harper, A.; Mustafee, N.; Yearworth, M. Facets of Trust in Simulation Studies. *Eur. J. Oper. Res.* **2021**, *289*, 197–213. [CrossRef]
21. Tako, A.A.; Kotiadis, K. PartiSim: A Multi-Methodology Framework to Support Facilitated Simulation Modelling in Healthcare. *Eur. J. Oper. Res.* **2015**, *244*, 555–564. [CrossRef]
22. Voinov, A.; Jenni, K.; Gray, S.; Kolagani, N.; Glynn, P.D.; Bommel, P.; Prell, C.; Zellner, M.; Paolisso, M.; Jordan, R.; et al. Tools and Methods in Participatory Modeling: Selecting the Right Tool for the Job. *Environ. Model. Softw.* **2018**, *109*, 232–255. [CrossRef]
23. O'Donnell, E.; Atkinson, J.-A.; Freebairn, L.; Rychetnik, L. Participatory Simulation Modelling to Inform Public Health Policy and Practice: Rethinking the Evidence Hierarchies. *J. Public Health Policy* **2017**, *38*, 203–215. [CrossRef] [PubMed]
24. Tian, Y.; Osgood, N.D.; Stempien, J.; Onaemo, V.; Danyliw, A.; Fast, G.; Osman, B.A.; Reynolds, J.; Basran, J. The Impact of Alternate Level of Care on Access Block and Operational Strategies to Reduce Emergency Wait Times: A Multi-Center Simulation Study. *Can. J. Emerg. Med.* **2023**, *25*, 608–616. [CrossRef] [PubMed]
25. Jun, J.B.; Jacobson, S.H.; Swisher, J.R. Application of Discrete-Event Simulation in Health Care Clinics: A Survey. *J. Oper. Res. Soc.* **1999**, *50*, 109–123. [CrossRef]
26. Fone, D.; Hollinghurst, S.; Temple, M.; Round, A.; Lester, N.; Weightman, A.; Roberts, K.; Coyle, E.; Bevan, G.; Palmer, S. Systematic Review of the Use and Value of Computer Simulation Modelling in Population Health and Health Care Delivery. *J. Public Health Med.* **2003**, *25*, 325–335. [CrossRef]
27. Morris, Z.S.; Boyle, A.; Beniuk, K.; Robinson, S. Emergency Department Crowding: Towards an Agenda for Evidence-Based Intervention. *Emerg. Med. J.* **2012**, *29*, 460–466. [CrossRef]
28. Günal, M.M.; Pidd, M. Discrete Event Simulation for Performance Modelling in Health Care: A Review of the Literature. *J. Simul.* **2010**, *4*, 42–51. [CrossRef]
29. Laker, L.F.; Torabi, E.; France, D.J.; Froehle, C.M.; Goldlust, E.J.; Hoot, N.R.; Kasaie, P.; Lyons, M.S.; Barg-Walkow, L.H.; Ward, M.J.; et al. Understanding Emergency Care Delivery Through Computer Simulation Modeling. *Acad. Emerg. Med.* **2018**, *25*, 116–127. [CrossRef]
30. Salmon, A.; Rachuba, S.; Briscoe, S.; Pitt, M. A Structured Literature Review of Simulation Modelling Applied to Emergency Departments: Current Patterns and Emerging Trends. *Oper. Res. Health Care* **2018**, *19*, 1–13. [CrossRef]
31. Hare, M. Forms of Participatory Modelling and Its Potential for Widespread Adoption in the Water Sector. *Environ. Policy Gov.* **2011**, *21*, 386–402. [CrossRef]
32. Boaz, A.; Borst, R.; Kok, M.; O'Shea, A. How Far Does an Emphasis on Stakeholder Engagement and Co-Production in Research Present a Threat to Academic Identity and Autonomy? A Prospective Study across Five European Countries. *Res. Eval.* **2021**, *30*, 361–369. [CrossRef]
33. Tako, A.A.; Kotiadis, K. Participative Simulation (Partisim): A Facilitated Simulation Approach for Stakeholder Engagement. In Proceedings of the 2018 Winter Simulation Conference (WSC), Göteborg, Sweden, 9–12 December 2018; pp. 192–206.
34. Voinov, A.; Kolagani, N.; McCall, M.K.; Glynn, P.D.; Kragt, M.E.; Ostermann, F.O.; Pierce, S.A.; Ramu, P. Modelling with Stakeholders—Next Generation. *Environ. Model. Softw.* **2016**, *77*, 196–220. [CrossRef]
35. Ulibarri, N. Collaborative Model Development Increases Trust in and Use of Scientific Information in Environmental Decision-Making. *Environ. Sci. Policy* **2018**, *82*, 136–142. [CrossRef]
36. Stave, K. Participatory System Dynamics Modeling for Sustainable Environmental Management: Observations from Four Cases. *Sustain. Sci. Pract. Policy* **2010**, *2*, 2762–2784. [CrossRef]
37. Beall, A.M.; Ford, A. Reports from the Field: Assessing the Art and Science of Participatory Environmental Modeling. *Int. J. Inf. Syst. Soc. Chang.* **2010**, *1*, 72–89. [CrossRef]
38. Richardson, G.P.; Andersen, D.F. Teamwork in Group Model Building. *Syst. Dyn. Rev.* **1995**, *11*, 113–137. [CrossRef]
39. Hovmand, P.S. *Community Based System Dynamics*; Springer: New York, NY, USA, 2014.
40. Adams, S.; Rhodes, T.; Lancaster, K. New Directions for Participatory Modelling in Health: Redistributing Expertise in Relation to Localised Matters of Concern. *Glob. Public Health* **2021**, *17*, 1827–1841. [CrossRef]
41. Seidl, R. A Functional-Dynamic Reflection on Participatory Processes in Modeling Projects. *Ambio* **2015**, *44*, 750–765. [CrossRef]
42. Freebairn, L.; Atkinson, J.-A.; Kelly, P.M.; McDonnell, G.; Rychetnik, L. Decision Makers' Experience of Participatory Dynamic Simulation Modelling: Methods for Public Health Policy. *BMC Med. Inform. Decis. Mak.* **2018**, *18*, 131. [CrossRef]
43. Freebairn, L.; Atkinson, J.-A.; Qin, Y.; Nolan, C.J.; Kent, A.L.; Kelly, P.M.; Penza, L.; Prodan, A.; Safarishahrbijari, A.; Qian, W.; et al. "Turning the Tide" on Hyperglycemia in Pregnancy: Insights from Multiscale Dynamic Simulation Modeling. *BMJ Open Diabetes Res. Care* **2020**, *8*, e000975. [CrossRef]
44. Frerichs, L.; Lich, K.H.; Dave, G.; Corbie-Smith, G. Integrating Systems Science and Community-Based Participatory Research to Achieve Health Equity. *Am. J. Public Health* **2016**, *106*, 215–222. [CrossRef] [PubMed]
45. Gerritsen, S.; Harré, S.; Rees, D.; Renker-Darby, A.; Bartos, A.E.; Waterlander, W.E.; Swinburn, B. Community Group Model Building as a Method for Engaging Participants and Mobilising Action in Public Health. *Int. J. Environ. Res. Public Health* **2020**, *17*, 3457. [CrossRef]
46. Augustsson, H.; Churruca, K.; Braithwaite, J. Re-Energising the Way We Manage Change in Healthcare: The Case for Soft Systems Methodology and Its Application to Evidence-Based Practice. *BMC Health Serv. Res.* **2019**, *19*, 666. [CrossRef] [PubMed]

47. Hovmand, P.S. Group Model Building and Community-Based System Dynamics Process. In *Community Based System Dynamics*; Springer: New York, NY, USA, 2014.
48. Reed, M.S. Stakeholder Participation for Environmental Management: A Literature Review. *Biol. Conserv.* **2008**, *141*, 2417–2431. [CrossRef]
49. Viswanathan, M.; Ammerman, A.; Eng, E.; Garlehner, G.; Lohr, K.N.; Griffith, D.; Rhodes, S.; Samuel-Hodge, C.; Maty, S.; Lux, L.; et al. Community-Based Participatory Research: Assessing the Evidence. *Evid. Rep. Summ.* **2004**, *18*, 1–8.
50. Checkland, P.; Poulter, J. Soft Systems Methodology. In *Systems Approaches to Making Change: A Practical Guide*; Reynolds, M., Holwell, S., Eds.; Springer: London, UK, 2020; pp. 201–253. ISBN 9781447174721.
51. Water, H.; van de Schinkel, M.; Rozier, R. Fields of Application of SSM: A Categorization of Publications. *J. Oper. Res. Soc.* **2007**, *58*, 271–287. [CrossRef]
52. Jones, W.; Kotiadis, K.; O'Hanley, J.R. Maximising Stakeholder Learning by Looping Again through the Simulation Life-Cycle: A Case Study in Public Transport. *J. Oper. Res. Soc.* **2021**, *73*, 2640–2659. [CrossRef]
53. Kotiadis, K.; Mingers, J. Combining Problem Structuring Methods with Simulation: The Philosophical and Practical Challenges. In *Discrete-Event Simulation and System Dynamics for Management Decision Making*; John Wiley & Sons Ltd.: Chichester, UK, 2014; pp. 52–75. ISBN 9781118762745.
54. Andersen, D.F.; Vennix, J.A.M.; Richardson, G.P.; Rouwette, E.A.J.A. Group Model Building: Problem Structuring, Policy Simulation and Decision Support. *J. Oper. Res. Soc.* **2007**, *58*, 691–694. [CrossRef]
55. Vennix, J.A.M. Group Model-Building: Tackling Messy Problems. *Syst. Dyn. Rev.* **1999**, *15*, 379–401. [CrossRef]
56. Esensoy, A.V.; Carter, M.W. Health System Modelling for Policy Development and Evaluation: Using Qualitative Methods to Capture the Whole-System Perspective. *Oper. Res. Health Care* **2015**, *4*, 15–26. [CrossRef]
57. Tako, A.A.; Kotiadis, K. Facilitated Conceptual Modelling: Practical Issues and Reflections. In Proceedings of the 2012 Winter Simulation Conference (WSC), Berlin, Germany, 9–12 December 2012; pp. 1–12.
58. Tako, A.A.; Vasilakis, C.; Kotiadis, K. A Participative Modelling Framework for Developing Conceptual Models in Healthcare Simulation Studies. In Proceedings of the 2010 Winter Simulation Conference, Baltimore, MD, USA, 5–8 December 2010; pp. 500–512.
59. Kotiadis, K.; Tako, A.A. Facilitated Post-Model Coding in Discrete Event Simulation (DES): A Case Study in Healthcare. *Eur. J. Oper. Res.* **2018**, *266*, 1120–1133. [CrossRef]
60. Tako, A.A.; Kotiadis, K.; Vasilakis, C.; Miras, A.; le Roux, C.W. Improving Patient Waiting Times: A Simulation Study of an Obesity Care Service. *BMJ Qual. Saf.* **2014**, *23*, 373–381. [CrossRef] [PubMed]
61. Brailsford, S.C.; Eldabi, T.; Kunc, M.; Mustafee, N.; Osorio, A.F. Hybrid Simulation Modelling in Operational Research: A State-of-the-Art Review. *Eur. J. Oper. Res.* **2019**, *278*, 721–737. [CrossRef]
62. Powell, J.H.; Mustafee, N. Widening Requirements Capture with Soft Methods: An Investigation of Hybrid M&S Studies in Health Care. *J. Oper. Res. Soc. Abingdon* **2017**, *68*, 1211–1222. [CrossRef]
63. Tolk, A.; Harper, A.; Mustafee, N. Hybrid Models as Transdisciplinary Research Enablers. *Eur. J. Oper. Res.* **2021**, *291*, 1075–1090. [CrossRef]
64. Gao, A.; Osgood, N.D.; An, W.; Dyck, R.F. A Tripartite Hybrid Model Architecture for Investigating Health and Cost Impacts and Intervention Tradeoffs for Diabetic End-Stage Renal Disease. In Proceedings of the Winter Simulation Conference 2014, Savannah, GA, USA, 7–10 December 2014; pp. 1676–1687.
65. Qin, Y.; Freebairn, L.; Atkinson, J.-A.; Qian, W.; Safarishahrbijari, A.; Osgood, N.D. Multi-Scale Simulation Modeling for Prevention and Public Health Management of Diabetes in Pregnancy and Sequelae. In *Proceedings of the Social, Cultural, and Behavioral Modeling*; Springer International Publishing: Berlin/Heidelberg, Germany, 2019; pp. 256–265.
66. Zhu, H.; Liu, S.; Li, X.; Zhang, W.; Osgood, N.; Jia, P. Using a Hybrid Simulation Model to Assess the Impacts of Combined COVID-19 Containment Measures in a High-Speed Train Station. *J. Simul.* **2023**, 1–25. [CrossRef]
67. Gao, A.; Osgood, N.D.; Jiang, Y.; Dyck, R.F. Projecting Prevalence, Costs and Evaluating Simulated Interventions for Diabetic End Stage Renal Disease in a Canadian Population of Aboriginal and Non-Aboriginal People: An Agent Based Approach. *BMC Nephrol.* **2017**, *18*, 283. [CrossRef]
68. Flynn, T.; Tian, Y.; Masnick, K.; McDonnell, G.; Huynh, E.; Mair, A.; Osgood, N. Discrete Choice, Agent Based and System Dynamics Simulation of Health Profession Career Paths. In Proceedings of the Winter Simulation Conference 2014, Savannah, GA, USA, 7–10 December 2014; pp. 1700–1711.
69. Vickers, D.M.; Osgood, N.D. A Unified Framework of Immunological and Epidemiological Dynamics for the Spread of Viral Infections in a Simple Network-Based Population. *Theor. Biol. Med. Model.* **2007**, *4*, 49. [CrossRef]
70. Mustafee, N.; Harper, A.; Fakhimi, M. From Conceptualization of Hybrid Modelling & Simulation to Empirical Studies in Hybrid Modelling. In Proceedings of the 2022 Winter Simulation Conference (WSC), Singapore, 11–14 December 2022; pp. 1199–1210.
71. Mustafee, N.; Harper, A.; Onggo, B.S. Hybrid Modelling and Simulation (M&S): Driving Innovation in the Theory and Practice of M&S. In Proceedings of the 2020 Winter Simulation Conference (WSC), Orlando, FL, USA, 14–18 December 2020.
72. Mustafee, N.; Powell, J.H. From Hybrid Simulation to Hybrid Systems Modelling. In Proceedings of the 2018 Winter Simulation Conference (WSC), Göteborg, Sweden, 9–12 December 2018.
73. McDonald, G.W.; Bradford, L.; Neapetung, M.; Osgood, N.D.; Strickert, G.; Waldner, C.L.; Belcher, K.; McLeod, L.; Bharadwaj, L. Case Study of Collaborative Modeling in an Indigenous Community. *Water* **2022**, *14*, 2601. [CrossRef]

74. Jiang, L.; Li, X.; Wang, M.C.; Osgood, N.; Whaley, S.E.; Crespi, C.M. Estimating the Population Impact of Hypothetical Breastfeeding Interventions in a Low-Income Population in Los Angeles County: An Agent-Based Model. *PLoS ONE* **2020**, *15*, e0231134. [CrossRef]
75. Tian, Y.; Hassmiller Lich, K.; Osgood, N.D.; Eom, K.; Matchar, D.B. Linked Sensitivity Analysis, Calibration, and Uncertainty Analysis Using a System Dynamics Model for Stroke Comparative Effectiveness Research. *Med. Decis. Mak.* **2016**, *36*, 1043–1057. [CrossRef] [PubMed]
76. Kreuger, L.K.; Qian, W.; Osgood, N.; Choi, K. Agile Design Meets Hybrid Models: Using Modularity to Enhance Hybrid Model Design and Use. In Proceedings of the 2016 Winter Simulation Conference (WSC), Washington, DC, USA, 11–14 December 2016; pp. 1428–1438.
77. Morley, C.; Unwin, M.; Peterson, G.M.; Stankovich, J.; Kinsman, L. Emergency Department Crowding: A Systematic Review of Causes, Consequences and Solutions. *PLoS ONE* **2018**, *13*, e0203316. [CrossRef] [PubMed]
78. Pines, J.M.; Griffey, R.T. What We Have Learned from a Decade of ED Crowding Research. *Acad. Emerg. Med.* **2015**, *22*, 985–987. [CrossRef]
79. Guttmann, A.; Schull, M.J.; Vermeulen, M.J.; Stukel, T.A. Association between Waiting Times and Short Term Mortality and Hospital Admission after Departure from Emergency Department: Population Based Cohort Study from Ontario, Canada. *BMJ* **2011**, *342*, d2983. [CrossRef]
80. Singer, A.J.; Thode, H.C., Jr.; Viccellio, P.; Pines, J.M. The Association between Length of Emergency Department Boarding and Mortality. *Acad. Emerg. Med.* **2011**, *18*, 1324–1329. [CrossRef]
81. Tekwani, K.L.; Kerem, Y.; Mistry, C.D.; Sayger, B.M.; Kulstad, E.B. Emergency Department Crowding Is Associated with Reduced Satisfaction Scores in Patients Discharged from the Emergency Department. *West. J. Emerg. Med.* **2013**, *14*, 11–15. [CrossRef]
82. Moskop, J.C.; Sklar, D.P.; Geiderman, J.M.; Schears, R.M.; Bookman, K.J. Emergency Department Crowding, Part 1—Concept, Causes, and Moral Consequences. *Ann. Emerg. Med.* **2009**, *53*, 605–611. [CrossRef]
83. Vogel, L. Canadians Still Waiting for Timely Access to Care. *Can. Med. Assoc. J.* **2017**, *189*, E375–E376. [CrossRef] [PubMed]
84. Pines, J.M.; Hilton, J.A.; Weber, E.J.; Alkemade, A.J.; Al Shabanah, H.; Anderson, P.D.; Bernhard, M.; Bertini, A.; Gries, A.; Ferrandiz, S.; et al. International Perspectives on Emergency Department Crowding. *Acad. Emerg. Med.* **2011**, *18*, 1358–1370. [CrossRef]
85. Bond, K.; Ospina, M.B.; Blitz, S.; Afilalo, M.; Campbell, S.G.; Bullard, M.; Innes, G.; Holroyd, B.; Curry, G.; Schull, M.; et al. Frequency, Determinants and Impact of Overcrowding in Emergency Departments in Canada: A National Survey. *Healthc. Q.* **2007**, *10*, 32–40. [CrossRef]
86. Saskatchewan ED Waits and Patient Flow Initiative Emergency Department Waits and Patient Flow Initiative Fall 2015 Newsletter. Available online: https://www.hqc.sk.ca/Portals/0/documents/ReducingERWaitsImprovingFlow/Emerg-Dept-Waits-Update-Fall-2015.pdf (accessed on 16 July 2017).
87. Saghafian, S.; Austin, G.; Traub, S.J. Operations Research/Management Contributions to Emergency Department Patient Flow Optimization: Review and Research Prospects. *IIE Trans. Healthc. Syst. Eng.* **2015**, *5*, 101–123. [CrossRef]
88. Paul, S.A.; Reddy, M.C.; DeFlitch, C.J. A Systematic Review of Simulation Studies Investigating Emergency Department Overcrowding. *Simulation* **2010**, *86*, 559–571. [CrossRef]
89. Zhang, X. Application of Discrete Event Simulation in Health Care: A Systematic Review. *BMC Health Serv. Res.* **2018**, *18*, 687. [CrossRef]
90. Rashwan, W.; Abo-Hamad, W.; Arisha, A. A System Dynamics View of the Acute Bed Blockage Problem in the Irish Healthcare System. *Eur. J. Oper. Res.* **2015**, *247*, 276–293. [CrossRef]
91. Vanderby, S.; Carter, M.W. An Evaluation of the Applicability of System Dynamics to Patient Flow Modelling. *J. Oper. Res. Soc.* **2010**, *61*, 1572–1581. [CrossRef]
92. Shi, P.; Chou, M.C.; Dai, J.G.; Ding, D.; Sim, J. Models and Insights for Hospital Inpatient Operations: Time-Dependent ED Boarding Time. *Manag. Sci.* **2016**, *62*, 1–28. [CrossRef]
93. Esensoy, A.V. Whole-System Patient Flow Modelling for Strategic Planning in Healthcare. Ph.D. Thesis, University of Toronto, Toronto, ON, Canada, 2016.
94. Rouwette, E.A.J.A.; Vennix, J.A.M.; van Mullekom, T. Group Model Building Effectiveness: A Review of Assessment Studies. *Syst. Dyn. Rev.* **2002**, *18*, 5–45. [CrossRef]
95. Robinson, S. Conceptual Modelling for Simulation Part II: A Framework for Conceptual Modelling. *J. Oper. Res. Soc. Abingdon* **2008**, *59*, 291–304. [CrossRef]
96. Institute for Healthcare Improvement. *Quality Improvement Essentials Toolkit*; Institute for Healthcare Improvement: Boston, MA, USA, 2017.
97. Feld, W.M. *Lean Manufacturing: Tools, Techniques, and How to Use Them*; CRC Press: Boca Raton, FL, USA, 2000; ISBN 9781420025538.
98. Hines, P.; Rich, N. The Seven Value Stream Mapping Tools. *Int. J. Oper. Prod. Manag.* **1997**, *17*, 46–64. [CrossRef]
99. Kinsman, L.; Rotter, T.; Stevenson, K.; Bath, B.; Goodridge, D.; Harrison, L.; Dobson, R.; Sari, N.; Jeffery, C.; Bourassa, C.; et al. "The Largest Lean Transformation in the World": The Implementation and Evaluation of Lean in Saskatchewan Healthcare. *Healthc. Q.* **2014**, *17*, 29–32. [CrossRef]

100. Saskatchewan Health Quality Council Health Care Leaders to Participate in Innovative Computer Modelling Boot Camp. Available online: https://www.saskhealthquality.ca/about-us/news/health-care-leaders-to-participate-in-innovative-computer-modelling-boot-camp/ (accessed on 30 April 2023).
101. Straus, S.E.; Tetroe, J.; Graham, I.D. *Knowledge Translation in Health Care: Moving from Evidence to Practice*, 2nd ed.; Wiley: Hoboken, NJ, USA, 2013; ISBN 9781118413548.
102. Komal, B.; Janjua, U.I.; Anwar, F.; Madni, T.M.; Cheema, M.F.; Malik, M.N.; Shahid, A.R. The Impact of Scope Creep on Project Success: An Empirical Investigation. *IEEE Access* **2020**, *8*, 125755–125775. [CrossRef]
103. Asplin, B.R.; Magid, D.J.; Rhodes, K.V.; Solberg, L.I.; Lurie, N.; Camargo, C.A., Jr. A Conceptual Model of Emergency Department Crowding. *Ann. Emerg. Med.* **2003**, *42*, 173–180. [CrossRef] [PubMed]
104. Hoot, N.R.; Aronsky, D. Systematic Review of Emergency Department Crowding: Causes, Effects, and Solutions. *Ann. Emerg. Med.* **2008**, *52*, 126–136. [CrossRef] [PubMed]
105. Doupe, M.B.; Chateau, D.; Chochinov, A.; Weber, E.; Enns, J.E.; Derksen, S.; Sarkar, J.; Schull, M.; Lobato de Faria, R.; Katz, A.; et al. Comparing the Effect of Throughput and Output Factors on Emergency Department Crowding: A Retrospective Observational Cohort Study. *Ann. Emerg. Med.* **2018**, *72*, 410–419. [CrossRef] [PubMed]
106. Asaro, P.V.; Lewis, L.M.; Boxerman, S.B. The Impact of Input and Output Factors on Emergency Department Throughput. *Acad. Emerg. Med.* **2007**, *14*, 235–242. [CrossRef] [PubMed]
107. Moineddin, R.; Meaney, C.; Agha, M.; Zagorski, B.; Glazier, R.H. Modeling Factors Influencing the Demand for Emergency Department Services in Ontario: A Comparison of Methods. *BMC Emerg. Med.* **2011**, *11*, 13. [CrossRef]
108. Forster, A.J.; Stiell, I.; Wells, G.; Lee, A.J.; van Walraven, C. The Effect of Hospital Occupancy on Emergency Department Length of Stay and Patient Disposition. *Acad. Emerg. Med.* **2003**, *10*, 127–133. [CrossRef]
109. Yarmohammadian, M.H.; Rezaei, F.; Haghshenas, A.; Tavakoli, N. Overcrowding in Emergency Departments: A Review of Strategies to Decrease Future Challenges. *J. Res. Med. Sci.* **2017**, *22*, 23. [CrossRef]
110. Moskop, J.C.; Sklar, D.P.; Geiderman, J.M.; Schears, R.M.; Bookman, K.J. Emergency Department Crowding, Part 2—Barriers to Reform and Strategies to Overcome Them. *Ann. Emerg. Med.* **2009**, *53*, 612–617. [CrossRef]
111. Mason, S.; Mountain, G.; Turner, J.; Arain, M.; Revue, E.; Weber, E.J. Innovations to Reduce Demand and Crowding in Emergency Care; a Review Study. *Scand. J. Trauma Resusc. Emerg. Med.* **2014**, *22*, 55. [CrossRef]
112. Saskatchewan Health Quality Council Connected Care: A Summary of Learnings from the Emergency Department Waits and Patient Flow Initiative. Available online: https://www.saskhealthquality.ca/wp-content/uploads/2021/06/Connected-Care-Summary-of-Learnings-from-ED-Waits-and-Patient-Flow-Initiative.pdf (accessed on 26 July 2021).
113. Khan, S.; Sanmartin, C. *LHAD research team Hospitalizations for Ambulatory Care Sensitive Conditions (ACSC): The Factors That Matter*; Statistics: Ottawa, ON, Canada, 2011.
114. Canadian Institute for Health Information. *Continuity of Care with Family Medicine Physicians: Why It Matters*; CIHI: Ottawa, ON, Canada, 2015.
115. Jones, W.; Kotiadis, K.; O'Hanley, J. Engaging Stakeholders to Extend the Lifecycle of Hybrid Simulation Models. In Proceedings of the 2019 Winter Simulation Conference (WSC), National Harbor, MD, USA, 8–11 December 2019; pp. 1304–1315.
116. Powell, J.; Mustafee, N. Soft OR Approaches in Problem Formulation Stage of a Hybrid M&S Study. In Proceedings of the Winter Simulation Conference 2014, Savannah, GA, USA, 7–10 December 2014; pp. 1664–1675.
117. Bal, A.; Ceylan, C.; Taçoğlu, C. Using Value Stream Mapping and Discrete Event Simulation to Improve Efficiency of Emergency Departments. *Int. J. Healthc. Manag.* **2017**, *10*, 196–206. [CrossRef]
118. Robinson, S.; Radnor, Z.J.; Burgess, N.; Worthington, C. SimLean: Utilising Simulation in the Implementation of Lean in Healthcare. *Eur. J. Oper. Res.* **2012**, *219*, 188–197. [CrossRef]
119. Robinson, S.; Worthington, C.; Burgess, N.; Radnor, Z.J. Facilitated Modelling with Discrete-Event Simulation: Reality or Myth? *Eur. J. Oper. Res.* **2014**, *234*, 231–240. [CrossRef]
120. Diallo, S.Y.; Gore, R.; Lynch, C.J.; Padilla, J.J. Formal Methods, Statistical Debugging and Exploratory Analysis in Support of System Development: Towards a Verification and Validation Calculator Tool. *Int. J. Model. Simul. Sci. Comput.* **2016**, *7*, 1641001. [CrossRef]

Disclaimer/Publisher's Note: The statements, opinions and data contained in all publications are solely those of the individual author(s) and contributor(s) and not of MDPI and/or the editor(s). MDPI and/or the editor(s) disclaim responsibility for any injury to people or property resulting from any ideas, methods, instructions or products referred to in the content.

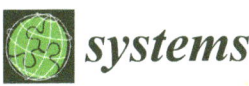

Article

Dynamic Optimization of Emergency Logistics for Major Epidemic Considering Demand Urgency

Jianjun Zhang [1], Jingru Huang [1], Tianhao Wang [1] and Jin Zhao [2,*]

[1] School of Economics and Management, Tongji University, Shanghai 200092, China
[2] Sino-German College of Applied Science, Tongji University, Shanghai 201804, China
* Correspondence: zj@tongji.edu.cn

Abstract: In recent years, epidemic disasters broke through frequently around the world, posing a huge threat to economic and social development, as well as human health. A fair and accurate distribution of emergency supplies during an epidemic is vital for improving emergency rescue efficiency and reducing economic losses. However, traditional emergency material allocation models often focus on meeting the amount of materials requested, and ignore the differences in the importance of different emergency materials and the subjective urgency demand of the disaster victims. As a result, it is difficult for the system to fairly and reasonably match different scarce materials to the corresponding areas of greatest need. Consequently, this paper proposes a material shortage adjustment coefficient based on the entropy weight method, which includes indicators such as material consumption rate, material reproduction rate, durability, degree of danger to life, and degree of irreplaceability, to enlarge and narrow the actual shortage of material supply according to the demand urgency. Due to the fact that emergency materials are not dispatched in one go during epidemic periods, a multi-period integer programming model was established to minimize the adjusted total material shortage based on the above function. Taking the cases of Wuhan and Shanghai during the lockdown and static management period, the quantitative analysis based on material distribution reflected that the model established in this paper was effective in different scenarios where there were significant differences in the quantity and structure of material demand. At the same time, the model could significantly adjust the shortage of emergency materials with higher importance and improve the satisfaction rate.

Keywords: major epidemic; demand urgency; emergency logistics; material distribution optimization

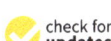

Citation: Zhang, J.; Huang, J.; Wang, T.; Zhao, J. Dynamic Optimization of Emergency Logistics for Major Epidemic Considering Demand Urgency. *Systems* **2023**, *11*, 303. https://doi.org/10.3390/systems11060303

Academic Editors: Andrew Page and Philippe J. Giabbanelli

Received: 25 February 2023
Revised: 16 May 2023
Accepted: 7 June 2023
Published: 13 June 2023

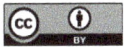

Copyright: © 2023 by the authors. Licensee MDPI, Basel, Switzerland. This article is an open access article distributed under the terms and conditions of the Creative Commons Attribution (CC BY) license (https://creativecommons.org/licenses/by/4.0/).

1. Introduction

The outbreak of COVID-19 caused huge disasters and heavy losses worldwide, which also triggered people's reflection and attention on the prevention and control of major epidemics and material support [1]. The issue of how to allocate scarce emergency materials reasonably has become a key concern for ensuring patient safety and reducing losses. Researchers [2–5] have addressed this issue from a variety of perspectives, primarily studying how to optimize the allocation of scarce emergency materials to reduce delivery times, reduce costs, and maximize demand satisfaction. The current research on emergency management material allocations still has limitations, as most models only focus on single-period allocations. However, for major public health events, as an epidemic develops, the demand for emergency materials will accordingly change dynamically [6]. Therefore, this study considered the demand characteristics of different periods of epidemic disasters and established a dynamic multi-period model to optimize material allocation.

During the outbreak of major epidemics, the supply of emergency materials often cannot meet the demand, and there is a serious of shortages of medical equipment, protective equipment, and daily necessities. The shortage of medical materials will lead to an increase in the spread of the epidemic. Therefore, this study took the shortage of materials as the optimization goal, aiming to improve the satisfaction rate of patients and further ensure their health.

Among the many shortages of emergency materials, different categories of materials have different demand characteristics. For example, consumables need to be delivered regularly to meet the needs of each person multiple times, but materials with high durability usually need to be delivered only once to each person [7]. Nevertheless, a low distribution efficiency will not only delay the delivery of emergency materials and increase the suffering of people affected, but for patients who rely on specific emergency materials, a shortage will directly endanger their lives, thus creating a greater social security risk [8]. However, research on the emergency material allocation of major public health events ignores the patients' subjective feelings. In this case, this study considered both the objective characteristics of scarce materials and the subjective urgency of patients' demand for materials and constructed an emergency material demand urgency index system to quantify and distinguish the urgency of different emergency materials.

To minimize casualties and property damage in disaster areas and to distribute emergency materials in the shortest time, emergency relief must simultaneously achieve the goal of efficiently, accurately, and equitably meeting the demand for emergency materials. Therefore, based on the proposed urgency of demand, this study designed a material shortage adjustment coefficient to adjust the amount of material shortage, reflecting not the traditional quantity of shortage, but taking into account the importance of materials, which is more in line with practical needs and achieving fair distribution.

Above all, this study took dynamic changes in emergency materials demand and differences in the urgency of emergency materials demand for various types of materials into consideration, to construct an index system indicating the urgency of emergency materials. Furthermore, this adjusted the goal of minimizing material shortage via the material shortage adjustment coefficient to develop a dynamic optimization model for emergency logistics with multi-period and multi-frequency distribution. This model ensured that high-importance emergency materials are distributed priority and that emergency materials are distributed fairly to improve emergency rescue.

This paper makes the following contributions:

(1) This paper proposes a dynamic optimization model for emergency logistics that takes multiple periods, frequencies, and types into account, in contrast to traditional emergency logistics, which only consider a single type of emergency material and a single period.
(2) Compared to the lack of research on patients' subjective feelings in the existing literature, this paper considers both the subjective feelings of patients towards the shortage of emergency materials, and the differences in the importance of different emergency materials, and establishes a demand urgency index system and numerical calculation method.
(3) Compared to existing models that focus on delivery time and cost as optimization objectives, the objective function of minimizing the total material shortage is improved by the material shortage adjustment coefficient, which is more in line with the fair distribution goal of balancing actual demand and material importance in reality.

The rest of this study is as follows. Section 2 presents the literature review. Section 3 introduces the assessment method of emergency material demand urgency. Section 4 constructs a dynamic distribution model of emergency materials that considers demand urgency. Section 5 presents an example analysis of two cities, Wuhan and Shanghai, at different stages of epidemic development. Section 6 presents the research conclusions and future research directions.

2. Literature Review

Generally, most researchers have studied emergency materials distribution by developing models and algorithms to provide decision-makers with solutions. Some researchers have focused on the improvement of emergency material distribution speed for vehicle routing problems. Xue et al. developed a multi-objective optimization model under capacity-constrained conditions, minimizing the shortest average waiting time for rescue at the affected point with access constraints [2]. Wang et al. proposed a scenario-specific emergency material distribution model with time windows to minimize emergency material loading and unloading time and distribution time [3]. Wang et al. developed a dual-objective mixed-integer programming model based on state–space–time networks with the minimum cost and the maximum emergency response speed to meet demands [9]. Wu et al. presented an emergency material dispatching model with a time window to satisfy the objective of minimum vehicle cost [10]. The above research shows that vehicle routing optimization is relatively rich for traditional emergency logistics in natural disasters.

Furthermore, to meet emergency relief needs more quickly, many researchers have studied the location problem of pre-disaster emergency facilities and post-disaster emergency facilities, as well as that of the emergency medical center. Boonmee and Kasemset proposed a decision model for locating, stocking, and distributing pre-disaster materials, which minimized response time as well as budget costs [4]. Ghasemi and Khalili-Damghani proposed a robust simulation optimization method to optimize the selection of emergency facility locations and material inventory during the planning stage [11]. Zhang et al. proposed a scenario-based stochastic planning method that integrated decisions on facility location, material inventory, and material distribution under different scenarios [12]. However, most of the models outlined above are single-period allocation models, which cannot be applied to the multi-period problem, where the demand amount changes dynamically over time. Only a few studies have explored multi-period models. Yang et al. proposed a robust optimization model, with a static pre-disaster phase and a dynamic post-disaster phase, for prepositioning the distribution of emergency supplies over multiple periods [13]. Wang et al. developed an optimization decision model for the dynamic distribution of emergency materials under fuzzy information conditions to minimize system loss and delay time [14]. While most of these studies focused on developing multi-period emergency logistics optimization under natural disasters, it was difficult to find emergency logistics studies that took into account how material demand changes with the spread of epidemics. Therefore, this paper focuses on the multi-period and multi-frequency allocation problem of emergency materials for major epidemics.

The main goal of the above studies was to design emergency logistics optimization strategies to improve the speed of material distribution and the efficiency of the allocation of relief facilities. However, it is also important to focus on the subjective perceptions of affected people regarding the effectiveness of humanitarian emergency relief, in addition to ensuring the efficiency of rescue [15]. Wang et al. designed a distress function to portray affected people's perceived distress costs using a numerical rating scale (NRS) and incorporated these factors into decision-making for the total costs of emergency response [16]. Zhu et al. measured psychological distress as an economic loss and developed a mathematical model to minimize total cost [17]. Sakiani et al. developed a mathematical model to minimize deprivation costs, fleet operation costs, and decision costs, solving a two-stage inventory routing problem [7]. Song et al. proposed an optimization model for the fair distribution of emergency supplies, which considered differentiated disaster classification, and aimed to minimize dispatching time and maximize fairness in emergency supplies distribution [18]. Zhan et al. designed a loss cost function to quantify the psychological tolerance of patients in case of a shortage of personal protective equipment; they then developed a location–allocation optimization model for emergency material distribution centers with the dual objective of minimizing loss cost and logistics cost [19]. According to the above research, the subjective feelings of disaster victims are usually quantified as costs to be modeled, but the internal connection between different materials shortages and the feelings of disaster victims is not taken into account, nor is the degree to which the materials affect their feelings.

Material allocation accuracy and fairness in emergency logistics optimization have been extensively studied [20–22]. When the pandemic occurs, the COVID-19 spreads very quickly. Accordingly, some scholars have introduced the concept of demand urgency to reduce the impact of different demand amounts on the fair distribution among different demand points. Hu et al. proposed a dynamic distribution model of emergency medical materials based on the demand urgency of materials, with the maximization of the weighted demand satisfaction rate as the main goal [5]. Zhao et al. constructed an evaluation index system for demand urgency and then developed a dual-objective model that minimizes distribution costs and prioritizes the distribution of demand points with the higher demand urgency [23]. Wang et al. developed a multi-objective optimization model that maximizes the satisfaction of affected people, minimizes the cost, and distributes fairly based on the demand urgency [24]. Liu et al. improved the index system for evaluating demand urgency and constructed a multi-objective model that maximizes both demand urgency and full load rate while minimizing the total cost of vehicle distribution [25]. Li et al. introduced the time penalty cost function to characterize the urgency of emergency material demand and proposed an uncertain location–allocation model for the emergency facility that minimizes time penalty cost, distribution cost, and carbon dioxide emissions [26]. Most studies suggest that introducing emergency material demand urgency can effectively improve material allocation fairness and accuracy. However, the urgency considerations for emergency material demand are not comprehensive. Therefore, this paper further improves the demand urgency indicator system.

The existing studies have laid a solid foundation for the research on the emergency material allocation problem. However, existing studies still have several gaps:

(1) There has been a lack of consideration for the dynamic change of emergency material demand during major epidemics. Currently, most research focuses on single-period material allocation models, which cannot be applied to the multi-period emergency material allocation problem.
(2) The relationship between the shortage of different types of materials and patients' pain perception was not fully considered in the modeling. It is not practical that regarding different types of materials as equally important.
(3) Current research on the urgency of emergency materials demand during major epidemics is not sufficient. In addition, the evaluation factors of demand urgency are not comprehensive.

The following contributions have been made to bridge the above research gap:

(1) Based on patients' subjective feelings towards different emergency materials and the differences in the importance of emergency materials, a more comprehensive demand urgency evaluation system was developed and the calculation of demand urgency was proposed accordingly.
(2) Integrating the urgency of material demand into dynamic emergency material allocation, a dynamic optimization model for emergency logistics was established, which minimizes the total amount of emergency material shortage over multi-period and multi-frequency distributions.
(3) Based on the demand urgency, the concept of material shortage adjustment coefficient was proposed for major epidemic emergency logistics. The objective of minimizing the total material shortage was adjusted by the material shortage adjustment coefficient to enhance the fairness of material allocation.

3. Demand Urgency Assessment of Emergency Material

In the context of emergency supply, demand urgency refers to the priority of satisfaction after the occurrence of demand. In the existing research, the demand urgency mainly has two connotations. The first connotation focuses on the categorization of the affected degree of the disaster areas, giving weights to different areas according to the severity of the disaster, such as increasing the priority of areas with greater weight and reducing the priority of areas with a smaller weight. The second connotation is to categorize the importance of different emergency materials, giving weights to different materials based on the importance of material; for example, increasing the priority of materials with high importance. The urgency of demand in this paper is consistent with the second connotation.

3.1. Index Selection and Description

During the outbreak of epidemics, on the demand side, the greater the rate of emergency material consumption, the greater the need for such materials in the same period, and the corresponding urgency [5,27]. On the supply side, the smaller the reproduction rate, the easier it is to increase the shortage of materials for the same demand, and therefore, the greater the urgency [23,27,28]. The sooner durable emergency materials arrive, the better the chances are of reducing the risk of delays in emergency rescue and improving emergency rescue efficiency [29]. If life-threatening or irreplaceable emergency supplies are not provided in a timely manner, it will increase the threat to the safety of the personnel [30]. Based on the above theoretical analysis and literature review, this paper summarizes the five main factors that affect the urgency of emergency material demand, as shown in Table 1.

Table 1. Urgency index system of emergency materials.

Indicator	Symbol	Indicator Description	Indicator Type	Relationship to Demand Urgency	Supporting Literature References
Material consumption rate	u_1	Average consumption per patient per unit of time	Exact real number	Positive correlation	[5,27,31]
Material reproduction rate	u_2	Supply volume per unit of time	Exact real number	Negative correlation	[23,25,27,28,32–34]
Durability	u_3	Whether it is a durable material	Binary	Positive correlation	[5,27,31,34,35]
Degree of danger to life	u_4	The degree to which the patient's risk of death increases in the absence of	Fuzzy number	Positive correlation	[30,35]
Degree of irreplaceability	u_5	Functional uniqueness and quantity of substitutable material	Fuzzy number	Positive correlation	[30,34,35]

The two indicators of *Material consumption rate* and *Material reproduction rate* are exact real numbers; that is, they measure the real situation of material use and supply. *Durability* means that the material can be repeatedly used. This variable is a binary variable, which is 1 when the material is durable and 0 otherwise. The *Degree of danger to life* and *Degree of irreplaceability* are fuzzy numerical variables that need to rely on subjective judgment. The two indicators are divided into five levels, and each level is scored 1–5, from low to high. The higher the score, the higher the importance of emergency material.

The above five indexes constitute the index system for measuring the urgency of different emergency materials.

3.2. Measurement of Demand Urgency

In order to ensure the objectivity of the calculation results, and that the weight of each factor is between 0 and 1 and the sum of the weights is equal to 1, this paper uses the entropy weight method to calculate the demand urgency. The entropy weight method is more objective than the Analytic Hierarchy Process (AHP) for the research problems in this paper. This is because the AHP quantifies the weight of the index according to the subjective analysis of the evaluator, but the entropy weight method determines weight using the discrete degree of the index value, which avoids human factors interfering with the weight calculation and is more objective. Furthermore, it is simpler and easier to understand than the TOPSIS method. In addition, many related studies [30,34,36] have also used the entropy weight method.

Step 1: Build the Normalized Matrix

From the above description, there are m types of materials and scores for each indicator. The score for a certain material on a certain indicator can be expressed as u_{mi}, wherein, i is the index of the indicator, m is the index of materials, and a two-dimensional list is formed by the scores for different materials on the above five indicators, which are expressed in the form of a matrix as follows:

$$A = \begin{pmatrix} u_{11} & u_{12} & \cdots & u_{15} \\ u_{21} & u_{22} & \cdots & u_{25} \\ \vdots & \vdots & \ddots & \vdots \\ u_{m1} & u_{m2} & \cdots & u_{m5} \end{pmatrix} \quad (1)$$

However, since the initial data for each index are inconsistent in dimension and unit, there is no comparability among the indexes, and the data cannot be directly compared. Therefore, the data need to be standardized. The specific formula is shown in Formula (2):

$$u^*_{mi} = \frac{u_{mi} - min\{u_{1i}, u_{2i}, \cdots, u_{mi}\}}{max\{u_{1i}, u_{2i}, \cdots, u_{mi}\} - min\{u_{1i}, u_{2i}, \cdots, u_{mi}\}} \quad (m = 1, 2, \cdots, M; i = 1, 2, \cdots, 5) \quad (2)$$

Thus, a normalized matrix is obtained $A = \begin{pmatrix} u^*_{11} & u^*_{12} & \cdots & u^*_{15} \\ u^*_{21} & u^*_{22} & \cdots & u^*_{25} \\ \vdots & \vdots & \ddots & \vdots \\ u^*_{m1} & u^*_{m2} & \cdots & u^*_{m5} \end{pmatrix}$. In this matrix, for the ith indicator, the greater the difference in the value u^*_{mi}, the greater the role of program evaluation, and the greater the weight of the index will be.

The normalized matrix is then normalized, and the specific formula is as shown in Formula (3):

$$u^{**}_{mi} = \frac{u^*_{mi}}{\sum_{m=1}^{M} u^*_{mi}}, m = 1, 2, \cdots, M; i = 1, 2, \cdots, 5 \quad (3)$$

Finally, the normalized matrix is obtained $A^{**} = \begin{pmatrix} u^{**}_{11} & u^{**}_{12} & \cdots & u^{**}_{15} \\ u^{**}_{21} & u^{**}_{22} & \cdots & u^{**}_{25} \\ \vdots & \vdots & \ddots & \vdots \\ u^{**}_{m1} & u^{**}_{m2} & \cdots & u^{**}_{m5} \end{pmatrix}$.

Step 2: Calculate the weight of each index l_m.

Based on the calculation of information entropy using the formula below, the entropy value of the ith index can be calculated:

$$o_i = \frac{\sum_{m=1}^{M} u^{**}_{mi} \cdot ln(u^{**}_{mi})}{ln(M)}, i = 1, 2, \cdots, 5 \quad (4)$$

If $u^{**}_{mi} = 0$, then define $\lim_{u^{**}_{mi} \to 0} (u^{**}_{mi} \cdot ln u^{**}_{mi}) = 0$.

Therefore, according to the calculated entropy value of each index, the weight of each index can be obtained by Formula (5):

$$l_i = \frac{1 - o_i}{5 - \sum_{i=1}^{5} o_i}, i = 1, 2, \cdots, 5 \quad (5)$$

Step 3: Determine the urgency of the demand for different materials

After the weight of each index is calculated in Step 2, the general weighted summation method is used to determine the calculation method of the comprehensive score of the demand urgency, as shown in Formula (6):

$$\varepsilon_m = l_1 u^{**}_{m1} + l_2 u^{**}_{m2} + l_3 u^{**}_{m3} + l_4 u^{**}_{m4} + l_5 u^{**}_{m5}, m = 1, 2, \cdots, M \quad (6)$$

3.3. Material Gap Adjustment Function

In the process of emergency rescue, the importance of different materials is also different. Therefore, when the infected population needs different materials at the same time, due to the limitations of distribution time and transportation capacity, it is necessary to give priority to the distribution of materials with higher importance. When considering the shortage degree of different materials in demand areas, it is not enough to measure the actual shortage of materials; the shortage of materials with different importance needs to be enlarged and narrowed according to the demand urgency score. When two emergency materials with different demand urgency have the same degree of shortage, due to the different importance, the material with high demand urgency will have a more severe impact on the epidemic.

Therefore, in order to achieve the goal of minimizing the total material shortage, it is necessary to adjust the shortage of different materials through certain methods, so that the higher the urgency of demand, the higher the priority of allocation. Based on the above discussion, this paper proposes the adjustment function of material shortage.

According to the demand urgency calculated above, the material shortage adjustment function is expressed in the following form:

$$\pi_m = e^{\varepsilon_m}, m = 1, 2, \cdots, M \tag{7}$$

where π_m is the shortage coefficient of emergency material m. Since the weight of each index is within 0–1, and the normalized value of each index is also within 0–1, the comprehensive score of demand urgency calculated by Formula (7) is also within 0–1. The relationship between the material shortage adjustment coefficient and the material demand urgency is shown in Figure 1.

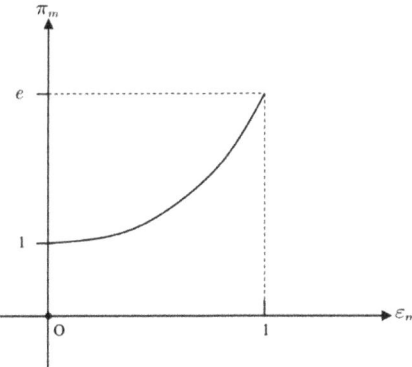

Figure 1. Adjustment function of material shortage.

If the demand urgency calculated by the method in Section 3.2 is 0, it is considered that the importance of the material is 0, so it is calculated by its actual shortage amount without adjustment; if the demand urgency is greater than 0, it is considered that the material has a certain importance, and its material shortage cannot be measured only by the actual amount, but it needs to be enlarged accordingly. When the demand urgency is greater than 0, the greater the value is, the more severe the impact of materials on epidemics and the higher the amplification ratio of the shortage, and the amplification trend becomes faster with the increase of the urgency value.

4. Dynamic Distribution Model of Emergency Materials Considering Demand Urgency
4.1. Problem Description and Model Assumptions

At the beginning of an outbreak, the virus spreads rapidly in a certain area, the number of infected people increases exponentially, and the emergency materials in stock in the area are consumed rapidly. In order to control the epidemic as soon as possible, the government will introduce strict quarantine measures and designate some medical institutions in the area as rescue centers. In order to meet the material needs of the rescue centers, it is necessary to transport materials from other areas to supplement the shortage. These transported materials are then stored in different temporary distribution centers, and the distribution centers accurately deliver the materials to the rescue centers according to demand. At the same time, considering the continuous development of the epidemic and in order to make distribution more accurate, the duration of the epidemic is divided into several equal periods, and distribution needs to be arranged according to the materials demand in each period

Figure 2 illustrates the problem graphically. In Figure 2, the large rectangle represents the area where the materials need to be distributed, and several irregular curves divide it into several independent areas with different shapes and sizes. Each region has a rescue center (represented by a small triangle), which is responsible for the treatment of infected patients in that area. There are also several distribution centers (represented by small squares) in the region, each with its own service area (represented by a dotted circle). Supplies are delivered from external areas (represented by solid circles) to temporary distribution centers, and then distributed from the temporary distribution centers to the rescue centers within the scope, according to their demands.

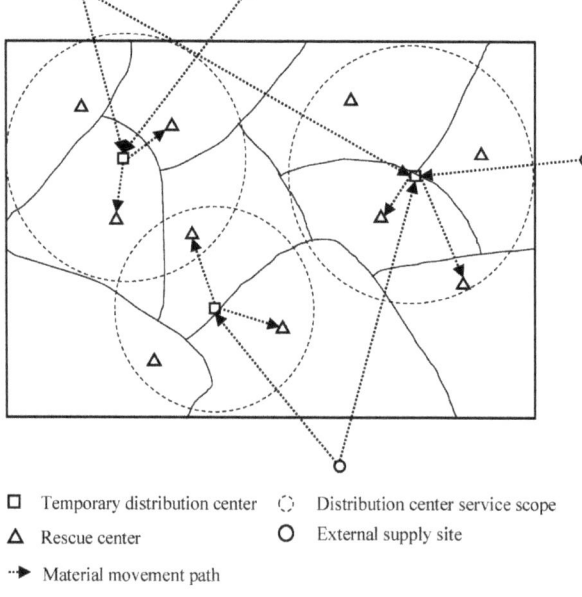

☐ Temporary distribution center ◌ Distribution center service scope
△ Rescue center ○ External supply site
┄▶ Material movement path

Figure 2. Emergency material distribution network diagram.

Some assumptions of this system are made as follows:
(1) Each rescue center is responsible for the treatment of infected patients in a certain scope, and there is no overlapping of the scopes of the rescue centers. Once the infected person is diagnosed, they will be sent to the nearest rescue center.
(2) The external supply sites are a kind of virtual node, which essentially have several possible channels for materials to enter the area. External emergency supply sites have no actual coordinates, but there are parameters such as supply volume, price, and so on. Accordingly, only the distribution of materials within the affected area is considered while the distribution of materials outside the affected area and the distance factor are not considered.

(3) The materials for each rescue center in one delivery can be provided by multiple distribution centers, and one distribution center can provide materials for different rescue centers in one delivery.
(4) Only the purchase cost of external material input (from the supply site to the distribution center) is considered, and the transportation cost of internal and external material (from the distribution center to the rescue center) and the storage cost in the distribution center are not considered.
(5) The volume difference is not considered, different materials can be loaded together, and the damage to road facilities and the limitations of road conditions are ignored.

4.2. Symbol Definition

(1) Sets

M: Set of emergency materials m = 1, 2, ..., M
T: Set of rescue periods t = 1, 2, ..., T
W: Set of emergency supply sites w = 1, 2, ..., W
J: Set of temporary distribution centers j = 1, 2, ..., J
K: Set of rescue centers k = 1, 2, ..., K

(2) Parameters

D_{jt}^m, D_{kt}^m: The volume of material m demanded by the temporary distribution center j and rescue center k in Period t, respectively.
ns_{wt}^m: The volume of the material m supplied from emergency supply site w in Period t.
c_{wt}^m: The price of the material m supplied from emergency supply site w in Period t.
Ω: Total budget during the epidemic.
P_{jt}^m: The volume of material m supplied by temporary distribution center j in Period t.
V_{jt}^m: The inventory of material m of temporary distribution center j in Period t.
V_{j0}^m: The initial inventory of material m of temporary distribution center j.
$\bar{V}_j^m$: The maximal inventory volume of material m of temporary distribution center j.
v_j^m: The safety inventory volume of material m of temporary distribution center j.
V_j: The total inventory capacity of temporary distribution center j.
ω_{kt}^m: The shortage volume of material m of rescue center k in Period t.
π^m: The shortage adjustment coefficient of material m.

4.3. Model Construction

The decision variables of the dynamic distribution model are:

x_{wjt}^m: The volume of material m transported from emergency supply site w to temporary distribution center j in Period t.

x_{jkt}^m: The volume of material m transported from temporary distribution center j to rescue center k in Period t.

p_{jkt}: Whether there is any material transported from temporary distribution center j to rescue center k in Period t.

p_{wjt}: Whether there is any material transported from emergency supply point w to temporary distribution center j in Period t.

In which, p_{jkt} and p_{wjt} are 0-1 variables, and when the event occurs, the variable is 1, otherwise 0.

Considering the importance of different materials, the total material shortage is characterized as an adjusted weighted shortage based on the material shortage adjustment coefficient. Taking the minimum total material shortage as the objective of the model, the corresponding integer linear programming model was established as follows:

$$\min \sum_{t=1}^{T} \sum_{k=1}^{K} \sum_{m=1}^{M} \pi^m \omega_{kt}^m \qquad (8)$$

s.t.

$$D_{kt}^m \geq \sum_{j=1}^{J} p_{jkt} x_{jkt}^m, t \in T, k \in K, m \in M \qquad (9)$$

$$P_{jt}^m \leq \sum_{k=1}^{K} p_{jkt} x_{jkt}^m, t \in T, j \in J, m \in M \tag{10}$$

$$P_{jt}^m \leq V_{j(t-1)}^m, t \in T, j \in J, m \in M \tag{11}$$

$$V_{jt}^m = V_{j(t-1)}^m - P_{jt}^m + \sum_{w=1}^{W} p_{wjt} x_{wjt}^m, t \in T, j \in J, m \in M \tag{12}$$

$$D_{jt}^m = V_j^m - V_{j(t-1)}^m + P_{jt}^m, t \in T, j \in J, m \in M \tag{13}$$

$$D_{jt}^m \geq \sum_{w=1}^{W} p_{wjt} x_{wjt}^m, t \in T, j \in J, m \in M \tag{14}$$

$$\sum_{j=1}^{J} p_{wjt} x_{wjt}^m \leq ns_{w(t-1)}^m, t \in T, w \in W, m \in M \tag{15}$$

$$V_{jt}^m \geq v_j^m, t \in T, j \in J, m \in M \tag{16}$$

$$V_{jt}^m \leq V_j^m, t \in T, j \in J, m \in M \tag{17}$$

$$\sum_{m=1}^{M} V_{jt}^m \leq V_j, t \in T, j \in J \tag{18}$$

$$\omega_{kt}^m = D_{kt}^m - \sum_{j=1}^{J} p_{jkt} x_{jkt}^m, t \in T, k \in K, m \in M \tag{19}$$

In the above Formulas (8)–(19), Formula (8) is the objective function of the model, which minimizes the material shortage after adjustment. Formula (9) reflects that during the rapid development of the epidemic, emergency materials are in short supply, so the total volume of supplies received by a single rescue center from the temporary distribution center in each period may not be able to meet all the needs, resulting in a certain material shortage.

Formulas (10) and (11) show that the goods shipped from a single distribution center are equal to the sum of the materials distributed to all the rescue centers and are less than the current inventory of the material. Formula (12) shows that the inventory of a certain material at the end of the current cycle is equal to the inventory at the end of the previous period minus the volume of materials transported in the current period plus those transported from the emergency supply site in the current period. Formulas (13)–(15) show that the demand of the temporary distribution center for a certain material is equal to the difference between the maximum storage capacity of the temporary distribution center and the current inventory, and is the same as the demand of the treatment center. The materials volume transported from the emergency supply site may not be able to meet the needs of the temporary distribution center, but it must not be larger than the total materials volume supplied by the supply site. Formulas (16)–(18) show that the inventory of materials should be less than the inventory capacity and greater than the safety inventory. Formula (19) defines the calculation method of the material shortage quantity of a single period in a certain rescue center.

5. Example Analysis

In order to verify the effectiveness of the model, this paper presents an example analysis of Wuhan and Shanghai under the background of city-wide lockdown and control at different stages of epidemic development. The computing environment was based on a personal computer (Intel Core I5 10210U 1.6 GHz CPU, 16 GB RAM, Windows 11 operating system), and Lingo 16 ExS was applied as the computing software. The parameters involved in the model were then adjusted, sensitivity analysis was carried out, and the impact of different parameter settings on the model results was compared. The details are as follows:

5.1. Relevant Background

At the end of 2019, the COVID-19 virus began to spread in Wuhan. In order to cut off the transmission of the virus and control the epidemic in a smaller range, Wuhan announced the "Lockdown" on 23 January 2020. In March 2022, the mutant strain of COVID-19, Omikron, began to break out in Shanghai, and the Shanghai Municipal Government executed the measure of "static management" on 1 April 2022.

5.2. Data Preparation

There are 13 and 16 administrative districts respectively in Wuhan and Shanghai, which are greatly different from each other. In order to improve the comparability of the solution results, the two cities were divided into five regions, respectively, according to the area and geographical location, as shown in Table 2.

Table 2. Regional division of cities.

	Wuhan		Shanghai	
Region	Contained Administrative Districts	Population Density (Person/km^2)	Contained Administrative Districts	Population Density (Person/km^2)
Region 1	Jiangan District, Jianghan District, Qiaokou District, Hanyang District, Wuchang District, Qingshan District, Hongshan District	7076	Huangpu District, Xuhui District, Changning District, Jing 'an District, Putuo District, Hongkou District, Yangpu District, Minhang District	14,161
Region 2	Dongxihu District, Hannan District, Caidian District	812	Pudong New Area, Fengxian District	3598
Region 3	Jiangxia District	489	Jiading District, Baoshan District	5531
Region 4	Huangpi District	456	Jinshan District, Songjiang District, Qingpu District	2148
Region 5	Xinzhou District	626	Chongming District	539

According to the existing literature, during the rapid development of the epidemic, Hubei Province designated five logistics parks as temporary transit stations for emergency materials, three of which were in Wuhan, located in Dongxihu District, Huangpi District, and Hannan District. In addition, according to the public data on the official website of the Hubei Provincial Health and Health Commission, during the epidemic period, all districts in Wuhan designated one or more hospitals to treat infected people. Therefore, after the re-division of the city, each region contained at least one designated rescue center. Shanghai has not released the information on the designated distribution centers.

This paper assumes that there were three different distribution centers (j_1, j_2, j_3) in the two cities and two emergency supply sites (w_1, w_2), which represented various ways for materials to enter the affected area. At the same time, each region had a corresponding rescue center, represented by (k_1, k_2, k_3, k_4, k_5).

All kinds of materials used during the epidemic can be divided into medical materials, protective materials, and living materials, according to the use classification. In addition, they can be divided into consumptive materials and durable materials, according to the consumption classification. In reality, during the outbreak of the epidemic in Wuhan, people paid more attention to the distribution of medical and protective materials, while in Shanghai, the distribution of living materials was a more important topic. Therefore, this study selected medicine, medical alcohol, ventilator, and pork as representative materials. Of these, medicines, medical alcohol, and pork are consumptive materials, and ventilators are durable materials. The time period unit in this study was days. Indeed, according to the actual situation, the time period can be taken from any other unit.

Based on the population density data in Table 2, according to epidemic development law, the material demand data for the two cities in the first 10 periods were set as shown in Tables 3 and 4 respectively.

Table 3. Demand data for emergency materials in Wuhan (unit: piece).

	Period	1	2	3	4	5	6	7	8	9	10
k = 1	Medicine	1218	1416	1836	2358	2910	3450	3948	4404	4806	5160
	Medical alcohol	406	472	612	786	970	1150	1316	1468	1602	1720
	Ventilator	174	174	194	214	227	231	227	218	204	188
	Pork	102	118	153	197	243	288	329	367	401	430
k = 2	Medicine	264	294	366	456	552	642	726	798	858	906
	Medical alcohol	88	98	122	152	184	214	242	266	286	302
	Ventilator	38	36	38	41	43	43	42	40	37	34
	Pork	22	25	31	38	46	54	61	67	72	76
k = 3	Medicine	174	192	234	294	354	414	462	510	546	582
	Medical alcohol	58	64	78	98	118	138	154	170	182	194
	Ventilator	25	24	25	27	28	28	27	26	24	22
	Pork	15	16	20	25	30	35	39	43	46	49
k = 4	Medicine	180	198	246	306	366	426	480	528	570	600
	Medical alcohol	60	66	82	102	122	142	160	176	190	200
	Ventilator	26	25	27	29	30	30	29	27	25	23
	Pork	15	17	21	26	31	36	40	44	48	50
k = 5	Medicine	162	180	222	276	330	384	432	480	516	546
	Medical alcohol	54	60	74	92	110	128	144	160	172	182
	Ventilator	23	22	23	25	26	26	25	24	22	20
	Pork	14	15	19	23	28	32	36	40	43	46

Table 4. Demand data for emergency materials in Shanghai (unit: piece).

	Period	1	2	3	4	5	6	7	8	9	10
k = 1	Medicine	5785	11,230	16,472	21,582	26,625	31,660	36,744	41,929	47,267	52,805
	Medical alcohol	1928	3743	5491	7194	8875	10,553	12,248	13,976	15,756	17,602
	Ventilator	48	47	34	22	14	8	5	3	2	1
	Pork	482	936	1373	1798	2219	2638	3062	3494	3939	4400
k = 2	Medicine	3317	6298	9022	11,520	13,826	15,966	17,967	19,850	21,635	23,339
	Medical alcohol	1106	2099	3007	3840	4609	5322	5989	6617	7212	7780
	Ventilator	28	27	19	12	7	4	2	1	1	1
	Pork	276	525	752	960	1152	1330	1497	1654	1803	1945
k = 3	Medicine	2040	3892	5599	7183	8663	10,059	11,385	12,656	13,884	15,081
	Medical alcohol	680	1297	1866	2394	2888	3353	3795	4219	4628	5027
	Ventilator	17	16	12	8	5	3	2	1	1	1
	Pork	170	324	467	599	722	838	949	1055	1157	1257
k = 4	Medicine	1842	3485	4973	6326	7562	8698	9748	10,727	11,645	12,512
	Medical alcohol	614	1162	1658	2109	2521	2899	3249	3576	3882	4171
	Ventilator	15	14	10	6	4	2	1	1	1	1
	Pork	154	290	414	527	630	725	812	894	970	1043
k = 5	Medicine	283	531	752	951	1131	1294	1443	1580	1706	1823
	Medical alcohol	94	177	251	317	377	431	481	527	569	608
	Ventilator	2	2	1	1	1	1	1	1	1	1
	Pork	24	44	63	79	94	108	120	132	142	152

The data for various urgency indexes of the given emergency materials are shown in Table 5.

Table 5. Score of each material in each indicator.

Name of Material	Symbol	Material Consumption Rate u_1	Material Reproduction Rate u_2	Whether It Is Durable Material u_3	Degree of Irreplaceability u_4	Insufficient Supply Endangers Life Level u_5
Medicine	m = 1	6	4	0	4	5
Medical alcohol	m = 2	2	1.5	0	2	1
Ventilator	m = 3	1	1	1	5	3
Pork	m = 4	0.5	3	0	1	2

5.3. Calculation and Result Analysis

According to the methods of calculating demand urgency and adjusting material shortage introduced in Section 3.3, the demand urgency and shortage adjustment coefficient of each material was obtained as shown in Table 6.

Table 6. Material demand urgency and material shortage adjustment coefficient.

Material m	Medicine m = 1	Medical Alcohol m = 2	Ventilator m = 3	Pork m = 4
Demand urgency ε_m	0.333	0.067	0.540	0.061
Material shortage adjustment coefficient π_m	1.395	1.069	1.716	1.062

After obtaining the shortage adjustment coefficient of each material, the solution for the model was obtained based on Lingo 16 software. The results of the materials accumulated in the first 10 periods from Wuhan emergency supply sites to temporary distribution centers are shown in Table 7, and those from Wuhan temporary distribution centers to various rescue centers are shown in Table 8. The results of the materials accumulated in the first 10 periods from Shanghai emergency supply sites to temporary distribution centers are shown in Table 9, and those from Shanghai temporary distribution centers to various rescue centers are shown in Table 10. Based on the model results, it was found that:

Table 7. Distribution results for emergency supply sites to temporary distribution centers in Wuhan (unit: piece).

Temporary Distribution Center	Emergency Materials	Emergency Supply Site	
		w = 1	w = 2
j = 1	Medicine	7410	3000
	Medical alcohol	4322	1780
	Ventilator	100	104
	Pork	958	136
j = 2	Medicine	10,548	4400
	Medical alcohol	2864	830
	Ventilator	187	15
	Pork	733	46
j = 3	Medicine	11,942	2300
	Medical alcohol	4064	850
	Ventilator	355	0
	Pork	1399	56

Based on the Shanghai data, the optimal value of the model was 111,794.9, and the transferred actual shortage was 88,636 pieces; therefore, the overall shortage rate was 10.18%. The specific shortage of different materials varies, and the specific shortage of each type of material is shown in Figure 3.

Table 8. Distribution results for temporary distribution centers to rescue centers in Wuhan (unit: piece).

Rescue Center	Emergency Materials	Temporary Distribution Center		
		j = 1	j = 2	j = 3
k = 1	Medicine	7726	9624	11,396
	Medical alcohol	4700	2172	3364
	Ventilator	304	300	394
	Pork	769	496	1155
k = 2	Medicine	1392	2754	798
	Medical alcohol	650	398	784
	Ventilator	0	2	37
	Pork	158	105	130
k = 3	Medicine	1482	684	696
	Medical alcohol	376	402	320
	Ventilator	0	0	24
	Pork	114	62	29
k = 4	Medicine	426	1314	1434
	Medical alcohol	162	508	426
	Ventilator	0	0	0
	Pork	44	88	112
k = 5	Medicine	384	1572	918
	Medical alcohol	414	414	220
	Ventilator	0	0	0
	Pork	59	78	79

Table 9. Distribution results for emergency supply sites to temporary distribution centers in Shanghai (unit: piece).

Temporary Distribution Center	Emergency Materials	Emergency Supply Site	
		w = 1	w = 2
j = 1	Medicine	3953	90,000
	Medical alcohol	39,000	22,600
	Ventilator	0	0
	Pork	6765	7300
j = 2	Medicine	54,405	13,000
	Medical alcohol	17,100	8000
	Ventilator	0	0
	Pork	3500	2400
j = 3	Medicine	130,047	0
	Medical alcohol	56,400	4000
	Ventilator	0	0
	Pork	19,635	0

Based on the Wuhan data, the results of the model show that the optimal value of the objective was 10,532.15, and the transferred actual average shortage of materials was 7805 pieces; therefore, the actual average shortage rate of materials was 10.84%. The shortage of different types of materials is shown in Figure 4.

In Figures 3 and 4, the blue rectangles represent the ideal shortage rates, that is, the shortage rate when all materials are used, while the orange rectangles represent the actual shortage rates, which is the result optimized by the model. It can be seen that although there was a significant difference in the absolute amount of material shortage between Shanghai and Wuhan, the overall shortage level was similar, as well as the shortage of each material, which indicates that the situation in the two cities is comparable.

Table 10. Distribution results for temporary distribution centers to rescue centers in Shanghai (unit: piece).

Rescue Center	Emergency Materials	Temporary Distribution Center		
		j = 1	j = 2	j = 3
k = 1	Medicine	99,263	76,054	105,552
	Medical alcohol	17,972	12,001	67,393
	Ventilator	40	45	44
	Pork	7882	1113	14,864
k = 2	Medicine	22,848	19,283	17,818
	Medical alcohol	20,981	6595	3007
	Ventilator	7	0	1
	Pork	3499	752	3288
k = 3	Medicine	0	2068	20,680
	Medical alcohol	21,651	5925	0
	Ventilator	0	5	4
	Pork	1257	1157	2483
k = 4	Medicine	1842	0	15,997
	Medical alcohol	10,996	10,052	0
	Ventilator	2	0	1
	Pork	2427	3878	0
k = 5	Medicine	0	0	0
	Medical alcohol	0	527	0
	Ventilator	1	0	0
	Pork	0	0	0

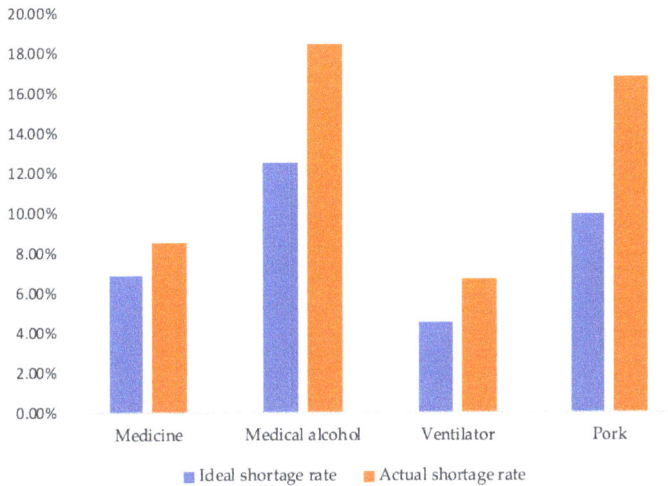

Figure 3. Material shortage of each type of material in Shanghai.

According to the demand urgency score for each material listed in Table 6, it can be seen that among the four materials, the importance of medicines and ventilators is higher, while the importance of the other two items is relatively lower. Figures 3 and 4 show that the actual shortage rate of medicines and ventilators was closer to the ideal shortage rate than the other two materials. These results show that the model established in this paper obviously adjusted the material distribution with higher importance, so the satisfaction of the more important materials reached a more ideal state. For the two kinds of materials, medicines belong to consumptive materials, while ventilators belong to durable materials. For the two types of materials, there was no significant difference in the optimization process.

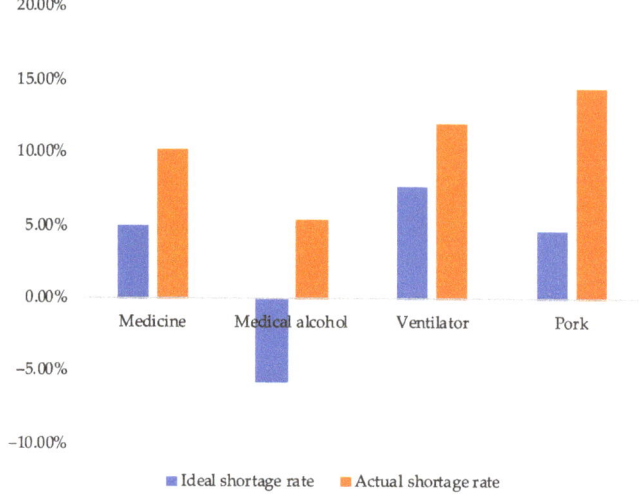

Figure 4. The shortage of each material in Wuhan.

5.4. Impact of Budget Funds

Based on the effective model established above, this section examines the impact of budget funds.

In reality, whether it is commercial logistics or emergency logistics, funds are always limited. Even for the emergency logistics led by the government, it is necessary to consider cutting costs and use limited funds as much as possible. The government needs to respond to emergency material demands in case of a shortage. Some of these materials are donated by society, while the majority come from government procurement. Government procurement is not unlimited, and the cost of purchasing emergency materials needs to be within a budget. This means that there is the following budget constraint in the model:

$$\sum_{t=1}^{T} \sum_{\omega=1}^{W} \sum_{j=1}^{J} \sum_{m=1}^{M} p_{wjt} c_{wt}^{m} x_{wjt}^{m} \leq \Omega \qquad (20)$$

where c_{wt}^{m} is the price of the material, and Ω is the government budget.

In Formula (20), the cost of emergency logistics is defined as the cost incurred in purchasing materials from suppliers, which must not be over budget. This paper divides budget funds into three grades: 10 million yuan, 50 million yuan, and 100 million yuan, which were substituted into the model, respectively, for a solution. The final results were analyzed based on the single objective solution without budget constraints, as shown in Table 11 and Figure 5.

As illustrated by Table 11 and Figure 5, when the budget funds were only 10 million yuan, the actual shortage of materials was 26,466 pieces, with a shortage rate of materials of up to 38.95%. With the increase of budget funds and the loosening of financial constraints, the shortage rate of materials gradually decreased. When the budget funds were 50 million yuan, the decrease in the shortage rate was the largest, with a decrease of over 14 percentage. This fully demonstrates that funds play an important role in the entire logistics, and if insufficient funds are invested, emergency logistics will not have a significant effect.

The shortage of three types of medical materials is shown in Figure 6. When the budget was between 10 million yuan and 50 million yuan, the shortage of medicines decreased the most significantly. However, when the budget was between 50 million yuan and 100 million yuan, the shortage of ventilators saw the biggest drop, while the shortage of medical alcohol remained at the same level. There are several possible reasons for this situation:

1. The demand for medicines was the highest. When the funding was only 10 million yuan, the shortage of medicines was much larger compared to the other two types of materials. Therefore, when the budget increased slightly, a large number of medicines were purchased to reduce the shortage.
2. The demand for ventilators was the lowest, but ventilators were the most expensive. When the financial constraint was tight, the limited funds were not used to purchase ventilators but first met the other two lower-priced and greater-demand materials. However, when the budget funds were sufficient, the importance of ventilators began to show, and more funds were used to purchase ventilators to meet the demand and reduce the shortage of this more important material.

Table 11. Sensitivity analysis results for budget funds.

Budget Constraints (Yuan)	10 Million	50 Million	100 Million	Unlimited
Objective function value	40,025.08	24,724.95	21,270.65	20,130.66
Actual shortage amount (piece)	26,466	16,722	14,617	13,830
Shortage rate	38.95%	24.61%	21.51%	20.35%

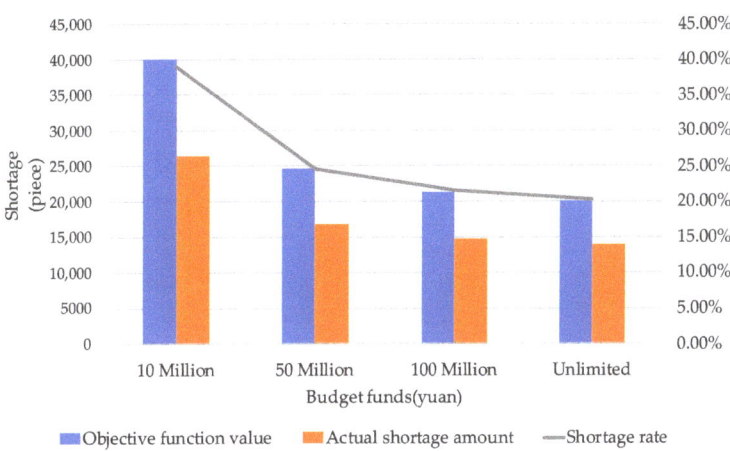

Figure 5. Sensitivity analysis results for budget funds.

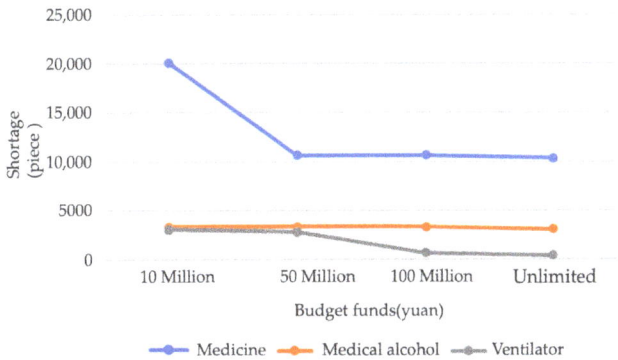

Figure 6. Material shortages under different budget constraints.

6. Conclusions

In the process of epidemic prevention and control, a perfect emergency logistics system is expected to be one the critical support to quickly control the epidemic and minimize casualties and losses. Emergency logistics not only needs to achieve the fastest distribution of materials, but it also needs to consider the accuracy and fairness of meeting the demand for materials in distribution. Therefore, in the context of the COVID-19 pandemic, this paper established a distribution model of emergency materials. In this model, the concept of demand urgency is introduced, and the importance of each material is measured through the demand urgency index system, to calculate the shortage adjustment coefficient of each material; furthermore, the shortage of the material is enlarged accordingly in the objective function, so that the material with higher importance is distributed more preferentially. Finally, the model was applied to study the cases of Wuhan and Shanghai, and it was found that, although there were differences in material demand volume and material demand structure between Shanghai and Wuhan, there were similar results for the two cities, indicating that the model can be applied to the emergency material distribution of major epidemics in a variety of situations.

Furthermore, there are some managerial implications:

(1) Medicines and ventilators were the two materials with higher demand urgency in this example, and the actual shortage rate was closer to the ideal state, which reflects the effectiveness of the model to some extent. Therefore, this proves that the shortage adjustment coefficient based on the demand urgency (material classification) had a more obvious adjustment effect on the distribution of more important materials.

(2) The effectiveness of emergency logistics increased with the increase of budget funds. When the budget funds were very limited, it resulted in a great shortage of emergency materials and a high shortage rate, regardless of the demand urgency. On the other hand, with the increase in budget funds, the demand urgency was clearly reflected in the allocation of funds. The more urgent materials received a larger share of finance, which means that increasing funds appropriately and conducting scientific allocation is an important strategy to improve the effectiveness of emergency rescue.

The considerations for follow-up studies are as follows:

(1) Although this paper considered multi-period emergency logistics dynamic planning, it simply divided the time into several equal small periods and gave a reasonable explanation for how to divide the periods. Therefore, in a follow-up study, we could carry out corresponding research on the reasonable division of the period, such as whether it is necessary to change the period into a random length, or the relationship between the division of the period and the development of the epidemic.

(2) In this paper, materials are divided into durable and consumable materials, but this division was too general to distinguish the differences between hundreds of materials in emergency logistics. Therefore, it is necessary to continue to study the division of emergency materials.

Author Contributions: Conceptualization, J.Z. (Jianjun Zhang); methodology, J.Z. (Jin Zhao); software, T.W.; writing—original draft preparation, J.H. and J.Z. (Jianjun Zhang); writing—review and editing, J.Z. (Jin Zhao). All authors have read and agreed to the published version of the manuscript.

Funding: This research was funded by the Sino-German Mobility Programme of the National Natural Science Foundation of China (No. M-0310), the Key Soft Science Project of Shanghai Municipal Science and Technology Commission (No. 23692109300, 22692108800), and Shanghai Philosophy and Social Sciences Project (No. 2022ZGL011).

Institutional Review Board Statement: Not applicable.

Informed Consent Statement: Not applicable.

Data Availability Statement: Not applicable.

Conflicts of Interest: The authors declare no conflict of interest.

References

1. Jiang, P.; Wang, Y.; Liu, C.; Hu, Y.-C.; Xie, J. Evaluating Critical Factors Influencing the Reliability of Emergency Logistics Systems Using Multiple-Attribute Decision Making. *Symmetry* **2020**, *12*, 1115. [CrossRef]
2. Xue, X.; Wang, X.; Han, T.; Ruan, J. Study on Joint Dispatch Optimization of Emergency Materials Considering Traffic Constraints and Capacity Limits. *Chin. J. Manag. Sci.* **2020**, *28*, 21–30.
3. Wang, S.R.; Huang, Q. A Hybrid Code Genetic Algorithm for VRP in Public-Private Emergency Collaborations. *Int. J. Simul. Model.* **2022**, *21*, 124–135. [CrossRef]
4. Boonmee, C.; Kasemset, C. The Multi-Objective Fuzzy Mathematical Programming Model for Humanitarian Relief Logistics. *Ind. Eng. Manag. Syst.* **2020**, *19*, 197–210. [CrossRef]
5. Hu, X.; Song, L.; Yang, B.; Wang, J. Optimal Matching of Urban Emergency Medical Supplies Under Major Public Health Events. *China J. Highw. Transp.* **2020**, *33*, 55–64.
6. Zhu, K.; Liang, Z.; Wang, X. Markov Decision Model of Emergency Medical Supply Scheduling in Public Health Emergencies of Infectious Diseases. *Int. J. Comput. Intell. Syst.* **2021**, *14*, 1155–1169. [CrossRef]
7. Sakiani, R.; Seifi, A.; Khorshiddoust, R.R. Inventory routing and dynamic redistribution of relief goods in post-disaster operations. *Comput. Ind. Eng.* **2020**, *140*, 106219. [CrossRef]
8. Zhao, Y.; Zhang, L. An Advanced Study of Urban Emergency Medical Equipment Logistics Distribution for Different Levels of Urgency Demand. *Int. J. Environ. Res. Public Health* **2022**, *19*, 11264. [CrossRef] [PubMed]
9. Wang, Y.; Peng, S.G.; Xu, M. Emergency logistics network design based on space-time resource configuration. *Knowl.-Based Syst.* **2021**, *223*, 107041. [CrossRef]
10. Wu, K.; Song, Y.; Lyu, W. Research on time window model for optimal scheduling on vehicle distribution of medical emergency materials. *J. Saf. Sci. Technol.* **2022**, *18*, 11–16.
11. Ghasemi, P.; Khalili-Damghani, K. A robust simulation-optimization approach for pre-disaster multi-period location-allocation-inventory planning. *Math. Comput. Simul.* **2021**, *179*, 69–95. [CrossRef]
12. Zhang, L.; Cui, N. Pre-Positioning Facility Location and Resource Allocation in Humanitarian Relief Operations Considering Deprivation Costs. *Sustainability* **2021**, *13*, 4141. [CrossRef]
13. Yang, M.; Liu, Y.; Yang, G. Multi-period dynamic distributionally robust pre-positioning of emergency supplies under demand uncertainty. *Appl. Math. Model.* **2021**, *89*, 1433–1458. [CrossRef]
14. Wang, Y.; Sun, B. Multi-period Optimization Model of Multi-type Emergency Materials Allocation Based on Fuzzy Information. *Chin. J. Manag. Sci.* **2020**, *28*, 40–51.
15. Holguin-Veras, J.; Perez, N.; Jaller, M.; Van Wassenhove, L.N.; Aros-Vera, F. On the appropriate objective function for post-disaster humanitarian logistics models. *J. Oper. Manag.* **2013**, *31*, 262–280. [CrossRef]
16. Wang, X.; Zhang, W.; Yu, Y.; Liu, B. An Optimization Model for Emergency Shelter Location and Relief Materials Allocation Considering Human Suffering. *Chin. J. Manag. Sci.* **2020**, *28*, 162–172.
17. Zhu, L.; Cao, J.; Gu, J.; Zheng, Y. Dynamic Routing-allocation Optimization of Post-disaster Emergency Resource Considering Heterogeneous Behaviors. *Chin. J. Manag. Sci.* **2020**, *28*, 151–161. [CrossRef]
18. Song, Y.; Bai, M.; Ma, Y.; Lyu, W.; Huo, F. Optimal model for fair dispatch of emergency materials considering regional disaster classification. *China Saf. Sci. J. CSSJ* **2022**, *32*, 172–179.
19. Zhan, S.-L.; Gu, X.; Ye, Y.; Chuang, Y.-C. The Allocation Method for Personal Protective Equipment in the Emerging Infectious Disease Environment. *Front. Public Health* **2022**, *10*, 904569. [CrossRef]
20. Wang, Y.; Bier, V.M.; Sun, B. Measuring and Achieving Equity in Multiperiod Emergency Material Allocation. *Risk Anal.* **2019**, *39*, 2408–2426. [CrossRef] [PubMed]
21. Zhu, L.; Gong, Y.; Xu, Y.; Gu, J. Emergency relief routing models for injured victims considering equity and priority. *Ann. Oper. Res.* **2018**, *283*, 1573–1606. [CrossRef]
22. Liu, K.; Zhang, H.; Zhang, Z.-H. The efficiency, equity and effectiveness of location strategies in humanitarian logistics: A robust chance-constrained approach. *Transp. Res. Part E Logist. Transp. Rev.* **2021**, *156*, 102521. [CrossRef]
23. Zhao, J.; Han, W.; Zheng, W.; Zhao, Y. Distribution of emergency medical supplies in cities under major public health emergency. *J. Traffic Transp. Eng.* **2020**, *20*, 168–177.
24. Wang, F.; Tang, T.; Li, Y.; Wang, X. Study on Optimal Allocation of Emergency Resources in Multiple Disaster Sites Under Epidemic Events. *Complex Syst. Complex. Sci.* **2021**, *18*, 53–62.
25. Liu, H.; Sun, Y.; Pan, N.; Li, Y.; An, Y.; Pan, D. Study on the optimization of urban emergency supplies distribution paths for epidemic outbreaks. *Comput. Oper. Res.* **2022**, *146*, 105912. [CrossRef]
26. Li, H.; Zhang, B.; Ge, X. Modeling Emergency Logistics Location-Allocation Problem with Uncertain Parameters. *Systems* **2022**, *10*, 51. [CrossRef]
27. Zhang, G.; Lu, S.; Su, Z.; Pan, G. Modeling and solving multi-objective emergency resource allocation in chemical industrial parks. *Control Decis.* **2022**, *37*, 962–972.
28. Chen, T.; Lin, Y. Typhoon Disaster Emergency Logistics Vehicle Dispatching Optimization Simulation under Big Data Background. *J. Catastrophol.* **2019**, *34*, 194–197.
29. Lei, L.; Pinedo, M.; Qi, L.; Wang, S.B.; Yang, J. Personnel scheduling and supplies provisioning in emergency relief operations. *Ann. Oper. Res.* **2015**, *235*, 487–515. [CrossRef]

30. Wang, Y.; Su, B.; Yan, P.; Guan, Y.; Deng, B.; Jia, L. Approach to the classification of the demand urgency of the affected points based on the improved TOPSIS. *J. Saf. Environ.* **2019**, *19*, 140–146.
31. Bodaghi, B.; Palaneeswaran, E.; Abbasi, B. Bi-objective multi-resource scheduling problem for emergency relief operations. *Prod. Plan. Control* **2018**, *29*, 1191–1206. [CrossRef]
32. Yang, Y.; Ma, C.X.; Zhou, J.B.; Dong, S.; Ling, G.; Li, J.C. A multi-dimensional robust optimization approach for cold-chain emergency medical materials dispatch under COVID-19: A case study of Hubei Province. *J. Traffic Transp. Eng. Engl. Ed.* **2022**, *9*, 1–20. [CrossRef]
33. Najafi, M.; Eshghi, K.; Dullaert, W. A multi-objective robust optimization model for logistics planning in the earthquake response phase. *Transp. Res. Part E Logist. Transp. Rev.* **2013**, *49*, 217–249. [CrossRef]
34. Ma, Z.; Zhang, J.; Gao, S. Research on emergency material demand based on urgency and satisfaction under public health emergencies. *PLoS ONE* **2023**, *18*, e0282796. [CrossRef] [PubMed]
35. Huang, L.D.; Shi, P.P.; Zhu, H.C. An integrated urgency evaluation approach of relief demands for disasters based on social media data. *Int. J. Disaster Risk Reduct.* **2022**, *80*, 103208. [CrossRef]
36. Zhang, L.; Zhang, H.; Liu, D.; Lu, Y. Particle Swarm Algorithm for Solving Emergency Material Dispatch Considering Urgency. *J. Syst. Simul.* **2022**, *34*, 1988–1998.

Disclaimer/Publisher's Note: The statements, opinions and data contained in all publications are solely those of the individual author(s) and contributor(s) and not of MDPI and/or the editor(s). MDPI and/or the editor(s) disclaim responsibility for any injury to people or property resulting from any ideas, methods, instructions or products referred to in the content.

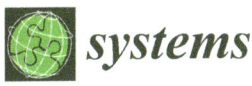

Article

Research on Intelligent Emergency Resource Allocation Mechanism for Public Health Emergencies: A Case Study on the Prevention and Control of COVID-19 in China

Ruhao Ma [1], Fansheng Meng [1,*] and Haiwen Du [2]

1. School of Economics and Management, Harbin Engineering University, Harbin 150001, China
2. School of Astronautics, Harbin Institute of Technology, Harbin 150001, China
* Correspondence: mfs_hrbeu@163.com

Abstract: The outbreak of COVID-19 posed a significant challenge to the emergency management system for public health emergencies, especially in China, where the epidemic began. As intelligent technology has injected new vitality into emergency management, applying intelligent technology to optimize emergency resource allocation (ERA) has become a focus of research in the post-epidemic era. Based on China's experience in preventing and controlling COVID-19, this paper first analyzes the characteristics and process of ERA in public health emergencies, and then synthesizes the relevant Chinese studies in recent years to identify the intelligent technologies affecting ERA in China using word frequency analysis technology. We also construct an intelligent emergency resource allocation mechanism in four areas: medical intelligence, management intelligence, decision-making intelligence, and supervision intelligence. Finally, we use the entropy-TOPSIS method to evaluate the impact of intelligent technologies on ERA, and we rank the criticality of intelligent technologies. The experimental results show that (i.) medical intelligence and management intelligence are the keys to developing intelligent ERA, and (ii.) among the identified essential intelligent technologies, artificial intelligence (AI), and big data technology have a more significant and critical role in emergency resource intelligence allocation.

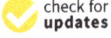

Citation: Ma, R.; Meng, F.; Du, H. Research on Intelligent Emergency Resource Allocation Mechanism for Public Health Emergencies: A Case Study on the Prevention and Control of COVID-19 in China. *Systems* **2023**, *11*, 300. https://doi.org/10.3390/systems11060300

Academic Editors: Philippe J. Giabbanelli and Andrew Page

Received: 9 May 2023
Revised: 29 May 2023
Accepted: 9 June 2023
Published: 11 June 2023

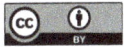

Copyright: © 2023 by the authors. Licensee MDPI, Basel, Switzerland. This article is an open access article distributed under the terms and conditions of the Creative Commons Attribution (CC BY) license (https:// creativecommons.org/licenses/by/ 4.0/).

Keywords: public health emergency; emergency resource allocation; intelligent technology

1. Introduction

Public health emergencies can profoundly impact public health, the environment, the economy, and even politics, and have therefore been the focus of attention from people and researchers in all walks of life and research. In early 2020, COVID-19 sent shockwaves throughout the economic and social order of countries around the world, greatly influencing emergency management systems and governance capacity worldwide [1].

When COVID-19 broke out, the best time for prevention and control was missed because of the delayed response of the Chinese government. This resulted in an inability to reasonably predict the extent of the damage [2], and this had at least two severe consequences: (i.) demand-supply imbalance on medical emergency resources (such as masks and rubbing alcohol, critical medical equipment, etc.) [3], and (ii.) the inaccurate demand information for emergency resources leading to unfair resource allocation, causing secondary harm to the people in the affected area. The isolation policy shortened human resources, increasing the pressure on medical care and epidemic prevention. The above-mentioned problems reflect the fact that the emergency resource allocation mechanism for public health emergencies in China still needs to be improved. There are loopholes in epidemic prediction and decision making, the supervision of information transmission, and ERA and transportation. The traditional way of allocating emergency resources based on human labour now faces significant challenges, and, indeed, COVID-19 has proved a challenge to the national governance system and capacity. It is necessary to improve the national emergency management mechanism in response to the shortcomings and deficiencies exposed during this epidemic.

Intelligent technology's high-performance computing and simulation capabilities as well as the idea of a "machine replacement" provide the direction for solving these problems. Intelligence has become a new approach for countries to solve resource allocation problems, which replaces traditional methods (such as manual labour). China has also made many attempts in this direction during the epidemic, such as online medical services, remote work policy, and infection control in public places through intelligent technologies. However, at this stage, research on the application of intelligent technologies in ERA needs to be improved [4]. As the normalized epidemic prevention and control significantly increases labour costs, the need to realize intelligent ERA is urgent. Therefore, constructing an intelligent emergency resource allocation mechanism for public health emergencies is of great theoretical significance and application value.

The key to solving the problems in ERA for public health emergencies is to use intelligent technology to improve ERA efficiency, which can fully leverage the role of emergency resources in epidemic prevention and control. Therefore, this article focuses on the intelligent technologies in ERA, and it answers the following research questions:

(i.) What are the essential intelligent technologies for intelligent ERA? We solved this problem in Section 3 by using word frequency analysis to extract essential intelligent technologies.

(ii.) How to intelligently allocate emergency resources for public health emergencies? We solved this problem in Section 4 by establishing an intelligent emergency resource allocation mechanism.

We constructed an evaluation index system for essential intelligent technologies through empirical methods in Section 5. The use of this evaluation system to rank the importance of essential intelligent technologies. Finally, Section 6 provides directions for further research on the application of intelligent technologies and suggestions for improving the efficiency of emergency management systems.

2. Related Works

Public health emergencies spread fast and cause significant losses. Since SARS in 2003, the construction of emergency management systems and related research in China has gradually increased [5]. The construction of the health emergency system in China has been significantly improved, but the efficiency in both resource dispatching and decision-making could still be higher [6]. Li et al. [7] have pointed out that the prevention and the control process of COVID-19 revealed many problems in China's emergency management system. These problems include the imperfect monitoring and early warning system, the unbalanced layout of emergency resources, insufficient storage of emergency supplies, and backward management.

2.1. Research on ERA

Before the COVID-19 pandemic, researchers mainly focused on optimizing the ERA decision-making process and site-path selection by constructing ERA models. Ge et al. [8] established a two-stage stochastic planning model for resource allocation in a complex disaster scenario. The model was used to make decisions under different disaster scenarios, such as the location of emergency facilities and the inventory of emergency materials. Peng et al. [9] established a robust site-path optimization model for multiple ERA types. It determines the optimal siting layout and distribution path for emergency resource supply points based on the uncertainty of emergency resource costs. Researchers also realize that emergency management of public emergencies is a complex project with multiple subjects and levels. The disaster situation, time-space distribution, and rescue costs are uncertain, so most studies construct scenarios with static demand for emergency resources. However, the actual ERA process is more complex. Therefore, some researchers studied ERA from the perspective of demand. Zhang et al. [10] established a demand-based emergency resources supply system by analyzing the characteristics of emergency demand

and constructing different emergency resource demand scenarios. Li et al. [11] established a multi-objective mixed integer planning model to solve the fairness problem of ERA among multiple subjects for the demand uncertainty situation. It uses min-max dissatisfaction as the fairness objective and the sum of system utilities as the utility objective. Yang et al. [12] construct an emergency resources demand strategy that can dynamically deploy resources for the demanding state of emergency relief materials. In addition to studying ERA, researchers realize that information resources participate in, guide, and supervise the process. This is vital to guaranteeing efficient ERA.

Digital and intelligent technologies lead the development of the fourth industrial revolution, and have revolutionized how things connect and interact with things, things with people, and people with each other. Therefore, the allocation of resources has undergone new changes. [13]. Researchers have begun to explore the relationship between intelligent technologies, such as AI, big data, and intelligent design, which significantly impact ERA strategy. On the one hand, some researchers believe that the characteristics of intelligent technologies are beneficial to improving the ERA process. For example, Akter et al. [14] argued that big data improves emergency management efficiency because it can visualize, analyze, and predict disasters. Deng et al. [15] proposed that AI can effectively alleviate the pressure of rising labour costs, compensate for the shortage of human labourers, and significantly reduce labour density. Dui et al. [4] argued that AI significantly accelerates epidemic data monitoring and prediction efficiency.

On the other hand, some researchers argue that environmental intelligence changes emergency resource allocation mechanisms to accommodate it. [16]. Chen et al. [17] argue that the big data environment brings increasing implications and challenges for effective data processing and decision-making. Therefore, intelligent techniques are critical in the emergency management life cycle. He et al. [18] argue that the convergence of the Internet, big data, machine learning, and AI has led to a consequent evolution of resource allocation mechanisms. Data intelligence has become the basis for resource allocation mechanisms in the Internet era. Despite the different motivations, both views recognize that ERA intelligence is the development trend of modern emergency management systems.

2.2. Research on the Intelligence of ERA

Most of the current academic research on the intelligence of ERA focuses on intelligent information management [19,20], intelligent decision-making of resource allocation [21–23], and intelligent medical applications [24,25]. Regarding the research on intelligent information management, Wang et al. [26] concluded that there are more severe data silos in Chinese public health information systems, which make it difficult to provide real-time data for handling large-scale public health emergencies. Shen et al. [27] argued that emergency response efficiency could be improved through two approaches. One is intelligent information management, while the other is optimizing and integrating various resources to obtain more reasonable decisions. Zeng et al. [28] constructed an intelligence mechanism for public health emergencies by analyzing the information needs of each wave of the epidemic. This mechanism collects, processes, and mines information for public health data intelligence. Liu et al. [29] constructed a mechanism for data collection and feature extraction of public opinion on emergencies on the Internet. They established a computer-aided warning system based on big data and distributed computing technology for network public opinion emergencies.

Regarding the research on intelligent decision-making for resource allocation, scholars believe that intelligent technologies can rapidly and accurately grasp and assess information under dynamic scenarios. Zhu et al. [30] proposed a demand prediction method based on machine learning, big data, and intelligent information processing technologies to assist in intelligent decision-making for ERA. Abdel et al. [31] constructed a novel intelligent healthcare decision support model based on soft computing and IoT techniques. The model facilitates the completion of continuous resource assessment in public health emergencies. Some researchers simulated the evolutionary patterns through intelligent algorithms for quantitative analysis to improve decision-making accuracy. For example, by analyzing the uncertain factors in the evolution, Chang et al. [32] used system dynamics theory and its related intelligent algorithms to simulate the evolutionary process of social security emergencies. Tian et al. [33] modelled different stages of the evolution of network public opinion emergencies as a "social burning life cycle". They simulated the evolution process of such emergencies using the generalized stochastic Petri net theory and its related intelligent algorithms.

For the research on intelligent medical applications, Wang et al. [34] analyzed the application of blockchain, the IoT, and other technologies in the supply chain management of medical supplies. He argued that intelligent technologies could provide a rapid and accurate supply of resources and realize the efficient operation of the emergency supply chain. Du [35] conducted an in-depth study on the regional collaborative emergency system based on big medical data. Chen et al. [36] established a "horizontal-vertical" model to integrate emergency medical resources. The model meets the needs of automatic information integration and intelligent analysis sharing, simplifying the medical process through emergency management visualization and digitizing medical information.

By analyzing related studies, we found that most researchers focus on the ERA from the following two aspects: (1) analyzing the impact of intelligent technologies, such as big data, AI, and information technology on ERA; (2) building intelligent mechanisms from each process of ERA. However, there are few works on quantitative analysis. Although China's public health emergency management capacity is increasing, ERA still has shortcomings. The most concerning factors are insufficient emergency resource reserves, unbalanced and inefficient allocation of emergency resources, and loopholes in the early warning system. This paper aims to optimize the emergency response system for public health emergencies in China and reduce the losses caused by public health emergencies such as COVID-19. We achieve it by taking the development of intelligent technology as an opportunity to build an intelligent emergency resource allocation mechanism and identify essential intelligent technologies. Our work is of great significance in promoting the development of intelligent ERA.

3. Allocation of Emergency Resources for Public Health Emergencies and Identification of Essential Intelligent Technologies

The traditional emergency resources are mainly summarized as material, human, scientific, and technological resources. Material resources include medical material resources for public health prevention and control, and material resources for people's livelihood to ensure the safety of life. Human resources include labour costs of medical, nursing, material production, transportation, and security costs in public health prevention and control. Scientific and technological resources guarantee high-tech public health prevention and treatment.

With the advent of the digital economy, information collection and delivery efficiency have increased dramatically. Information resources (including big data, information, and related facilities and equipment) have become an emerging active element in emergency resources.

3.1. Characteristics of ERA for Public Health Emergencies

Due to the diverse, regional, and unpredictable characteristics of public health emergencies, ERA is a dynamic and complex project. It has multiple supply points, demand points, emergency supplies, and transportation modes. The active information resources also give new characteristics to it:

(1) A multi-subject, multi-level super-network system. Firstly, multiple subjects are involved in ERA for public health emergencies. It requires the support and cooperation of multiple parties, such as the government, market and civil organizations, and the public. Second, because public health emergencies often involve a wide geographical area, the affected areas may be from the provinces, cities, villages, and towns. There-

fore, from the government's perspective, the resource allocation process cascades upward from lower government levels. The ERA system shows multi-level characteristics. At the same time, at least three levels of the deployment network exist from the supply point to the transit point and then to the demand point. The boundaries between supply, staging, and demand points are not apparent for significant public health emergencies. The point of supply for one resource may also be the point of demand for another. Physical networks, financial networks, and information networks are interwoven in the supply-and-demand networks to form a hyper-network system for ERA.

(2) The disaster situation, resource needs, and priorities are dynamic. The initial transmission location of public health emergencies cannot be predicted. Different urban areas have differences in population density, economic level, road network, information communication, and other conditions. Therefore, there are differences in the emergency capacity and supply of emergency resources among different regions. The spread and destructiveness of viruses are not constant. Furthermore, medical resources are time-sensitive and often difficult to replace. Emergency resource needs and priorities change with the dynamics of an epidemic. It requires that each relief department be able to develop strategies and make timely allocation decisions in response to changes in the epidemic. Emergency resource allocation mechanisms must be well adapted to the dynamic variability of the epidemic, and they should also be able to make timely adjustments in response to dynamic demands in time and space.

(3) The role of information resources. The rapid development of information technology has led to changes in the primary way of allocating emergency resources for public health emergencies. Mobile communications and the Internet have accelerated the speed of access and dissemination of information resources. However, due to the multiple sources of emergency information and non-uniform data formats, most demand-related information cannot be accessed timely. It makes the emergency information construction with information silos, information coupling, and poor information communication. Therefore, timely information response, fast transmission, and good analysis capabilities are the key issues to improving the efficiency of ERA. Building an emergency information management platform is a crucial way to improve emergency information management capability.

3.2. ERA Process for Public Health Emergencies

The dynamic variability of emergency resources should change with the status of public health emergencies. The focus of public health prevention and control differs in different development parses. Therefore, to build an intelligent emergency resource allocation mechanism for public health emergencies, we need to clarify: (i.) the cyclical changes in emergency resource demand for public health emergencies, and (ii.) the characteristics of emergency resource types and the demand characteristics of different periods.

The development cycle of the epidemic is mainly divided into the early phase, rising phase, outbreak phase, and stable phase. As the epidemic enters different stages of development, the need for emergency resources changes dynamically. (i.) In the early stage of epidemic spread, information resources still need to be provided. The trend of epidemic changes still needs to be clarified, and the regional information interconnection network has not yet been formed. Therefore, the responses of managers are slow, and the demand for emergency resources is in a more subdued early warning period. (ii.) The risk level is elevated when the epidemic moves into the rising stage. Relevant departments start to pay attention to and adopt prevention and control strategies and mobilize emergency resources, and the demand for emergency resources is in the start-up period. (iii.) The epidemic's severity climbs when the outbreak period is entered. The number of cases increases, epidemic information resources surge, and prevention and control efforts are in full swing. The demand for emergency resources dramatically increases and enters the treatment period of emergency resource supply. (iv.) As the epidemic moves from the end of the outbreak phase to the stable phase, hospital admissions are gradually cleared. The urgent demand for emergency resources decreases, and the demand enters the reserve period. On the one hand, the production department adjusts the resource production plan to the normal production and living level. On the other hand, the management keeps an eye on the epidemic situation to prevent a second outbreak, and the priority of various resource needs changes.

The ERA process should include resource information management, resource allocation plan design, resource distribution plan decision, and resource allocation supervision (see Figure 1). (i.) Emergency resource information management refers to collecting information during the emergency resource preparation phase of a public health emergency. The information is related to the quantity and supply location of all emergency resources (including reserve resources, resources that can be raised, and resources that can be produced). Information management facilitates understand the distribution, supply quantity, and supply speed of various resource supplies in a short period, and target the distributed mobilization efforts. (ii.) The design of the resource allocation plan decides when and where to use the type and quantity of emergency resources and makes a reasonable resource distribution plan. It collects information on the demand for emergency resources and considers the distance from the supply point to the demand point, the transportation environment, and the degree of urgency. Finally, responsible decisions are made by combining emergency resource management information during a public health event. (iii.) The resource distribution plan decision is to consider the transportation route and mode of transportation for emergency resource distribution and to choose the optimal plan. (iv.) Resource allocation supervision ensures that ERA information is fair and open, and that resources are distributed in place. It also ensures that each emergency point's needs meet the maximum extent in order to avoid resource misallocation and omission.

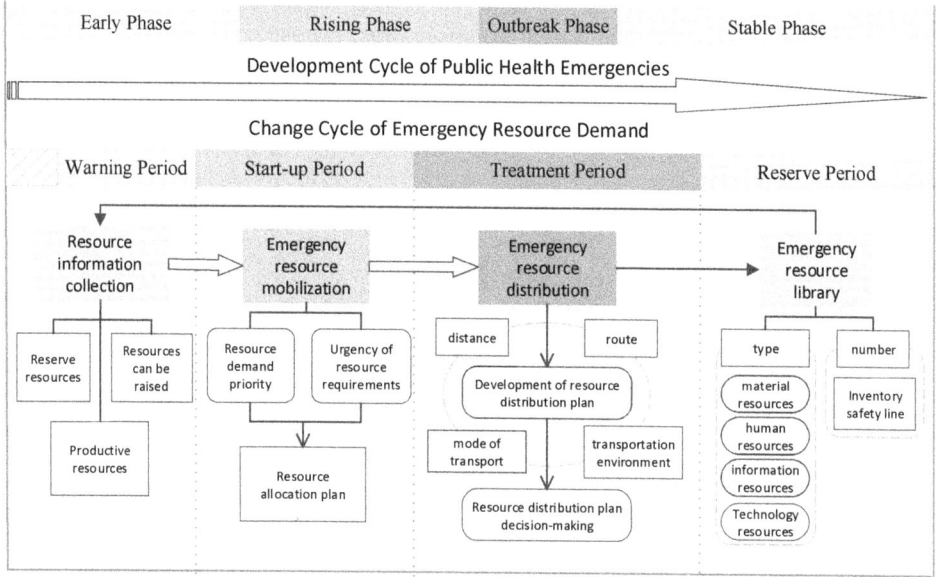

Figure 1. ERA process for public health emergencies.

After analyzing ERA's demand characteristics and process for public health emergencies, we believe that the essential intelligent technologies for ERA should achieve the following functions: (i) to assist public health prevention and relief work; (ii) to improve the efficiency and effectiveness of information management and decision making; (iii.) to reduce human labour force participation rate and time cost; and (iv.) to achieve intelligent supervision of the allocation process and reduce the occurrence of the unreasonable allocation of resources. Clarifying the need for intelligent technology for ERA is a guarantee for identifying vital, intelligent technologies.

3.3. Essential Intelligent Technology Identification

Intelligence is the property of making objects with functions, such as sensing, judging, learning, and executing, with the support of the Internet, big data, IoT, and AI. Intelligence is the goal of digitization, informatization, and networking, while intelligent technology is the deep integration and subsequent extension of digital, information, and Internet technology.

The development of intelligent technology has brought significant changes to people's lives. During the COVID-19 pandemic, intelligent technology has come to the forefront of practical operations to control the spread of the virus. For example, intelligent robots distribute daily medicines and supplies to isolated patients. Big medical data and information systems are also used to trace the route of patients' journeys. Moreover, technologies such as AI and expert systems assist researchers in virus tracing to discover the virus's causes, transmission routes, and hazards. Advanced intelligent technology not only simplifies the treatment process and its difficulty but also helps to improve the accessibility of emergency resources. For example, e-commerce logistics, which has gradually emerged due to epidemic control, provides security for transporting and supplying medical and household materials. Features such as work-from-home, online conferences, and online business processing ensure that people's lives and work are orderly during an epidemic.

Word frequency analysis (WFA) is a text analysis method used to calculate the frequency of each word in a text and to conduct statistics and analysis based on these frequencies. WFA can quickly extract the most widely-used intelligent technology in allocating emergency resources for public health emergencies. It provides a research foundation for constructing an intelligent emergency resource allocation mechanism. This paper used the China National Knowledge Infrastructure (CNKI) as the source of statistical data. We selected years from 2012 to 2022 and searched the journal literature for "intelligent", "intelligent technology", "resource allocation", "emergency public health event", and other related terms. A total of 309 results were obtained by searching the journal literature using "public health emergencies" and other related terms as subject terms. Through further screening and manual removal of non-academic journal literature, such as no-authors and correspondence, we obtained 253 highly relevant works on this topic. We exported sample data in EndNote text format and analyzed the keywords of the sample data using SATI [37], ultimately generating a keyword matrix (see Figure 2). In the keyword matrix, we used "intelligent" as the core related vocabulary of research hotspots in this field. We manually merged synonyms, removed unintentional words, and then sorted the frequency of popular keywords. Finally, we extracted ten intelligent technologies that benefit ERA in public health emergencies. (See Table 1 below.)

Table 1. List of Intelligent Technology Applications for Emergency Resource Management.

No	Name of Intelligent Technology	Application Description of Intelligent Technology in Medical and Resource Allocation
1	Artificial Intelligence	AI technologies can simulate, extend, and expand human intelligence to achieve functions, such as medical imaging-assisted diagnosis, intelligent drug development, intelligent health management, and assisted resource allocation decisions.
2	Internet	The Internet as a carrier and technical means can inform the process of ERA, realize instant communication, remote consultation, online consultation, etc.
3	(Medical) Information System	The Medical Information System can realize the storage, collection and query of information related to ERA. The information system assists emergency resource information management and conducts resource allocation planning.

Table 1. *Cont.*

No	Name of Intelligent Technology	Application Description of Intelligent Technology in Medical and Resource Allocation
4	Information Technology	The use of Information Technology can make the acquisition, transmission, processing, control, display, and storage of resource allocation information intelligent, such as radio frequency identification technology (RFID), sensing technology, network communication technology, etc.
5	The Internet of Things (IoT)	The Internet of Things (IoT) is to connect material resources with the network, exchange communication through information dissemination medium, and complete intelligent identification, positioning, tracking, supervision, and other functions.
6	Big Data	Big Data application technologies include data collection, data pre-processing, distributed storage, machine learning, etc. The deep combination of big data and cloud computing technology can realize functions such as epidemic prediction, intelligent medical care, resource management, and logistic network optimization.
7	Expert System	An Expert System is used to address problems in the field using the knowledge and the problem-solving methods of human experts, and it can assist in clinical medical diagnosis and ERA program decisions.
8	Intelligent Design	Intelligent Design is the application of modern information technology and computer simulation of human thinking activities, combined with neural networks and machine learning technology to assist in the automation of the design process.
9	Wearable Technology	Wearable technology is the embedding of multimedia, sensors, and wireless communication technologies into clothing and software support for data interaction and cloud interaction in order to help achieve real-time monitoring of the health status of a patient.
10	Machine Replacement Technology	Machine Replacement Technology is the use of robotic hands, automated control equipment, or assembly line automation for intelligent technology transformation of enterprises in order to achieve the purpose of reducing staff, increasing efficiency, improving quality, and ensuring safety.

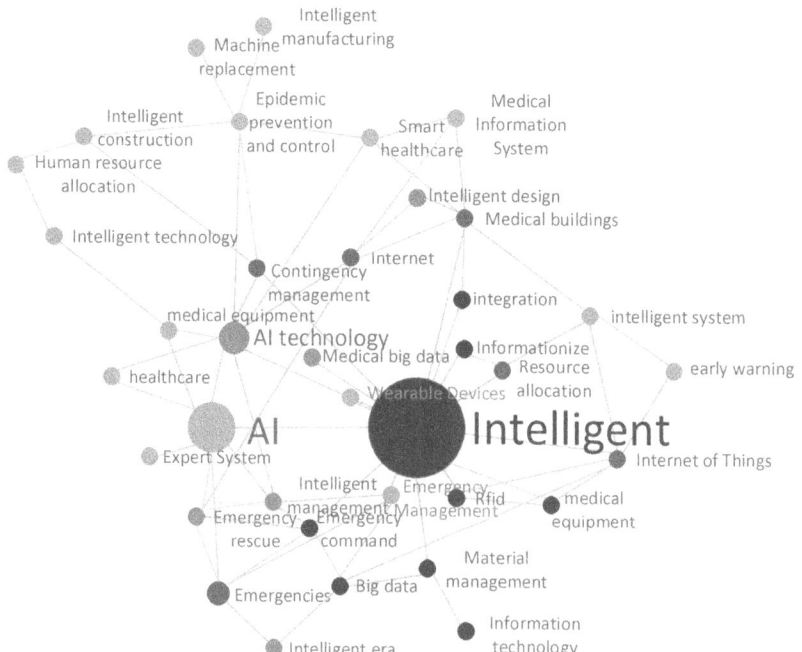

Figure 2. Keyword Matrix Graph of Intelligent Technology for ERA.

4. Intelligent Emergency Resource Allocation Mechanism

Different from the general resource allocation process, intelligent ERA should achieve three targets: (i.) meet the emergency resource demand, (ii.) improve resource allocation efficiency, and (iii.) save resource allocation costs using intelligent technology. Therefore, this study builds an information platform for ERA based on identifying intelligent technologies that combine public health emergencies' characteristics and the ERA process. We also established an intelligent emergency resource allocation mechanism for public health emergencies, including medical intelligence, management intelligence, decision-making intelligence, and supervision intelligence (see Figure 3).

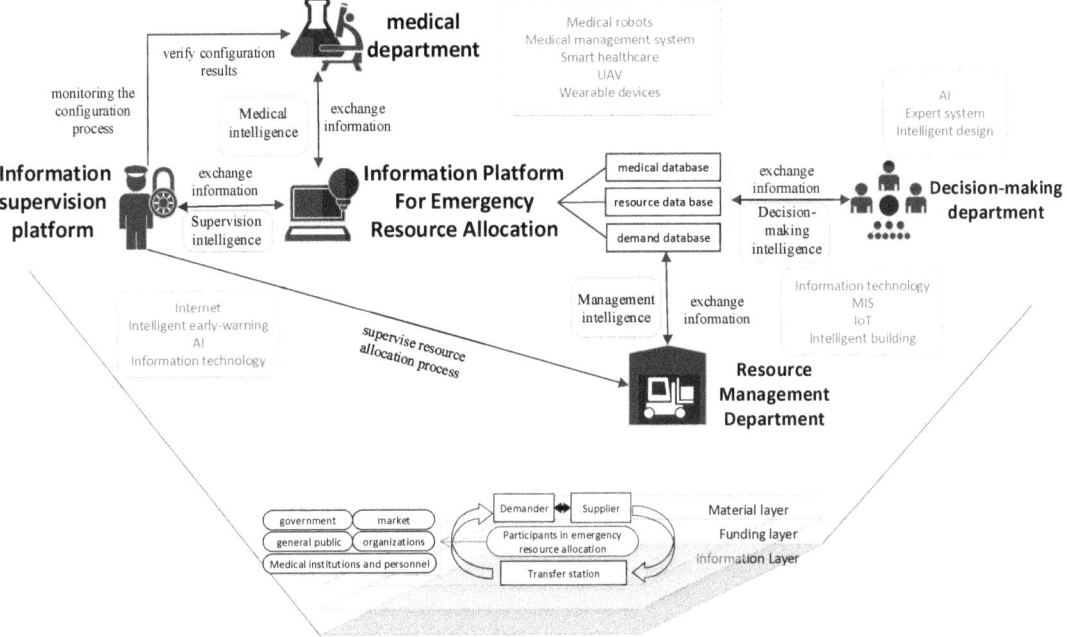

Figure 3. Intelligent emergency resource allocation mechanism for public health emergencies.

(1) Information platform for ERA. The information platform for ERA is a comprehensive platform that realizes the functions of information collection, screening and filtering, identification and error correction, sorting and classification, and transmission and feedback in ERA. It is the central hub of ERA and can store, process, and transmit data. The information platform for ERA comprises a regional interconnection network and database. The regional interconnection network connects the affected areas and supply points horizontally while connecting the management and decision-making departments at all levels vertically. It uses Information Technology and the Internet to form a "horizontal-vertical" interlocking information transmission network to realize information exchange between subjects. The information base includes medical databases, resource databases, and demand databases. Among them, the medical database mainly stores information related to IPC and assists in researching the outbreak of diseases. The resource information base covers the status of emergency resource storage, including (i.) the type and quantity of reserve resources, (ii.) the person-hours and expected quantity of productive resources, and (iii.) the source and quantity of preparable resources. The demand database collects and stores information at each demand point during an epidemic, and updates it instantly to provide a basis for ERA management and decision-making. As the data and information in public health emergencies are complicated, ERA needs the support of an integrated,

networked, and intelligent information platform. Therefore, establishing an information platform for ERA is the cornerstone of the intellectual development of ERA.

(2) Medical Intelligence. Medical intelligence is the most direct manifestation of intelligent ERA during an epidemic. Based on the data support of the Medical Information systems, modern digital medical treatment is realized using the IoT and Internet+. It also creates intelligent medical treatment with online and offline interaction. Therefore, it can improve the sharing of medical resources, simplify time-consuming and labour-intensive manual medical processes, and reduce costs. With the development of intelligent technology, innovative medicine is gradually being realized. It can use intelligent auxiliary medical devices to complete medical work with a high degree of difficulty. Further, it can also realize the interaction between patients and medical personnel, medical institutions, and medical equipment by establishing a regional medical information cloud platform. Medical intelligence reduces medical congestion, shortens the practice of waiting for treatment, and expands medical coverage.

(3) Management Intelligence. Management Intelligence simplifies the management process through intelligent technology and fully uses the information to help achieve the integrated use of resources. Management Intelligence is not simply system software applications for repetitive data processing and exchange. Instead, emergency resource management is based on intelligent buildings to manage people and equipment better, achieving human-machine coordination. It manifests using information management systems and robots instead of traditional human work. The resource information database can control the inventory of resources and then transmit and process resource shipment and inventory information in real time. It uses sensors and other equipment to automate instruction transmission. In addition, it can also intelligently perceive, recognize, and process instruction information and respond. Meanwhile, intelligent warehousing and logistics methods are labour-saving, thereby reducing the risk of infection. Intelligent technology can thus help people achieve efficient resource allocation with less human resource investment, and it is therefore a necessary means for improving the efficiency of ERA.

(4) Decision-Making Intelligence. Decision-Making Intelligence means using the advantages of AI and expert systems to help managers solve complex decision-making problems in collaboration with human intelligence. Due to the dynamic complexity of ERA information, relying on the traditional human and computer approaches for decision-making takes both time and effort. This can easily cause huge losses due to untimely actions during epidemic prevention and control. AI, as an intelligent auxiliary technology, can realize functions such as analyzing the current epidemic situation, optimizing and calculating resource allocation schemes, and predicting the epidemic's trend. Furthermore, the program's feasibility is tested by simulations, which shows that decision-making intelligence saves human resources and improves decision-making efficiency. It also reduces the risk of decision making and reduces the waste of resources.

(5) Supervision intelligence. The timely acquisition, transmission, and management of epidemic information is the key to reducing the harm of public health emergencies. During COVID-19, information is often transmitted through the sequence of "front-line workers and epidemic prevention agencies" ("lower-level managers") and "higher-level managers and research institutions". Due to the vast geographical area and complex administrative divisions involved in the epidemic, information acquisition, analysis, and feedback are prone to delayed transmission, mismatch, and incorrect or missing communications. Therefore, an intelligent supervision mechanism for intelligent ERA should be established to strengthen the supervision and management guaranteeing information security. First, the intelligence of the supervision platform should be realized. Large data centres and information supervision platforms should be built to intelligently supervise various application scenarios, thereby improving the allocation risk prevention and control system. Secondly, intelligent supervision should be realized, i.e., using AI to improve management efficiency through digital management, and achieve rapid risk warnings and alarms through the

Internet of Things data collection and intelligent technology analysis. Finally, to achieve an intelligent regulatory process, the Internet and Information Technology should achieve instant information transfer and feedback, which can promote effective and intelligent data transfer between departments, and which can also help to build a perfect closed loop of active discovery, automatic instructions, rapid processing, real-time feedback, and risk prevention and control.

5. Evaluation of Essential Intelligent Technologies for ERA

5.1. Indicator System Construction

The lack of a mature scale for evaluating essential technologies in ERA makes it hard to build the indicator system. To address this problem, we borrowed indicators from existing works to construct the evaluation index system for essential technologies in ERA. Among them, essential technology evaluation indicators are from [38–40], while medical resource evaluation indicators are from [41]. This evaluation index system combines the characteristics of ERA and intelligent technology for public health emergencies. We integrate relevant research results to construct the system from four aspects: medical intelligence [42,43], management intelligence [35,44], decision-making intelligence [17,45,46], and supervision intelligence [47,48]. The content and description of evaluation indicators are shown in Table 2.

Table 2. Essential Intelligent Technology evaluation index system.

Primary Indicators	Secondary Indicators	Tertiary Indicators	Indicator Description	Indicator Attribute
Medical intelligence A1	Medical resource savings B1	Occupancy of medical devices C1	The impact of intelligent technology on reducing medical device congestion	Positive
		Waiting time savings C2	The impact of intelligent technology on reducing unnecessary waiting time for medical treatment	Positive
		Human resource savings C3	The impact of intelligent technology on reducing the demand for medical personnel	Positive
	Use value B2	Reaction time C4	The reaction time consumed when intelligent technology provides interactive functions	Opposite
		Consultation time C5	The time spent on diagnosis and treatment using intelligent technology	Opposite
		Operational difficulty C6	The operational difficulty of intelligent technology, i.e., the ability requirements for relevant operators	Opposite
		Cure rate C7	The impact of intelligent technology on improving the cure rate	Positive
	Economic benefits B3	Technology maturity C8	The impact of intelligent technology on the accuracy and risk of medical diagnosis	Positive
		Application breadth C9	The application scope and popularity of intelligent technology in medical institutions	Positive
		Additional services C10	The possibility of intelligent technology providing additional services	Positive
Management intelligence A2	Management cost savings B4	Time-cost savings C11	Quantitative indicators of time-cost savings in ERA using intelligent technology	Positive
		Manpower cost savings C12	Quantitative indicators of manpower costs for ERA that can be saved by utilizing intelligent technology	Positive
	Management effectiveness B5	Reduction of resource mismatch C13	The impact of intelligent technology on reducing adverse phenomena such as resource mismatch and missed allocation	Positive
		Managing information security C14	The impact of using Intelligent Technology on resource management information security	Positive

Table 2. Cont.

Primary Indicators	Secondary Indicators	Tertiary Indicators	Indicator Description	Indicator Attribute
Decision-making intelligence A3	Decision-making efficiency B6	Information transmission speed C15	The Impact of intelligent technology on the Transmission Speed of Decision Information and Decision Instructions	Positive
		Decision duration C16	The reduction in decision-making time caused by intelligent technology	Positive
	Effects on decision-making B7	Fault tolerance of decision-making C17	The impact of intelligent technology on improving scheme fault tolerance and reducing decision risks	Positive
		Effectiveness of decision-making C18	The impact of intelligent technology on improving the effectiveness of decision-making plans	Positive
Supervision intelligence A4	Regulatory timeliness B8	Alert response time C19	The impact of intelligent technology on reducing the early warning response time of resource allocation regulation	Opposite
		Inspection time C20	The impact of intelligent technology on reducing the inspection time of resource allocation supervision	Opposite
		Correction time C21	The impact of intelligent technology on reducing error correction time for resource allocation supervision	Opposite
	Social benefit B9	Social stability C22	The impact of intelligent technology on improving social stability	Positive
		International image C23	The impact of intelligent technology on improving a country's international image	Positive

5.2. Evaluation Model of Essential Intelligent Technologies for ERA Based on Entropy Value-TOPSIS Method

In this paper, medical practitioners, emergency resource managers, and intelligent manufacturing-related researchers were selected to score the evaluation indexes of each Intelligent Technology. The research subjects are from major cities in China, such as Beijing, Harbin, and Wuhan. This selection aims to reduce individual experts' subjectivity in determining indicator weights and ensure the comprehensiveness and professionalism of the evaluation results as much as possible. The scores are from 0 to 9, representing the importance of the technology to the evaluation index from low to high. For the reverse index, the higher the score, the lower the importance of the technology. We distributed seven questionnaires, all of which were returned, and we obtained the original evaluation data.

5.2.1. Entropy Power Method

The basic idea of assigning weights using the entropy method is to determine the objective weights according to the magnitude of the variability of the indicators. If the information entropy E_j of the indicator is small, its weight will be larger, indicating that the indicator value plays a more significant role in the comprehensive evaluation. Experts are susceptible to subjective factors such as experience, interest preference, and personal habits. Combining the entropy method to assign the index weights can weaken the influence of subjective factors to a certain extent. The evaluation data are normalized to obtain the standardization matrix $E = \{Y_{ij}\}$, based on determining the specific indicators of essential Intelligent Technology evaluation. Y_{ij} denotes the value of the jth index of the ith technology after standardization. According to the information entropy to determine the formula (Equation (1)):

$$E_j = -\frac{1}{\ln n} \sum_{n=1}^{n} p_{ij} \ln p_{ij} \quad E_j \geq 0$$
$$p_{ij} = Y_{ij} / \sum_{i=1}^{n} Y_{ij} \quad ,$$

(1)

where if $p_{ij} = 0$, then $\lim_{p_n \sim 0} p_{ij} \ln p_{ij} = 0$ is defined. The weight of each indicator is then calculated by the formula:

$$w_i = \frac{1 - E_i}{k - \sum E_i} \ (i = 1, 2, \cdots, k), \tag{2}$$

According to the formula, the information entropy and weight values of each essential Intelligent Technology evaluation index are obtained (see Table 3).

Table 3. Information entropy and weight of essential Intelligent Technology evaluation index.

Index	Entropy	Weight (%)
C1 Occupancy of medical devices	0.903	4.16
C2 Waiting time savings	0.909	3.91
C3 Human resource savings	0.907	3.99
C4 Reaction time	0.926	3.20
C5 Consultation time	0.903	4.17
C6 Operational difficulty	0.912	3.77
C7 Cure rate	0.814	8.00
C8 Technology maturity	0.871	5.57
C9 Application breadth	0.896	4.50
C10 Additional services	0.920	3.44
C11 Time-cost savings	0.932	2.94
C12 Manpower cost savings	0.865	5.82
C13 Reduction of resource mismatch	0.853	6.32
C14 Managing information security	0.907	4.00
C15 Information transmission speed	0.914	3.69
C16 Decision duration	0.929	3.05
C17 Fault tolerance of decision-making	0.903	4.19
C18 Effectiveness of decision-making	0.869	5.62
C19 Alert response time	0.917	3.57
C20 Inspection time	0.926	3.19
C21 Correction time	0.907	4.00
C22 Social stability	0.865	5.82
C23 International image	0.929	3.07

From the calculation results, it can be concluded that the top five indicators in the weight of the 23 indicators are: C7, C13, C12, C22, and C18. Intelligent Technology significantly impacts the ERA for public health emergencies in these five aspects. Moreover, these five indicators are mainly distributed in medical and decision-making intelligence, indicating that medical and management intelligence is essential for developing intelligent ERA.

5.2.2. Use TOPSIS Method to Identify Essential Intelligent Technologies

TOPSIS is an approaching ideal point ranking method that can rank a finite number of evaluation objects according to their relative proximity to the ideal solution. The evaluation object selected by this method should be as close as possible to the positive ideal solution and as far as possible from the negative ideal solution. TOPSIS can fully use the original data information to reflect each intelligent technology's gaps accurately. It can rank the degree of influence of Intelligent Technology on intelligent ERA. The research steps are as follows:

(1) Create the original decision matrix A:

$$A = \begin{array}{c} \\ x_1 \\ x_2 \\ \vdots \\ x_m \end{array} \begin{array}{cccc} o_1 & o_2 & \cdots & o_n \\ \begin{bmatrix} x_{11} & x_{12} & \cdots & x_{1n} \\ x_{21} & x_{22} & \cdots & x_{2n} \\ \vdots & \vdots & & \vdots \\ x_{m1} & x_{m2} & \cdots & x_{mn} \end{bmatrix} \end{array}, \tag{3}$$

where x_m is the mth intelligent technology, o_n is the nth evaluation index, and x_{mn} is the numerical result of the nth evaluation index of the mth intelligent technology.

(2) Normalize each numerical result by converting the decision matrix A into a canonical decision matrix $E = \{u_{ij}\}$, i.e.,

$$u_{ij} = \frac{x_{ij}}{\sqrt{\sum_{i=1}^{m} x_{ij}^2}}, \qquad (4)$$

For the inverse indicators, the data are reversed before the normalization process in order to ensure the consistency of the evaluation data.

(3) Construct a weighted decision matrix based on the index weights determined by the entropy weighting method.

The weights w are assigned according to the degree of importance of each evaluation attribute, and the formula is:

$$\overline{F} = (\overline{X}_{ij})_{m \times n} = w \cdot F, \qquad (5)$$

The weighted decision matrix is obtained.

(4) Define the positive ideal solution as x^+ and the negative ideal solution as x^-, then $\overline{x}_j^+, \overline{x}_j^-$ are, respectively:

$$\begin{cases} \overline{x}_j^+ = \max\{x_{1j}, x_{2j}, \cdots x_{mj}\} \\ \overline{x}_j^- = \min\{x_{1j}, x_{2j}, \cdots x_{mj}\} \end{cases} (j = 1, 2, \cdots n), \qquad (6)$$

The positive and negative ideal solutions for the 23 indicators are shown in Table 4.

Table 4. Ideal solution for evaluation indicators.

Index	Positive Ideal Solution	Negative Ideal Solution
C1 Occupancy of medical devices	0.016	0.008
C2 Waiting time savings	0.016	0.007
C3 Human resource savings	0.017	0.010
C4 Reaction time	0.012	0.008
C5 Consultation time	0.016	0.011
C6 Operational difficulty	0.014	0.009
C7 Cure rate	0.031	0.020
C8 Technology maturity	0.022	0.012
C9 Application breadth	0.018	0.011
C10 Additional services	0.013	0.008
C11 Time-cost savings	0.011	0.007
C12 Manpower cost savings	0.020	0.016
C13 Reduction of resource mismatch	0.027	0.013
C14 Managing information security	0.015	0.010
C15 Information transmission speed	0.014	0.010
C16 Decision duration	0.013	0.007
C17 Fault tolerance of decision-making	0.018	0.008
C18 Effectiveness of decision-making	0.024	0.012
C19 Alert response time	0.014	0.008
C20 Inspection time	0.013	0.007
C21 Correction time	0.016	0.010
C22 Social stability	0.022	0.014
C23 International image	0.012	0.008

(5) The Euclidean distances of each intelligent technique from the positive ideal solution x^+ and the negative ideal solution x^- are defined as:

$$D_i^+ = \sqrt{\sum_{j=1}^{n}\left(\overline{x}_{ij} - x_j^+\right)^2} \quad (i = 1, 2, \cdots, m), \tag{7}$$

$$D_i^- = \sqrt{\sum_{j=1}^{n}\left(\overline{x}_{ij} - x_j^-\right)^2} \quad (i = 1, 2, \cdots, m) \tag{8}$$

(6) Calculate the relative closeness of each intelligent technique to the positive ideal solution, which can be defined as:

$$\varphi_i = \frac{D_i^-}{D_i^+ + D_i^-} \quad (i = 1, 2, \cdots, m), \tag{9}$$

$\varphi_i \in [0, 1]$. Moreover, the larger φ_i is, the more significant the contribution of its corresponding Intelligent Technology to the intelligence of ERA in public health emergencies.

5.2.3. Experimental Results

(1) Based on the above experimental process, the evaluation results of essential intelligent technologies were obtained (see Table 5). The experimental results show that AI technology significantly impacts the intelligent ERA for public health emergencies, with a TOPSIS closeness of 0.766. They were followed by Big Data technology and expert systems, with a TOPSIS closeness of 0.683 and 0.529, respectively. In contrast, wearable technology has a negligible impact, with a TOPSIS closeness of 0.276.

Table 5. Evaluation Results of Essential Intelligent Technologies.

Intelligent Technology	Di+	Di-	TOPSIS Closeness φ_i	Sort
AI	0.009	0.030	0.766	1
Internet	0.021	0.020	0.485	7
Information System	0.020	0.022	0.518	4
Information Technology	0.020	0.020	0.497	6
The Internet of Things	0.020	0.021	0.513	5
Big Data	0.013	0.027	0.683	2
Expert System	0.020	0.022	0.529	3
Intelligent Design	0.027	0.016	0.367	9
Wearable Technology	0.029	0.011	0.276	10
Machine Replacement Technology	0.026	0.017	0.405	8

The chart shows the experimental results (see Figure 4). AI and big data technology in Intelligent Technology are the most critical. Moreover, the positive ideal solution closeness of the expert system, Internet, information system, information technology, and IoT technology is around 0.5, which are more critical and less different. Machines for human technology, intelligent design, and wearable technology have a lower degree of positive ideal solution closeness. They are less critical to intelligent ERA than other intelligent technologies.

(2) Combining the weight data in Tables 2 and 3, and further processing the experimental results resulted in Table 6. To compare the contributions of A1–A4 to the intelligence of ERA, we obtain the weights of A1–A4 by adding the weights of the corresponding tertiary indicators. However, the number of tertiary indicators corresponding to each primary indicator differs. We average the weights of primary indicators to eliminate the impact of the number of tertiary indicators on indicator weights. According to the calculation results (see Table 6), it can be concluded that the average weight of A1 and A2 is higher. It indicates that the relevant indicators of medical intelligence and management intelligence significantly impact the intelligent ERA for public health emergencies.

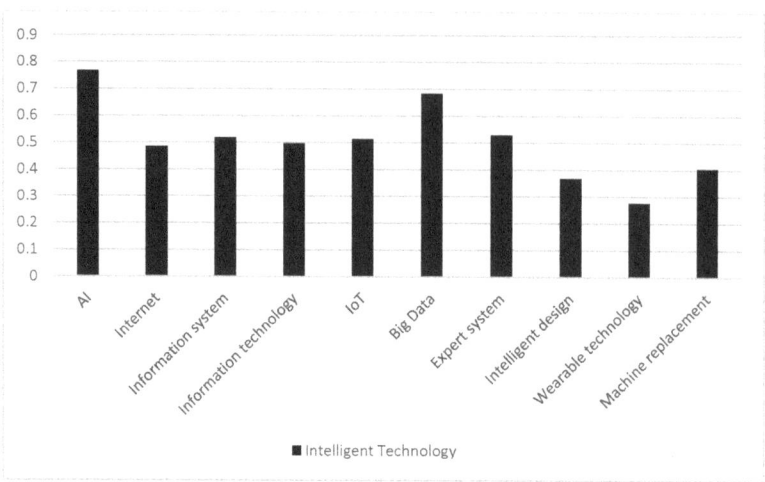

Figure 4. TOPSIS closeness of essential intelligent technologies.

Table 6. Average Weight of Primary Indicators.

Primary Indicators	Medical Intelligence A1		Management Intelligence A2		Decision-Making Intelligence A3		Supervision Intelligence A4	
Secondary Indicators	Medical resource savings B1	12.06	Management cost savings B4	8.76	Decision-making efficiency B6	6.74	Regulatory timeliness B8	10.76
	Use value B2	19.14	Management effectiveness B5	10.32	Effects on decision-making B7	9.81	Social benefit B9	8.89
	Economic benefits B3	13.51						
Weight	44.71		19.08		16.55		19.65	
Average Weight	4.47		4.77		4.13		3.93	

6. Conclusions

This section may be divided by subheadings. It should provide a concise and precise description of the experimental results, their interpretation, and the experimental conclusions that can be drawn.

6.1. Research Findings

With the development of the digital economy, intelligent technology, and the influence of the normalization of COVID-19 prevention and control, intelligence becomes the future development direction of ERA for public health emergencies. Therefore, this paper constructs an intelligent emergency resource allocation mechanism for public health emergencies. It identifies the essential intelligent technologies affecting intellectual development, and conducts an essential evaluation. Firstly, we determined essential intelligent technologies' evaluation indicators and weights through expert consultation and the entropy weight method. Then, the TOPSIS method was used to evaluate the criticality of Intelligent Technology in ERA. This method considers the distance between Intelligent Technology and ideal points as the essential criterion. It combines objective analysis with experts' subjective judgments, which makes the evaluation results more scientific and reliable. The main conclusions drawn from the study are as follows:

(1) ERA for public health emergencies is a multi-subject, multi-level super network-system, and the demand and priority of emergency resources change with the devel-

opment of the epidemic. This paper categorizes emergency resources into material, human, information, and scientific and technological resources, and it focuses on the role of information resources. Information resources meet resource needs in ERA for public health emergencies while also playing the role of central control and auxiliary supervision. Intelligent emergency resource allocation mechanism gives full play to the characteristics of information resources. Based on establishing an information platform for ERA, this paper uses Intelligent Technology to make each allocation link intelligent, including medical intelligence, management intelligence, decision-making intelligence, and supervision intelligence, in order to achieve efficient resource allocation and cost savings.

(2) We conclude essential intelligent technologies through word frequency analysis of research on ERA for public health emergencies. Intelligent technologies include AI, the Internet, information systems, information technology, the Internet of Things, big data technology, etc. These intelligent technologies all play an essential role in developing intelligent ERA for public health emergencies.

(3) This study establishes an evaluation index system for the essential intelligent technologies of ERA in four aspects: medical intelligence, management intelligence, decision-making intelligence, and supervision intelligence. We used the entropy weight and TOPSIS methods to build the evaluation model for each intelligent technology. The results show that the evaluation indexes with greater weights are in medical intelligence and management intelligence. This indicates that medical intelligence and management intelligence are the focus of developing ERA intelligence. Furthermore, AI and big data technology have a significant key role in the ERA intelligence.

6.2. Key Research Insights

The development of intelligent technology has brought significant changes to ERA for public health emergencies, providing new possibilities to improve efficiency and reduce the cost of resource allocation. During the COVID-19 pandemic, the application of intelligent technology has emerged, but there is still room for optimization. We focus on essential intelligent technologies for ERA for public health emergencies. Therefore, our study can also provide directions and suggestions for further research on the application of intelligent technology in emergency resource management. We proposed the following management insights:

(1) Pay attention to the role of information resources. Applying intelligent technology to acquiring, screening, storing, processing, and transmitting information resources in ERA is essential. This can help reduce the flow time of information resources and the response time of management departments, speed up the interaction rate, and ensure information security and timeliness. An information platform for ERA should be established promptly during the prevention and treatment of public health emergencies. All entities and levels should improve their information infrastructure and strengthen the application of big data, information systems, and information technology, forming a multi-level and regional information interconnection network crisscrossed vertically and horizontally. The management department should fully utilize intelligent devices for resource management and decision making. Intelligent decision making can enable all departments to respond quickly to changes in the epidemic.

(2) Medical intelligence is the focus of ERA intelligence. Accelerating the process of intelligence in medical institutions and building intelligent buildings can help alleviate the phenomenon of medical resource tension, medical equipment congestion, and lack of medical personnel. Medical building intelligence is the introduction of Intelligent Technology and facilities and the improvement of internal organizational structure. The intelligence of medical buildings refers to the management style and the intelligence of management personnel. It is necessary to popularize the concept of competent healthcare, fully leverage the advantages of AI and logistics network technology, and improve the efficiency of medical resource utilization.

(3) The resource management department should strengthen the application of information technology in intelligent resource management, and should use information systems to simplify management processes. "Machines replace humans" can reduce the labour-cost and block infection channels to the maximum extent. Departments related to decision making should use AI and expert systems to make ERA decisions, which can improve effectiveness and reduce the risks of decision making. The government should establish a specialized supervisory agency and use information technology to monitor the ERA process in real-time. This can ensure that resources are allocated and emergency resource needs are met, it can avoid problems such as information mismatch, allocation omission, or unfair allocation of resources.

Simultaneously conducting the intelligent allocation of emergency resources for public health emergencies is needed as China possesses a high level of research and development in intelligent technology. China's vast territory and large population present both a disadvantage and an advantage when distributing emergency resources for public health emergencies. The government should integrate the capabilities of scientific research institutions, enterprises, the public, and other subjects, and should give full play to the advantages of a large country. This can help to form an intelligent system of ERA that is suitable for the conditions of China.

6.3. Boundedness and Future Works

The word frequency analysis method only considers the frequency of words appearing in the text while ignoring the semantic and contextual information of the words. Words with the same frequency may have different meanings in different contexts, and word frequency analysis cannot capture this difference. Therefore, the essential intelligent technology extracted solely through word frequency analysis technology cannot reflect the importance of this technology, and so we further obtained the evaluation index system for key intelligent technologies through the entropy weight TOPSIS method. We have obtained the importance ranking of intelligent technologies through essential technology evaluation, making the research results more comprehensive.

Based on existing research on public health emergencies, we identified essential intelligent technologies for ERA using word frequency techniques, and we ranked their importance. The importance ranking reflects the degree of attention paid by researchers to each intelligent technology in ERA, which is somewhat subjective. The importance of intelligent technologies in ERA will change as intelligent technologies are continuously updated. Therefore, the essential intelligent technologies identified in this paper only apply to the post-epidemic era and the development stage of the digital economy.

We propose an intelligent direction for ERA in public health emergencies. After empirical research, we find that medical intelligence and management intelligence are the keys to intelligence. Therefore, future works will focus on (1) the specific application of key intelligent technologies in ERA, such as the study of medical building intelligence, and (2) research on intelligent management processes, emergency resource allocation mechanisms, etc.

Most of the research data in this article comes from China. The experience of ERA adopted by China in epidemic prevention and control may have particular reference value, but its applicability depends on the specific situation. There are several factors to consider here. (1) Differences in countries and regions. Each country and region's social, economic, and healthcare systems have different characteristics. When applying China's ERA experience to other countries and regions, it is necessary to consider particular local circumstances and actual needs. (2) Types of public health emergencies. The research experience of this paper focuses on the prevention and the control of COVID-19. If faced with other types of public health emergencies, such as natural disasters, infectious diseases, etc., adjustments and adaptations must be made according to the specific situation. (3) Policy and institutional environment. China has taken strict measures and actions in epidemic prevention and control, which involve government leadership, resource allocation, social cooperation, and other aspects. The policy and institutional environment of other countries and regions may differ, so it is unsuitable to apply China's experience directly elsewhere.

Nevertheless, China's experience in epidemic prevention and control can provide some helpful guidance and inspiration. Other countries and regions can learn from China's practices. However, they must adjust and customize according to the local environment and needs. International cooperation and experience sharing can also promote countries and regions to better respond to public health emergencies.

Author Contributions: Conceptualization, methodology, and validation, R.M.; supervision and project administration, F.M.; formal analysis, H.D. All authors have read and agreed to the published version of the manuscript.

Funding: This research was funded by Harbin Engineering University Central University Basic Research Business Fund Project, grant number 3072020CFT0901.

Data Availability Statement: The data presented in this study are available on request from the corresponding author. The data are not publicly available due to the data privacy policy implemented by the organization that funded the research.

Conflicts of Interest: The authors declare no conflict of interest.

References

1. Ouyang, T.H.; Zheng, S.W.; Cheng, Y. The Construction of a Governance System for Large-scale Public Health Emergency, A Case Study Based on the Chinese Scenario. *J. Manag. World* **2020**, *36*, 19–32.
2. Chu, J.W.; Guo, C.X. Data Management Practice and Thinking on Outbreak of Major Infectious Diseases, A Case Study of COVID-19. *Inf. Stud. Theory Appl.* **2020**, *43*, 1–8.
3. Jiang, Y.S.; Li, Y.; Zhao, Y.P. Mask Dilemma and Innovation for Production and Operation Mode of Public Health Products. *Sci. Res. Manag.* **2020**, *41*, 37–46.
4. Qu, S.N.; Yang, D.H. Intelligent Response to Public Health Emergencies, Theoretical Retrospection and Trend Analysis. *Reform* **2020**, *3*, 14–21.
5. Shan, C.C.; Zhou, L.; Qin, X.K. The Status Quo and Problems with and Solutions to Chinas National Emergency Management System. *China Public Adm. Rev.* **2020**, *2*, 5–20.
6. Qu, T.J.; Gu, S.Y.; Li, M.Z.; Zhang, X.L.; Sun, M.J.; He, Z.S. Status and Challenges of Public Health Emergency Management in China. *Chin. J. Public Health Manag.* **2019**, *35*, 433–435+440.
7. Li, Z.G.; Qian, Y.Y. The Research on Improving National Modern Emergency Management System under Epidemic Situation. *Rev. Econ. Manag.* **2020**, *36*, 17–24.
8. Ge, H.L.; Liu, N. A Stochastic Programming Model for Relief Resources Allocation Problem Based on Complex Disaster Scenarios. *Syst. Eng. Theory Pract.* **2014**, *34*, 3034–3042.
9. Peng, C.; Li, J.L.; Wang, S. Multiple Relief Resources Robust Location-Routing Optimization. *Chin. J. Manag. Sci.* **2017**, *25*, 143–150.
10. Zhang, Y.L.; Chen, L. Construction of Emergency Resources Demand Scenarios for Unconventional Emergencies. *Soft Sci.* **2014**, *28*, 50–55.
11. Li, D.; Liu, X. Emergency Resources Allocation with Fair Considerations under Uncertain Demand. *Ind. Eng. Manag.* **2013**, *18*, 54–60+90.
12. Yang, F.; Ye, C.M.; Chong, D.S. Decision Model of Rescue Demand in Urban Emergency Based on Accident Evolution and Its Optimization Solution. *Oper. Res. Manag. Sci.* **2020**, *28*, 79–88.
13. Liu, G. Resource Allocation Mode Reform Based on Cyberspace (2). *Shanghai J. Econ.* **2019**, *6*, 38–48.
14. Akter, S.; Wamba, S.F. Big Data and Disaster Management, a Systematic Review and Agenda for Future Research. *Ann. Oper. Res.* **2019**, *283*, 939–959. [CrossRef]
15. Deng, Z. Promoting the Deep Integration of Artificial Intelligence and Manufacturing Industry, Difficulties and Policy Suggestions. *Econ. Rev. J.* **2018**, *8*, 41–49.
16. Sahoh, B.; Choksuriwong, A. Smart Emergency Management Based on Social Big Data Analytics, Research Trends and Future Directions. In Proceedings of the 2017 International Conference on Information Technology, Singapore, 27–29 December 2017.
17. Chen, N.; Liu, W.; Bai, R.; Chen, A. Application of Computational Intelligence Technologies in Emergency Management, a Literature Review. *Artif. Intell. Rev.* **2019**, *52*, 2131–2168. [CrossRef]
18. He, D.A.; Ren, X. The Evolution and Prospect of Resource Allocation Mechanism in the Internet Age. *Economist* **2018**, *10*, 63–71.
19. Luo, Y.M.; Liu, W.; Yue, X.G.; Rosen, M.A. Sustainable Emergency Management Based on Intelligent Information Processing. *Sustainability* **2020**, *12*, 1081. [CrossRef]

20. Chu, J.W.; Zhu, L.L. Research on the Network Public Opinion Warning of Emergencies Based on Big Data Analysis. *Inf. Stud. Theory Appl.* **2017**, *40*, 61–66.
21. Haghighi, P.D.; Burstein, F.; Zaslavsky, A.; Arbon, P. Development and Evaluation of Ontology for Intelligent Decision Support in Medical Emergency Management for Mass Gatherings. *Decis. Support Syst.* **2013**, *54*, 1192–1204. [CrossRef]
22. Sharma, G.; Lee, J.E. Role of Artificial Intelligence in Crisis and Emergency Management. *JSCM (J. Saf. Crisis Manag.)* **2019**, *9*, 1–6. [CrossRef]
23. Augusto, V.; Murgier, M.; Viallon, A. A Modelling and Simulation Framework for Intelligent Control of Emergency Units in the Case of Major Crisis. In Proceedings of the 2018 Winter Simulation Conference (WSC), Gothenburg, Sweden, 9–12 December 2018; pp. 2495–2506.
24. Oueida, S.; Aloqaily, M.; Ionescu, S. A Smart Healthcare Reward Model for Resource Allocation in Smart City. *Multimed. Tools Appl.* **2019**, *78*, 24573–24594. [CrossRef]
25. Sirisha, G.; Reddy, A.M. Smart Healthcare Analysis and Therapy for Voice Disorder using Cloud and Edge Computing. In Proceedings of the 2018 4th International Conference on Applied and Theoretical Computing and Communication Technology (iCATccT), Mangalore, India, 6–8 September 2018; pp. 103–106.
26. Wang, Q.L.; Wang, Z.; Qu, Q. The Construction of New National Public Health Information System, Reflections on Improving the System Resilience. *Reform* **2020**, *4*, 17–27.
27. Shen, H.; Liu, Z.M. Intelligent Management of Data Source in Disaster Medical Emergency Rescue. *J. Tongji Univ. (Med. Sci.)* **2018**, *39*, 1–4.
28. Zeng, Z.M.; Huang, C.Y. Research on the Intelligence System of Public Health Emergencies with an Epidemic Control Orientation. *J. Intell.* **2017**, *36*, 79–84.
29. Liu, J.; Li, L. Analysis of Intelligent Early Warning Mechanism of Network Public Opinion in the Background of Big Data. *J. Intell.* **2019**, *38*, 92–97+183.
30. Zhu, X.; Zhang, G.; Sun, B. A Comprehensive Literature Review of the Demand Forecasting Methods of Emergency Resources from the Perspective of Artificial Intelligence. *Nat. Hazards* **2019**, *97*, 65–82. [CrossRef]
31. Abdel-Basset, M.; Manogaran, G.; Gamal, A.; Chang, V. A Novel Intelligent Medical Decision Support Model Based on Soft Computing and IoT. *IEEE Internet Things J.* **2019**, *7*, 4160–4170. [CrossRef]
32. Chang, D.; Gui, H.Y.; Fan, R. Situational Evolution and Simulation Research of Social Security Emergency in Megacities, Taking Beijing as an Example. *J. Beijing Jiaotong Univ. (Soc. Sci. Ed.)* **2020**, *19*, 86–97.
33. Tian, S.H.; Sun, M.Q.; Zhang, J.Y. Evolution Model of Website Public Opinion in Emergency Based on Generalized Stochastic Petri Nets. *Inf. Sci.* **2018**, *36*, 106–111.
34. Wang, Y.J.; Tang, X.B.; Chen, X.H. Development Opportunities and Strategies for the Digital Economy Industry in China under the Influence of New Coronavirus Pneumonia. *Sci. Res. Manag.* **2020**, *41*, 157–171.
35. Du, L. Research on Key Technologies of Regional Synergy Emergency System Based on Medical Data Center. *Procedia Comput. Sci.* **2019**, *154*, 732–737. [CrossRef]
36. Chen, S.; Chen, Y.Q.; Cheng, S.W.; Luo, Z.Q.; Zhang, W.; Cao, Z.L.; Wang, J.Z.; Lv, C.Z. An Overview of the Construction of Emergency and Pre-hospital First Aid Platform. *J. Acute Dis.* **2018**, *7*, 1–4.
37. Liu, Q.Y.; Ye, Y. A Study on Mining Bibliographic Records by Designed Software SATI, Case Study on Library and Information Science. *J. Inf. Resour. Manag.* **2012**, *1*, 50–55.
38. Liu, S.F.; Jian, L.R. Research on the Index System for Evaluating Key Technologies in Regional International Cooperation. *Sci. Technol. Prog. Policy* **2009**, *26*, 126–129.
39. Wang, S.; Zhu, G.L. Research on Tracking and Evaluating the Benefits of National Key Technologies. *Sci. Res. Manag.* **1998**, *4*, 3–5.
40. Weiss, B.A.; Schmidt, L.C. The multi-relationship evaluation design framework: Creating evaluation blueprints to assess advanced and intelligent technologies. In *Proceedings of the 10th Performance Metrics for Intelligent Systems Workshop*; Association for Computing Machinery: New York, NY, USA, 2010; pp. 136–145.
41. Budarin, S.S.; Boichenko, I.I.; Nikonov, E.L.; Elbek, I.V. The planning of values of indices of quality of resource management in medical organizations of the Moscow state medical care system. *Probl. Sotsial'noi Gig. Zdr. I Istor. Meditsiny* **2019**, *27*, 303–307.
42. Chu, J.F.; Li, X.X.; Zhe, Y. Emergency medical resource allocation among hospitals with non-regressive production technology: A DEA-based approach. *Comput. Ind. Eng.* **2022**, *171*, 108491. [CrossRef]
43. Wang, F.Y.; Xie, Z.; Liu, H.; Pei, Z.; Liu, D. Multiobjective emergency resource allocation under the natural disaster chain with path planning. *Int. J. Environ. Res. Public Health* **2022**, *19*, 7876. [CrossRef]
44. Meng, Q. A Study on the Urban Emergency Management System Based on the Internet of Things. In *Proceedings of the Thirteenth International Conference on Management Science and Engineering Management*; Springer International Publishing: Cham, Switzerland, 2020; Volume 1, pp. 645–655.
45. Wang, L. Research on distributed emergency resource scheduling system based on Internet of Things. In Proceedings of the 2016 Chinese Control and Decision Conference (CCDC), Yinchuan, China, 28–30 May 2016; pp. 3707–3711.
46. Sun, F.Q.; Yu, X.; Liu, S.; Lu, F. Urban emergency intelligent decision system in rough set on two universes. In Proceedings of the 26th Chinese Control and Decision Conference (2014 CCDC), Changsha, China, 31 May–2 June 2014; pp. 4904–4907.

47. Yin, S.; Zhang, N.; Xu, J.F. Information fusion for future COVID-19 prevention: Continuous mechanism of big data intelligent innovation for the emergency management of a public epidemic outbreak. *J. Manag. Anal.* **2021**, *8*, 391–423. [CrossRef]
48. Jia, D.; Wu, Z.Y. Intelligent evaluation system of government emergency management based on BP neural network. *IEEE Access* **2020**, *8*, 199646–199653. [CrossRef] [PubMed]

Disclaimer/Publisher's Note: The statements, opinions and data contained in all publications are solely those of the individual author(s) and contributor(s) and not of MDPI and/or the editor(s). MDPI and/or the editor(s) disclaim responsibility for any injury to people or property resulting from any ideas, methods, instructions or products referred to in the content.

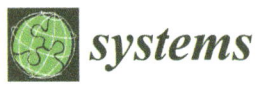 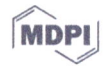

Article

Strategies to Prevent Suicide and Attempted Suicide in New South Wales (Australia): Community-Based Outreach, Alternatives to Emergency Department Care, and Early Intervention

Eileen Goldberg [1], Cindy Peng [1,*], Andrew Page [2], Piumee Bandara [2] and Danielle Currie [1]

[1] The Sax Institute, Glebe, NSW 2037, Australia; eileen.goldberg@saxinstitute.org.au (E.G.); danielle.currie@saxinstitute.org.au (D.C.)
[2] Translational Health Research Institute, Western Sydney University, Penrith, NSW 2571, Australia; a.page@westernsydney.edu.au (A.P.); bandarap@who.int (P.B.)
* Correspondence: cindy.peng@saxinstitute.org.au; Tel.: +61-02-9188-9500

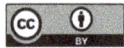

Citation: Goldberg, E.; Peng, C.; Page, A.; Bandara, P.; Currie, D. Strategies to Prevent Suicide and Attempted Suicide in New South Wales (Australia): Community-Based Outreach, Alternatives to Emergency Department Care, and Early Intervention. *Systems* 2023, *11*, 275. https://doi.org/10.3390/systems11060275

Academic Editor: Wayne Wakeland

Received: 24 April 2023
Revised: 19 May 2023
Accepted: 26 May 2023
Published: 31 May 2023

Copyright: © 2023 by the authors. Licensee MDPI, Basel, Switzerland. This article is an open access article distributed under the terms and conditions of the Creative Commons Attribution (CC BY) license (https://creativecommons.org/licenses/by/4.0/).

Abstract: Background: This study describes the development of a system dynamics model to project the potential impact of a series of proposed suicide prevention interventions in New South Wales (NSW, Australia) over the period 2016 to 2031. Methods: A system dynamics model for the NSW population aged ≥ 20 years which represented the current incidence of suicide and attempted suicide in NSW was developed in partnership with a consortium of stakeholders, subject matter experts, and consumers with lived experience. Scenarios relating to current suicide prevention initiatives were investigated to identify the combination of interventions associated with the largest reductions in the projected number of attempted suicide and suicide cases for a 5-year follow-up period (2019–2023). Results: The largest proportion of cases averted for both suicide and attempted suicide over the intervention period was associated with community-based suicide prevention outreach teams and peer-led drop-in facilities (6.8% for attempted suicide, 6.4% for suicide). A similar proportion of potential cases averted of both attempted suicide and suicide (6.4%) was evident for targeted interventions focusing only on those in the population with suicidal thoughts and a previous history of attempted suicide. Conclusion: Initiatives that are characterised by the short-term stabilisation of suicidal distress at the point of crisis, averting the need for a hospital encounter, and the referral of individuals to non-acute community-based care were associated with the largest potential reductions in suicidal behaviour in NSW.

Keywords: suicide prevention; suicide; self-harm; systems modelling; simulation

1. Introduction

Suicide and self-harm are major public health issues worldwide. Suicide is the leading cause of death among Australians aged 15–44 years. In 2019, over 3318 people died by suicide in Australia, 29% of which were from New South Wales (NSW), Australia's most populous state [1,2]. Despite consistent efforts to reduce suicide in Australia, the suicide rate has remained relatively stable over the last two decades, with evidence of a recent increase [3].

Within Australia, there has been growing attention to and investment in suicide prevention. The Prime Minister's National Suicide Prevention Advisor has led a new focus on a whole-of-government approach for suicide prevention to comprehensively address the social, economic, health, cultural, and environmental factors contributing to suicide risk in the population [4]. Within NSW, targeted suicide prevention investments have been made in order to reach the goal of a 20 per cent reduction in the rate of suicide [5]. As part of this initiative, vulnerable populations including rural communities and those who have previously self-harmed and/or are in suicidal crisis have been identified as priority populations for intervention.

Suicide prevention strategies for priority populations are typically classified as selective interventions or indicated interventions. Selective interventions are directed towards individuals who are at greater risk for suicidal behaviour and may include training frontline workers and gatekeepers for the early detection of suicide risk or tailored psychosocial or peer support [6]. Indicated interventions are targeted towards individuals who are already displaying signs of suicidal behaviour. These interventions are more timely and assertive in managing suicide risk through active follow-up, often referred to as "aftercare" following a suicide attempt. Aftercare typically includes case management, referral to psychiatric treatment, psychosocial support, and skill-building exercises [6].

Evidence for selective and indicated interventions is still emerging. Existing data suggest that psychosocial treatment and management and aftercare interventions are effective in reducing suicidal behaviour [7–9]. There is also a growing body of evidence showing that gatekeeper training could prevent suicides [8,10]. More recently, peer support groups led by people with lived experience have also emerged as an alternative non-clinical strategy for suicide prevention; however, evidence to date on their effectiveness is limited [11]. Collectively, a "systems approach" to suicide prevention, one that delivers a combination of evidence-based interventions simultaneously, spanning the spectrum of prevention, is recognised internationally as having the best chance to reduce population suicide rates [12,13]. However, measuring the impact of multiple interventions over time and in varying contexts presents a challenge, and identifying which interventions have the most impact is also difficult.

System dynamics modelling has recently emerged as one means of addressing the complexities of evaluating multi-component public health interventions, particularly with respect to suicide prevention [14,15], and it provides policymakers with decision support tools to consider the likely impacts of interventions within complex social and health systems. Using the best available evidence, system dynamics modelling allows for an assessment of the potential impacts of different interventions at a population level, and for the identification of those interventions likely to have the greatest impact in reducing suicidal behaviour [15]. Unlike traditional analytic approaches that are typically static and independent, systems modelling can identify drivers of population-level outcomes, including changes in service interactions, workforce capacity, and the combined effects of multiple interventions [14].

Accordingly, using population-based data for NSW, we developed a system dynamics model to project the impact of a series of suicide prevention interventions on suicidal behaviour in NSW in order to assist policy decision making. Specifically, the objectives of this study were to: (1) identify suicide prevention activities likely to deliver the greatest reductions in self-harm hospitalisations and suicide deaths for NSW and (2) identify system-level factors driving population-level changes in suicide and self-harm outcomes following the implementation of suicide prevention interventions.

2. Methods

2.1. Study Context

New South Wales is the most populous state in Australia, with a population of 8,072,163 according to the 2021 Census, and represents approximately one third of the Australian population [16]. In 2017, the age-standardised rate of suicide in NSW was 10.6 per 100,000, and 76.8 per 100,000 for hospital-treated self-harm [17]. These rates are below national rates, which, in 2021, were 12.0 per 100,000 for suicide and 116.3 per 100,000 for hospital-treated self-harm [17]. Targeted suicide prevention investments have been made in NSW [5,18], and the current study focuses on a selection of these initiatives and related investments, as outlined in detail below.

2.2. Model Development

A participatory approach was adopted to develop the dynamic simulation model iteratively in partnership with NSW Health and in collaboration with a consortium of stakeholders with knowledge of or experience with suicide and/or suicide prevention in the local context. The consortium consisted of government and non-government health service providers, health policy agencies, academics, and consumers with lived experience. A core team with expertise in dynamic modelling, systems thinking, and research facilitated and provided oversight of model development. This process was informed by published research, administrative data, two participatory online workshops, out-of-session stakeholder consultations, and two demonstration forums held between October 2020 and June 2021.

Two online workshops were held via Zoom using Group Model Building techniques [19–22] adapted for the online environment with the use of a cloud-based visual collaboration platform (https://miro.com/ accessed on 25 September 2020). The first workshop (held over two days in October 2020) introduced the consortium of stakeholders to system dynamics modelling methodology and included the conceptual mapping of and collaborative discussion on the population-level factors contributing to the increasing rate of suicide over time. The stages of the lived experience of suicide were identified and mapped, noting critical points of potential intervention in preventing suicidal thinking and suicide attempt and re-attempt. Stakeholders mapped key existing suicide and mental health services and support pathways available in NSW and factors influencing the flow of the population along these pathways, and considered gaps and limitations in the system.

The second online workshop (held over two days in February 2021) focused on participants' feedback on the model structures included in a first draft of the conceptual model, and they hypothesised effects of the selected suicide prevention initiatives in the system (Table 1, and as described below). A conceptual diagram based on these participatory mapping exercises and discussions undertaken by the consortium of stakeholders was subsequently developed (Supplementary Figure S1), with model sub-sectors relating to "Stages of Suicidal Behaviour" (Supplementary Figure S2a), "Non-acute Community Support" (Supplementary Figure S2b), and "Crisis and Acute Care" (Supplementary Figure S2c).

Table 1. Suicide prevention interventions included in the system dynamics model.

Intervention	Description
Early identification and intervention	
Community-based suicide prevention outreach teams	A service provided in a community-based setting using clinical and non-clinical models of care. Mobile teams made accessible to people in suicidal crisis who would not usually contact mental health services for help. The primary purpose is the stabilisation of individuals experiencing suicidal crisis and provision of onward referral to suicide-specific community-based care.
Peer-led drop-in facilities	Peer-led drop-in facilities based in the community in proximity to emergency departments to provide a non-clinical alternative to presenting to an emergency department for people experiencing suicidal crisis. The facilities to be staffed by peer workers with lived experience of suicide and/or self-harm and supported by mental health clinicians. The service to include crisis risk assessment/screening, psychosocial support, and safety planning for suicidal behaviours to aid de-escalation and recovery.
Gatekeeper training	Provision of evidence-based suicide prevention training in the NSW community to increase the number of key community members with the skills and confidence to safely speak with and support individuals at increased risk of suicidal ideation and behaviour.
Post-attempt indicated intervention	
Post-suicide attempt aftercare support	Immediate and assertive follow-up with individuals discharged from hospital to increase access to and engagement with community-based treatment services to prevent repetition of suicidal behaviour. To include the provision of safety planning, non-clinical psychosocial support and encouragement to adhere to treatment, and problem-solving counselling with links to practical support including housing, finances, relationships. The average duration of support is assumed to be 3 months post-discharge.

Table 1. Cont.

Intervention	Description
Peer support groups	Provision of appropriate peer-facilitated support for people experiencing suicidal ideation and/or for people who have attempted suicide. Encourages empathetic talking about suicide combined with exploring alternative coping strategies, facilitated by people with lived experience of suicide.
Selective mental health intervention	
Expansion of clinical counselling workforce in rural communities	Expansion of clinical counselling workforce in rural and remote NSW that would provide wider access to appropriate psychological and emotional support for people at high risk of suicidality (suicidal thoughts and behaviours) in regional areas.

2.3. Model Structure

The construction, quantification, calibration, and validation of the computational model (main structure in Figure 1; see Supplementary Materials for further detail) was undertaken using standard approaches for system dynamics models [19,23–27], and developed using Stella Architect® software (version 2.1.1) (www.iseesystems.com/ accessed on 27 November 2020). The system dynamics model was initialised using 2016 local administrative data and model time units are in years, and projects to 2031.

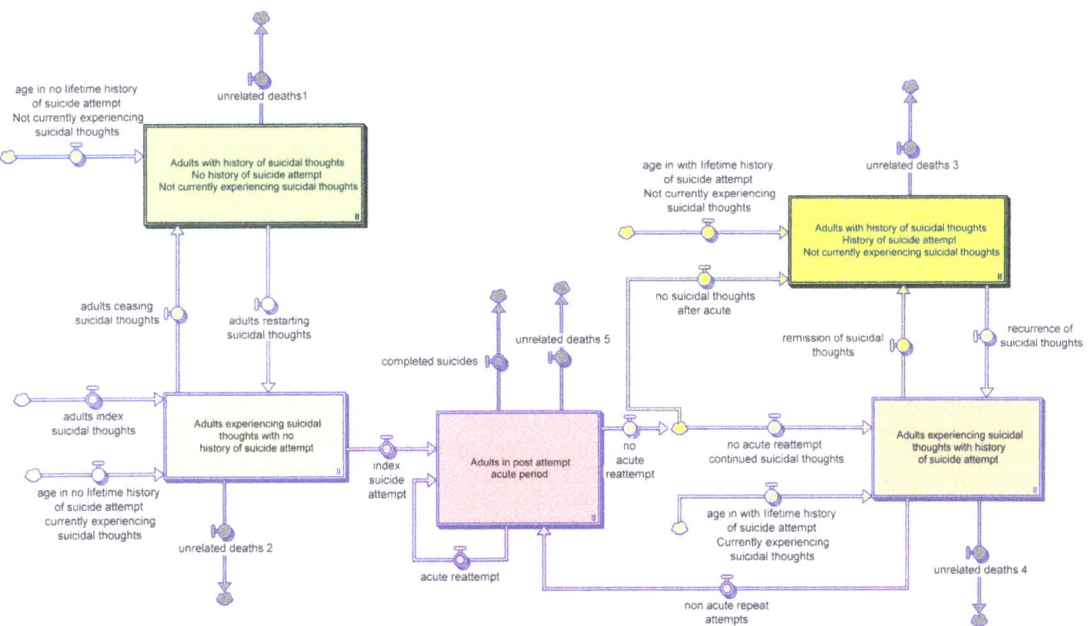

Figure 1. Main model structure representing stages of suicidal thoughts and behaviour.

The model consists of the following interacting components: (a) population dynamics; (b) stages of suicidal thoughts and behaviour (including incidence of suicidal thoughts, suicidal crisis, suicide attempt, and suicide); (c) crisis and acute care (including occurrences of acute formal stabilisation and/or social support); (d) non-acute community support and service access (including occurrences of non-acute community-based care and service access); (e) non-acute community support and service effects (relating to the probability of transition to remission from suicidal thoughts, given service access and ability of service to meet consumer's perceived needs); and (f) initiatives and scenarios (further detail on each of the core components is provided in Supplementary Materials).

Parameter values for the model were informed by published research, local administrative data, and expert consensus (Supplementary Table S1). The model is based on the population of NSW aged $\geq$ 20-years, and the model validity was tested by comparing outputs from 2016 to 2021 with trends in routinely reported suicide deaths and hospital presentations for suicide attempt/non-fatal suicide behaviour in NSW (obtained from the NSW Suicide Monitoring System death data, NSW Combined Admitted Patient Epidemiology Data, and ABS population estimates).

The model also allowed for time to scale up to achieve targets for intervention uptake and population reach. Due to the limited evidence base for some of the proposed intervention activities, services, and programmes, the model incorporated the ability to change intervention parameters to reflect new evidence on the effectiveness of specific interventions in the future. Thus, the final model allows for "what-if" analyses of the potential impact of combinations of key suicide prevention interventions to inform priority areas for future investment and public health programmes.

2.4. Suicide Prevention Interventions Modelled

Six identified interventions were included in the model (Table 1). These interventions were: (i) post-suicide attempt aftercare support, (ii) gatekeeper training, (iii) peer-led drop-in facilities, (iv) expansion of clinical counselling workforce in rural communities, (v) community-based suicide-prevention outreach teams, and (vi) broader enhancements in peer support and peer-led initiatives. Interventions were identified on the basis of current policy priorities identified by stakeholders during the participatory design phase of the model, and related to suicide prevention initiatives that are currently being implemented as part of the "Towards Zero Suicide" initiatives [18] and other population-based multi-component interventions, such as the Lifespan initiative [28] and the National Suicide Prevention Trial [29,30]. All interventions were simulated for the period of calendar year 2019 to 2023 (inclusive), in line with an evaluation time frame of the NSW Towards Zero Suicides Initiative [18], and then onto 2031. Effects of interventions were assessed as differences between outcomes from simulated scenarios (i.e., one initiative or combinations of initiatives were run) and a "business as usual" comparator. Descriptions, default values, and assumptions for the base-case are further detailed in the Supplementary Materials.

3. Results

3.1. Baseline Estimates of Suicide and Attempted Suicide

Between 2019 and 2023, under a "business-as-usual" baseline scenario, the model projected that the number of people in NSW who attempted suicide was expected to increase by 13% to approximately 32,300 over the 5-year period, and it projected the number of people who died by suicide to increase by 11%, to approximately 930 persons per annum. Over the same time period, the model projected an 11.8% increase in annual suicide-related hospital encounters, and a 10.6% increase in the annual number of people engaged in community-based care due to suicidality. The projections for suicide equate to a projected age-standardised rate of 12.1 per 100,000 people for suicide-related deaths in NSW at the end of 2023. At the same rate over 10 years, 2019–2030, the model projected that the cumulative number of suicide-related deaths would be 11,520, a 29% increase in annual suicide attempts, and 25% increase in annual suicide-related deaths.

3.2. Impact of Targeted Interventions

The potential impact of early and indicated interventions suggested that 6.3% of cases of attempted suicide and 6.8% of cases of suicide could be averted (Table 2). The largest potential contributions of individual interventions were for community-based suicide prevention outreach teams and peer-leddrop-in facilities, for both attempted suicide and suicide (Table 2). A similar number of potential cases averted for both attempted suicide and suicide (6.4%) was evident for targeted interventions focusing on only those in the population with suicidal thoughts and a previous history of attempted suicide (Table 2, Figures 2 and 3).

Table 2. Modelled cumulative cases of averted suicide and attempted suicide from 2019 to 2023.

	Suicide Attempts			Suicides		
	Cumulative Cases	Cases Averted	% Reduction	Cumulative Cases	Cases Averted	% Reduction
Early identification and intervention						
Base run	148,831			4354		
Suicide prevention outreach teams	144,960	3871	2.6	4230	124	2.8
Peer-led drop-in facilities	144,344	4488	3.0	4212	142	3.3
Gatekeeper training	148,530	301	0.2	4348	6	0.1
Post-attempt indicated interventions						
Expanding aftercare	148,462	370	0.2	4346	8	0.2
Expanding peer support	148,249	582	0.4	4338	16	0.4
Expanding rural counsellors	148,196	636	0.4	4337	17	0.4
Aftercare and expanding rural counsellors	148,103	729	0.5	4332	22	0.5
Early and indicated interventions combined	139,504	9327	6.3	4059	295	6.8
Targeted interventions for people with suicidal thoughts (a)						
No history of suicide attempts (b)	145,539	3293	2.2	4268	86	2.0
No history of suicide attempts (c)	147,790	1041	0.7	4310	44	1.0
Previous suicide attempt (last 12 months)	141,148	7683	5.2	4096	258	5.9
Previous suicide attempt	139,273	9558	6.4	4077	277	6.4

(a) Targeting people with suicidal thoughts with suicide prevention outreach and peer-led drop-in facilities. (b) For index year of suicidal thoughts. (c) For non-index year of suicidal thoughts.

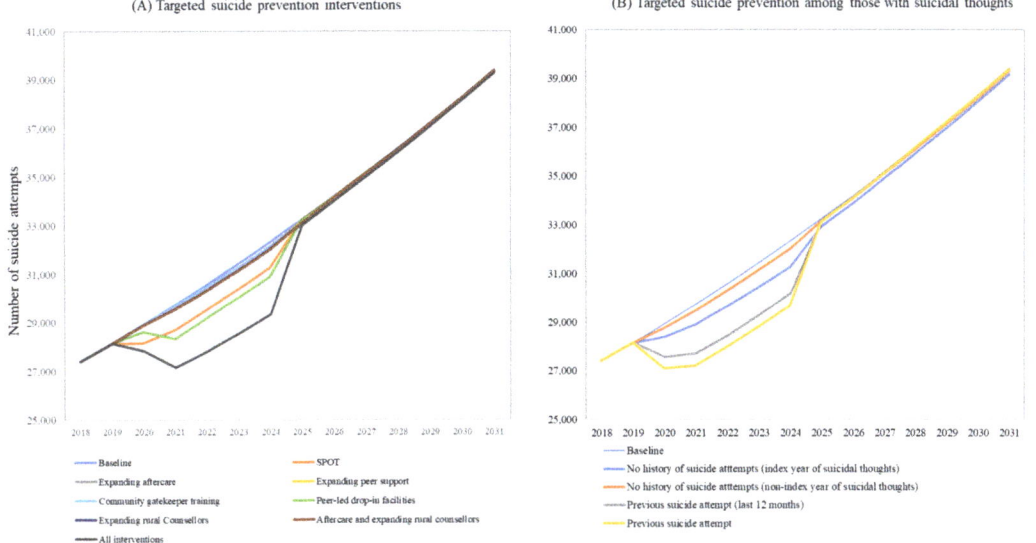

Figure 2. Modelled impact of targeted suicide prevention interventions on NSW suicide attempts (2019–2023) for (**A**) the general population, and (**B**) those with suicidal thoughts. See Table 1 for description of suicide prevention interventions included in this figure.

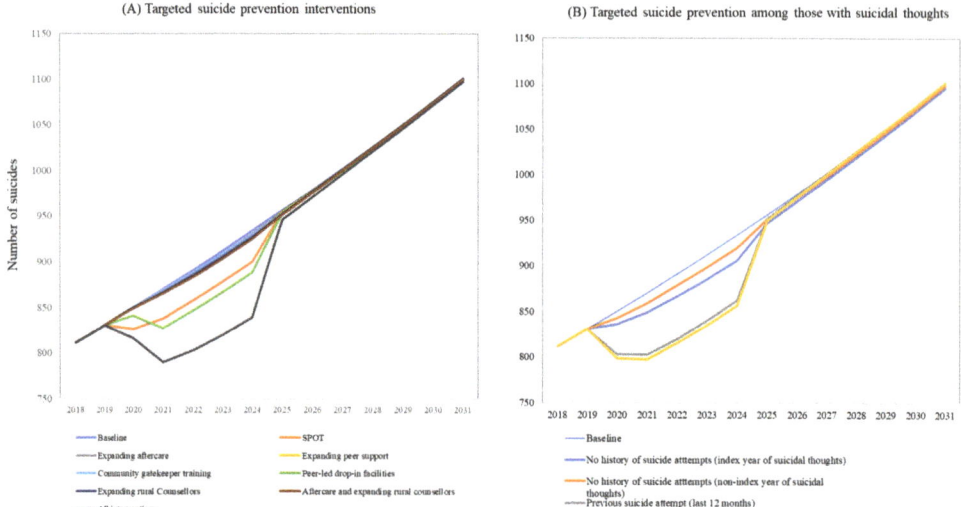

Figure 3. Modelled impact of targeted suicide prevention interventions on NSW suicide (2019–2023) for (**A**) the general population, and (**B**) those with suicidal thoughts. See Table 1 for description of suicide prevention interventions included in this figure.

If a target of a 20% reduction in suicide-related deaths is used for the NSW population aged $\geq$ 20 years, then the model projects that these initiatives would contribute 48% toward this reduction (an equivalent rate per 100,000 of 12.7 by 2023). In combination, these two interventions would also divert approximately 8.7% of individuals away from hospital encounters, and an additional 1.3% of individuals would be referred to non-acute community-based care (compared to the business-as-usual scenario over the five-year period).

4. Discussion

This study describes the co-design, development, and application of a system dynamics model that aims to inform the optimal combination of suicide prevention activity in New South Wales (Australia). Of the range of initiatives included in the model, the two initiatives projected to be the most effective at preventing suicide-related deaths and suicide attempts were community-based suicide prevention outreach teams and peer-led drop-in facilities. Community-based outreach was estimated to avert 2.6% of attempted suicides and 2.8% of suicides over the 5-year projection period. Peer-led drop-in facilities were estimated to avert 3.0% of attempted suicides and 3.3% of suicides over the 5-year projection period. Both these types of initiatives are characterised by the short-term stabilisation of suicidal distress at the point of crisis, averting the need for a hospital encounter and the referral of individuals to non-acute community-based care. The combined potential effect of all early and indicated interventions was estimated to avert ~6% of attempted suicides and ~7% of suicides over the intervention period.

Importantly, model findings also suggest that while greater short-term reductions in suicide-related deaths were demonstrated when interventions target individuals at high risk of experiencing a suicide re-attempt (i.e., post-suicide aftercare support), this will be at the expense of potential longer-term reductions in suicide that could be achieved by targeting interventions towards individuals who have yet to experience a suicide attempt, particularly those in the index year of experiencing suicidal thoughts. The implication of this finding is that modifying intermediary risk factors associated with subsequent suicidal behaviour (psychological distress, mental disorder, and social and economic stressors) among those in the general community may be an additional strategy for early intervention to prevent hospital-treated self-harm and suicide.

There are a number of limitations for consideration when interpreting the findings of this paper. Firstly, the system dynamics model described in the current study models populations in aggregate and is limited in providing insights into individual-level impacts, or for specific population subgroups. The model captures population and behavioural dynamics that impact mental health service capacity, and the uptake and scaling of suicide prevention activity. However, agent-based models are better placed to capture complex individual-level behaviours and sociodemographic characteristics [31]. A system dynamics modelling approach is perhaps more appropriate in the current context, given the need for policymakers to understand the likely population-level impacts of proposed interventions to prevent suicide, and the need for timely insights for responsive decision making.

Secondly, there is potential measurement bias in the secondary data used to parameterise the model, and the extent to which estimates identified from the literature, or sourced from other populations, may be generalisable to the NSW context. Population-based data relating to mental health services (such as hospitalisations, workforce information, and service capacity), population-level psychological distress, and suicidal behaviour (suicide and hospital-treated intentional self-harm) were based on routinely collected datasets. It is acknowledged that there is potential under-enumeration of suicide and attempted suicide, due to misclassification (for events of "undetermined intent"), and attempted suicides represent only those cases that present to services (and not the total population burden associated with suicidal behaviour). Some estimates for parameters were not available from secondary datasets, and in these instances, a combination of estimation and stakeholder consensus was used to establish parameter values. Additionally, the model interface incorporated a series of "sliders" for a selection of parameters to allow for stakeholders to investigate the impact of alternative assumptions for parameters on the model projections of suicide and attempted suicide.

Thirdly, the model considered a limited set of interventions and scenarios. Selected interventions were based on stakeholder priorities in the context of current prominent suicide prevention initiatives such as the NSW Health Towards Zero Suicide initiatives [18], and related initiatives relating to population-level multi-component interventions [28–30]. Other potentially relevant interventions, for example, relating to social determinants associated with suicidal behaviour [32] and the provision of psychosocial or economic interventions to modify intermediary risk factors [33], may also be important for consideration. Alternative scenarios and combinations of interventions may result in a different set of findings.

Fourthly, the model was developed for the NSW population, which may affect the generalisability of the findings. However, while the model was developed for a specific population, the insights are based upon generically framed suicide prevention initiatives that are not based on a specific prescribed approach to design, implementation, and resourcing. The findings are likely applicable to other high-income country contexts with a similar epidemiology of suicide, and where there are coordinated aftercare strategies that are planned for those at suicidal risk in publicly funded health systems that provide (nominally) universal healthcare.

A key strength of the modelling approach in the current study was the quantitative approach to capture the complexity of suicidal behaviour and the mental health system, in combination with the participatory approach that involved stakeholders and subject matter experts in mapping the underlying structure of the system, and in the critical appraisal of model inputs. This is distinct from the more qualitative, non-evidence-based approaches that can sometimes be associated with the prioritisation of suicide prevention policies and interventions.

This study suggests that the combination of community-based suicide prevention outreach teams and peer-led drop-in facilities was associated with the greatest potential reductions in both suicides and attempted suicides over the selected 5-year intervention period. However, model findings also suggest that while short-term reductions in suicide can be achieved by focusing on individuals at high risk of experiencing a suicide re-attempt (that is, via aftercare support services), this will be at the expense of potential longer-term reductions in suicide that could be achieved by targeting interventions towards individuals who have yet to experience a suicide attempt. These findings emphasise the immediate and longer-term benefits of targeting early intervention among individuals who may be experiencing psychological distress in the general community, as well as those at higher risk, in order to achieve the greatest reductions in suicides and attempted suicides and optimise mental health services for the NSW population.

Supplementary Materials: The following supporting information can be downloaded at: https://www.mdpi.com/article/10.3390/systems11060275/s1, Figure S1: Conceptual model of the stages of suicidal behaviour; Figure S2: Refined conceptual diagram of proposed model sectors; Description of system dynamics model components available with Figures S3–S7; Figure S3: Population Dynamics Sector; Figure S4: Stages of suicidal behaviour sector; Figure S5: Crisis and acute care sector; Figure S6: Non-acute community support sector; Figure S7: Non-acute community support and service effect sector; Table S1: Numerical Input and Data Sources.

Author Contributions: Conceptualization, E.G., C.P., A.P., P.B. and D.C.; methodology, D.C.; validation, D.C.; formal analysis, C.P., A.P. and D.C.; writing—original draft preparation, E.G. and P.B.; writing—review and editing, E.G., C.P., A.P., P.B. and D.C.; project administration, C.P. and E.G. All authors have read and agreed to the published version of the manuscript.

Funding: Health Administration Corporation for and on behalf of NSW Health; The Australian Prevention Partnership Centre.

Data Availability Statement: The data presented in this study are available on request from the corresponding author.

Acknowledgments: We would like to acknowledge the contribution of Shallu Sharma, Decision Analytics, Sax Institute, who provided inputs into the system dynamics model. We also acknowledge and thank the broader modelling consortium stakeholder group members for providing their perspectives and expertise to the core model-building team to inform the design of the system dynamics model. This project is an excellent example of a successful collaboration between the Sax Institute, NSW Health, and other not-for-profit and research organisations working to improve the lives of individuals, families, and communities impacted by suicide in NSW and Australia.

Conflicts of Interest: The authors declare no conflict of interest that are relevant to the content of this article. This research is based on a system dynamics model developed as part of work commissioned by the Health Administration Corporation for and on behalf of NSW Health undertaken by the Sax Institute. The NSW Ministry of Health specified the scope and objectives of the model, and the model structure was developed by Dr Danielle Currie, Senior Systems Dynamic Modeller, Sax Institute, on the basis of inputs and content expertise as part of a participatory-design model-building process facilitated by the Sax Institute. The funder had no role in the collection, analyses, or interpretation of data reported in this manuscript, in the writing of the manuscript, or in the decision to publish the results.

References

1. Australian Bureau of Statistics. Causes of Death. Australian Bureau of Statistics. 2020. Available online: https://www.abs.gov.au/statistics/health/causes-death/causes-death-australia/2019#intentional-self-harm-suicides-key-characteristics (accessed on 25 May 2023).
2. NSW Health. NSW Suicide Monitoring System—Report 1 October 2020: NSW Health. 2020. Available online: https://www.health.nsw.gov.au/towardszerosuicides/Pages/suicide-monitoring-system.aspx (accessed on 25 May 2023).
3. Jorm, A.F. Lack of impact of past efforts to prevent suicide in Australia: Please explain. *Aust. N. Z. J. Psychiatry* **2019**, *53*, 379–380. [CrossRef] [PubMed]
4. Australian Government Department of Health. National Suicide Prevention Adviser—Final Advice. 2020. Available online: https://www.health.gov.au/resources/publications/national-suicide-prevention-adviser-final-advice (accessed on 25 May 2023).
5. NSW Health. Strategic Framework for Suicide Prevention in NSW 2018–2023—Implementation Plan NSW Health. 2020. Available online: https://www.health.nsw.gov.au/mentalhealth/resources/Pages/strategic-framework-implementation-plan.aspx (accessed on 25 May 2023).

6. Wasserman, D.; Iosue, M.; Wuestefeld, A.; Carli, V. Adaptation of evidence-based suicide prevention strategies during and after the COVID-19 pandemic. *World Psychiatry* **2020**, *19*, 294–306. [CrossRef] [PubMed]
7. Hawton, K.; Witt, K.G.; Salisbury, T.L.T.; Arensman, E.; Gunnell, D.; Hazell, P.; Townsend, E.; van Heeringen, K. Psychosocial interventions following self-harm in adults: A systematic review and meta-analysis. *Lancet Psychiatry* **2016**, *3*, 740–750. [CrossRef]
8. Mann, J.J.; Michel, C.A.; Auerbach, R.P. Improving suicide prevention through evidence-based strategies: A systematic review. *Am. J. Psychiatry* **2021**, *178*, 611–624. [CrossRef] [PubMed]
9. Zalsman, G.; Hawton, K.; Wasserman, D.; van Heeringen, K.; Arensman, E.; Sarchiapone, M.; Carli, V.; Höschl, C.; Barzilay, R.; Balazs, J.; et al. Suicide prevention strategies revisited: 10-year systematic review. *Lancet Psychiatry* **2016**, *3*, 646–659. [CrossRef] [PubMed]
10. Isaac, M.; Elias, B.; Katz, L.Y.; Belik, S.-L.; Deane, F.P.; Enns, M.W.; Sareen, J. Gatekeeper training as a preventative intervention for suicide: A systematic review. *Can. J. Psychiatry* **2009**, *54*, 260–268. [CrossRef] [PubMed]
11. Schlichthorst, M.; Ozols, I.; Reifels, L.; Morgan, A. Lived experience peer support programs for suicide prevention: A systematic scoping review. *Int. J. Ment. Health Syst.* **2020**, *14*, 65. [CrossRef]
12. Baker, S.T.; Nicholas, J.; Shand, F.; Green, R.; Christensen, H. A comparison of multi-component systems approaches to suicide prevention. *Australas. Psychiatry* **2018**, *26*, 128–131. [CrossRef]
13. Krysinska, K.; Batterham, P.J.; Tye, M.; Shand, F.; Calear, A.L.; Cockayne, N.; Christensen, H. Best strategies for reducing the suicide rate in Australia. *Aust. N. Z. J. Psychiatry* **2016**, *50*, 115–118. [CrossRef]
14. Atkinson, J.-A.; Skinner, A.; Hackney, S.; Mason, L.; Heffernan, M.; Currier, D.; King, K.; Pirkis, J. Systems modelling and simulation to inform strategic decision making for suicide prevention in rural New South Wales (Australia). *Aust. N. Z. J. Psychiatry* **2020**, *54*, 892–901. [CrossRef]
15. Page, A.; Atkinson, J.-A.; Campos, W.; Heffernan, M.; Ferdousi, S.; Power, A.; McDonnell, G.; Maranan, N.; Hickie, I. A decision support tool to inform local suicide prevention activity in Greater Western Sydney (Australia). *Aust. N. Z. J. Psychiatry* **2018**, *52*, 983–993. [CrossRef] [PubMed]
16. Australian Bureau of Statistics. Population: Census. 2021. Available online: https://www.abs.gov.au/statistics/people/population/population-census/latest-release (accessed on 25 May 2023).
17. Australian Institute of Health and Welfare. Suicide and Self-Harm Monitoring. 2022. Available online: https://www.aihw.gov.au/suicide-self-harm-monitoring/data/suicide-self-harm-monitoring-data (accessed on 25 May 2023).
18. NSW Health. Towards Zero Suicide Initiatives. NSW Health. 2022. Available online: https://www.health.nsw.gov.au/towardszerosuicides/Pages/initiatives.aspx (accessed on 25 May 2023).
19. Hovmand, P.S.; Hovmand, P.S. *Group Model Building and Community-Based System Dynamics Process*; Springer: Berlin/Heidelberg, Germany, 2014.
20. Rouwette, E.A.; Korzilius, H.; Vennix, J.A.; Jacobs, E. Modeling as persuasion: The impact of group model building on attitudes and behavior. *Syst. Dyn. Rev.* **2011**, *27*, 1–21. [CrossRef]
21. Seidl, R. A functional-dynamic reflection on participatory processes in modeling projects. *AMBIO* **2015**, *44*, 750–765. [CrossRef] [PubMed]
22. Ulrich, W. Operational research and critical systems thinking—An integrated perspective: Part 1: OR as applied systems thinking. *J. Oper. Res. Soc.* **2012**, *63*, 1228–1247. [CrossRef]
23. Andersen, D.F.; Richardson, G.P. Scripts for group model building. *Syst. Dyn. Rev. J. Syst. Dyn. Soc.* **1997**, *13*, 107–129. [CrossRef]
24. Bérard, C. Group model building using system dynamics: An analysis of methodological frameworks. *Electron. J. Bus. Res. Methods* **2010**, *8*, 35–45.
25. Vennix, J.A.; Andersen, D.F.; Richardson, G.P.; Rohrbaugh, J. Model-building for group decision support: Issues and alternatives in knowledge elicitation. *Eur. J. Oper. Res.* **1992**, *59*, 28–41. [CrossRef]
26. Voinov, A.; Gaddis, E.B. Values in participatory modeling: Theory and practice. In *Environmental Modeling with Stakeholders: Theory, Methods, and Applications*; Springer: Cham, Switzerland, 2017; pp. 47–63.
27. Voinov, A.; Kolagani, N.; McCall, M.K.; Glynn, P.D.; Kragt, M.E.; Ostermann, F.O.; Pierce, S.A.; Ramu, P. Modelling with stakeholders—Next generation. *Environ. Model. Softw.* **2016**, *77*, 196–220. [CrossRef]
28. Shand, F.; Torok, M.; Cockayne, N.; Batterham, P.J.; Calear, A.L.; Mackinnon, A.; Martin, D.; Zbukvic, I.; Mok, K.; Chen, N.; et al. Protocol for a stepped-wedge, cluster randomized controlled trial of the LifeSpan suicide prevention trial in four communities in New South Wales, Australia. *Trials* **2020**, *21*, 332. [CrossRef]
29. Currier, D.; King, K.; Oostermeijer, S.; Hall, T.; Cox, A.; Page, A.; Pirkis, J. *National Suicide Prevention Trial: Final Evaluation Report (Version 2)*; University of Melbourne: Parkville, Australia, 2022.
30. Page, A.; Pirkis, J.; Bandara, P.; Oostermeijer, S.; Hall, T.; Burgess, P.M.; Harris, M.; Currier, D. Early impacts of the 'National Suicide Prevention Trial' on trends in suicide and hospital admissions for self-harm in Australia. *Aust. N. Z. J. Psychiatry* **2023**. [CrossRef] [PubMed]
31. Page, A.; Diallo, S.Y.; Wildman, W.J.; Hodulik, G.; Weisel, E.W.; Gondal, N.; Voas, D. Computational Simulation Is a Vital Resource for Navigating the COVID-19 Pandemic. *Simul. Healthc.* **2022**, *17*, e141–e148. [CrossRef] [PubMed]

32. Knipe, D.; Padmanathan, P.; Newton-Howes, G.; Chan, L.F.; Kapur, N. Suicide and self-harm. *Lancet* **2022**, *14*, 1903–1916. [CrossRef]
33. Machado, D.B.; Williamson, E.; Pescarini, J.M.; Alves, F.J.O.; Castro-De-Araujo, L.F.S.; Ichihara, M.Y.; Rodrigues, L.C.; Araya, R.; Patel, V.; Barreto, M.L. Relationship between the Bolsa Família national cash transfer programme and suicide incidence in Brazil: A quasi-experimental study. *PLoS Med.* **2022**, *19*, e1004000. [CrossRef] [PubMed]

Disclaimer/Publisher's Note: The statements, opinions and data contained in all publications are solely those of the individual author(s) and contributor(s) and not of MDPI and/or the editor(s). MDPI and/or the editor(s) disclaim responsibility for any injury to people or property resulting from any ideas, methods, instructions or products referred to in the content.

Article

An Agent-Based Social Impact Theory Model to Study the Impact of In-Person School Closures on Nonmedical Prescription Opioid Use among Youth

Narjes Shojaati and Nathaniel D. Osgood *

Department of Computer Science, University of Saskatchewan, Saskatoon, SK S7N 5C9, Canada
* Correspondence: nathaniel.osgood@usask.ca

Abstract: Substance use behavior among youth is a complex peer-group phenomenon shaped by many factors. Peer influence, easily accessible prescription opioids, and a youth's socio-cultural environment play recognized roles in the initiation and persistence of youth nonmedical prescription opioid use. By altering the physical surroundings and social environment of youth, in-person school closures may change risk factors for youth drug use. Acknowledging past research on the importance of the presence of peers in youth substance use risk behavior, this paper reports the findings from the use of an agent-based simulation grounded in social impact theory to investigate possible impacts of in-person school closures due to COVID-19 on the prevalence of nonmedical prescription opioid use among youth. The presented model integrates data from the Ontario Student Drug Use and Health Survey and characterizes the accessibility of within-home prescription opioids. Under the status quo, the lifting of in-person school closures reliably entails an increase in the prevalence of youth with nonmedical prescription opioid use, but this effect is ameliorated if the prescription opioids are securely stored during the in-person school closures period.

Keywords: agent-based modeling; social impact theory; cellular automata; youth; nonmedical prescription opioid use; in-person school closures; COVID-19-related public health order

1. Introduction

Youth are among the high-risk population for substance use behaviors [1,2]. Substance use behavior among youth is a complex phenomenon and involves diverse influential factors including the socio-cultural environment [3,4], substance-using peers, and personal network characteristics [5–7]. Some youth initiate drug use because of friends and continue it to fit in with their social network and environment. Such initiation is of particular significance in that many adults have initiated substance use during their teen and young adult years [8,9]. With growing appreciation for the impact of peers, families, and communities on youth substance use, schools are also recognized as important social environments affecting student knowledge, attitudes, and behavior toward substance use [10].

One of the initial actions taken during the COVID-19 pandemic to lower mortality and avoid unsustainable acute care service utilization was the implementation of public health orders that frequently included partial or full in-person school closures, and sometimes encouraged families to minimize socialization and remain at home where possible [11]. In Ontario, the first school closure was announced on 12 March 2020, in effect from 14 March 2020, and continued with several gradual and staggered reopening and closures throughout the course of the following two years, as shown in Figure 1 [12]. Finally, Ontario schools reopened for in-person learning on 17 January 2022 [13].

The presence of youth at home during in-person school closures may have positive and negative implications for their mental health and propensity to use substances. While a lack of in-person contact with classmates and instructors is likely to produce elevated anxiety, boredom, and discontent in some young people, others may have welcomed less stressful peer interaction and a temporary decline in bullying and other forms of unpleasant experiences associated with in-person learning [14]. Among youth, the adoption of unhealthy coping mechanisms, such as substance use, as a result of pandemic-related stress, are of particular concern, since they are less likely to consider the negative consequences of their action [15]. The increased risk of opioid use among youth could result from elevated accessibility of prescription opioids due to unsafe medication storage practices by family members at home [16–18], witnessing elevated parental nonmedical prescription opioid use [19], and increased alcohol and cannabis consumption among youth during the pandemic [20–22]. Such regularities and the prospects of requiring in-person school closures as part of future public health orders suggest the importance of understanding the impact of in-person school closures on substance use among young Canadians during and after the COVID-19 pandemic.

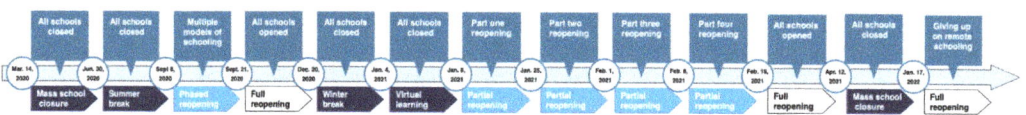

Figure 1. Ontario-level in-person school closures and reopening timeline. This figure is based on Gallagher et al. [12] licensed under CC BY 4.0 (https://creativecommons.org/licenses/by/4.0/).

There is a body of research applying social network analysis to secure insights into substance use behavior among youth [23–25]. Although social network analysis can offer enormous insights into the social context of and influence on the use of drugs, reducing an individual to a node in a network limits the integration of personal characteristics [26]. While incorporating such representation of network structures, an agent-based modeling approach can more deeply analyze individual affiliative structures in the context of evolving and actively interacting agents with varying characteristics [27,28].

To explore fundamental elements of substance use among youth, different agent-based models have been built [29–36]. These models highlight the use of the computational modeling method as a possible way to explore the complex concept of substance use amongst youth. One little-explored approach to study the possible association between social influence and substance use amongst youth is through opinion dynamics computational models. Opinion dynamics computational models can highlight mechanisms underlying the convergence of behaviors and theoretical implications for imitator behaviors. There is a substantial body of literature on opinion dynamics models, with model formulations having been contributed from domains as varied as social psychology, statistical physics, mathematics, and computer science. These varying angles of contributions have led to a vast and diverse body of research [37–39]. Despite the breadth of past applications of opinion dynamics models, there are few computational modelling studies that employ the opinion dynamics model to study addictive behaviors [40,41], and none of them devote particular attention towards how in-person school closures may affect youth nonmedical prescription opioid use.

Broadly, opinion formation models can be categorized into discrete and continuous models. Discrete models permit an agent to hold one of a finite set of opinions, whereas continuous models allow for a real-valued opinion [38]. Below, we informally characterize eight prominent subgroups in the opinion dynamics models within the literature [37], recognizing that the taxonomy employed here is not a canonical one and that other forms of classification of opinion dynamics models can be seen within the literature [38].

One of the earliest dichotomous discrete opinion dynamics models to simulate how people's attitudes evolve over time is the voter model. Each individual inside an arbitrary network is selected randomly and adopts the state of a randomly chosen neighbor. Arrival at a consensus is the main feature of the voter model [42]. Many variants of the voter model have been examined, including a nonlinear formulation [43], alternative starting network configurations [44], the impacts of "zealots" carrying invariant beliefs [45], and those reflecting various co-evolutionary principles [46]. A second discrete model of opinion dynamics —the majority rule model—considers a set of agents who have discrete opinions and selects alternatives that enjoy majority support [47,48]. Third, the Sznajd model provides a discrete model of opinion dynamics and implements a rule in which a pair of neighbors is randomly chosen to change their nearest neighbor's opinion; if that pair of close neighbors agree, their nearest neighbors will eventually agree. By contrast, if the pair disagree, the opinion of the nearest neighbors remains unchanged, with no common opinion developing among their nearest neighbors [49–51]. Fourth, the bounded confidence model was developed by Deffaunt et al. and consists of a stochastic model for the evolution of continuous-valued opinions within a finite group of peers [52]. Fifth, the relative agreement model is a variant of the bounded confidence model that uses individual uncertainty as the criterion for deciding whether two agents can interact; uncertainty, as well as opinion, can be modified by interactions within this model [53]. Sixth, the continuous opinions and discrete actions model describes a situation in which agents hold real-valued opinions yet may only express themselves in discrete terms [54]. Seventh, the social judgment-based opinion model shares certain features with the continuous opinions and discrete actions model with two alternative structures: one in which agents can express their opinion as a real number and another in which they are restricted to one of a set of discrete possibilities [55,56]. A final class of opinion dynamics models are those employing the social impact theory model, which offers a discrete model of opinion dynamics based on social impact theory in psychology [57]. Social impact theory associates each agent with three variables—a level of persuasiveness, a level of supportiveness, and a binary opinion. The model further presents a set of formulae to characterize the total impact on each agent based on the number, strength, and immediacy of its neighbors [58]. This work employs this final class of opinion dynamics models as an established theory of clear relevance to study the impact on youth drug use of direct (in-person) peer influences at school and indirect perceived norms from the socio-cultural environment.

The COVID-19 pandemic has had a profound impact on the lives of people around the world, including youth. In particular, the closure of in-person schools has raised questions about the potential impact on nonmedical prescription opioid use among youth. The current study centers on the question of how in-person school closures during and after the COVID-19 pandemic affect nonmedical prescription opioid use among youth, and what measures can be taken to alleviate any potential risks or improve the situation. The findings of this research can be utilized to develop policies and interventions aimed at decreasing the risk of nonmedical prescription opioid use among youth during and after in-person school closures. This study is one of the first to investigate the impact of in-person school closures on nonmedical prescription opioid use among youth during and after the COVID-19 pandemic in Canada. To support this investigation, this work employed an agent-based model formulated based on the social impact model of opinion formation [59,60], and was calibrated to reflect data from the Ontario Student Drug Use and Health Survey (OSDUHS) [61,62].

The remainder of this paper is organized as follows: Section 2 describes the model, including the agent-based formulation and the social impact theory implementation, cellular automata spatial structure, and the experimental design. Section 3 elucidates the results. Section 4 includes the corresponding discussion and concludes the paper.

2. Materials and Methods

Within this work, the influences of peers, families, and socio-cultural environment on nonmedical prescription opioid use among youth are investigated using an agent-based model (ABM) operating within a spatial grid-based network structure in accordance with cellular automata (CA) principles. The data on the prevalence of nonmedical prescription opioid use among youth, as well as the frequency and sources of use reported in the Ontario Student Drug Use and Health Survey (OSDUHS) [61,62], were used to parameterize and calibrate the ABM. The selection of the most appropriate agent-based modeling toolkit for this project was based on a variety of factors, including the programming experience and abilities of the individuals involved, the activity of the toolkit's community and the availability of specialized resources, the scalability and adaptability of the platform, and the built-in visualization options. Two separate reports [63,64] evaluated various agent-based modeling toolkits against different criteria and offered recommendations based on specific needs. For this study, the model was created using simulation software AnyLogic Version 8.8.1 [65] and the model was run for a time horizon from 2017 to 2025.

The design of the agent-based model drew on the social impact model of opinion formation [59,60]. The agent-based model was created, parameterized, calibrated, and used to investigate the prevalence of nonmedical prescription opioid use among youth, their prescription opioids resources, and the frequency of nonmedical prescription opioid use within the past year when varying peer influence, youth exposure to prescription opioids at home, and the influence of the socio-cultural environment. To support this investigation, the peer network context, families, and the socio-cultural environment shaping nonmedical prescription opioid use in youth were captured within a three-level CA context (corresponding to peers, families, and the socio-cultural environment), where each youth's nonmedical prescription opioid use evolved according to the social impact theory of opinion formation.

2.1. Agent-Based Modeling

The use of agent-based modeling in this study supports the analysis of changes in the prevalence of nonmedical prescription opioid use among youth and the characterization of the effects of their peers, families, and socio-cultural environment. Hence, the model features three type of agents: youth, family, and socio-cultural environment. Youth behavior is governed by three different state charts depicted in Figure 2. These state charts collectively characterize the possible state-space for a single youth and the events that lead to transitions from one state to another.

The logic for transitions between states within the Youth Drug Use Opinion Evidence state chart was informed by social impact theory. At the topmost level, the Youth Drug Use state chart characterizes whether the individual currently uses nonmedical prescription opioids. Youth who are not currently using nonmedical prescription opioids are divided into two groups: youth who have never used nonmedical prescription opioids and youth who previously used but have since quit by electing not to use nonmedical prescription opioids when the opportunity arose. Youth who currently use nonmedical prescription opioids are also divided into two groups: youth who are within their initial period of nonmedical prescription opioids use and youth who relapsed after previously quitting.

The Frequency of Drug Use in the past year state chart represents the number of times that youth used nonmedical prescription opioids during the past year, and it is updated as time passes and as youth use nonmedical prescription opioids.

The Drug Sources state chart depicts two important sources for the most recent prescription opioids use for youth: family and friends. Youth are considered to have a possible opportunity to obtain opioids from family when their family includes at least one person with an opioid prescription. In the absence of a family source, youth can seek available prescription opioids amongst their close friends (considered to be those within their range 1 Moore neighborhood; see below); based on a probability, youth can obtain prescription opioids from friends who are themselves nonmedical prescription opioid users. The unspecified state reflects other sources of opioids.

Each youth is associated with a family, as represented by a family agent. Each such family agent has a family size parameter, which is drawn from a Poisson distribution to represent the empirical data that the average family size in Canada was 2.9 in 2019 [66]. The probability of filling an opioid prescription per week for each family member previously without an opioid prescription and the per week probability of ending opioid prescription treatment for each family member with prescription opioids are calibrated to represent the 12.7% of Canadians who reported having used opioids pain relief medications in 2018 [67].

If a member of any family has been prescribed an opioid, a child in the family might be exposed to prescription opioids, with the level of exposure differing between families. The child exposure to opioids parameter is calibrated to represent the 49.3% of Ontario youth who reported using nonmedical prescription opioids, obtaining them from a parent, sibling, or someone else with whom they live [61,62].

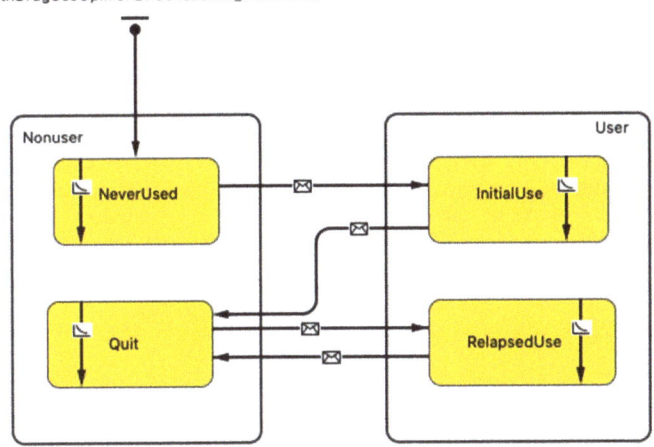

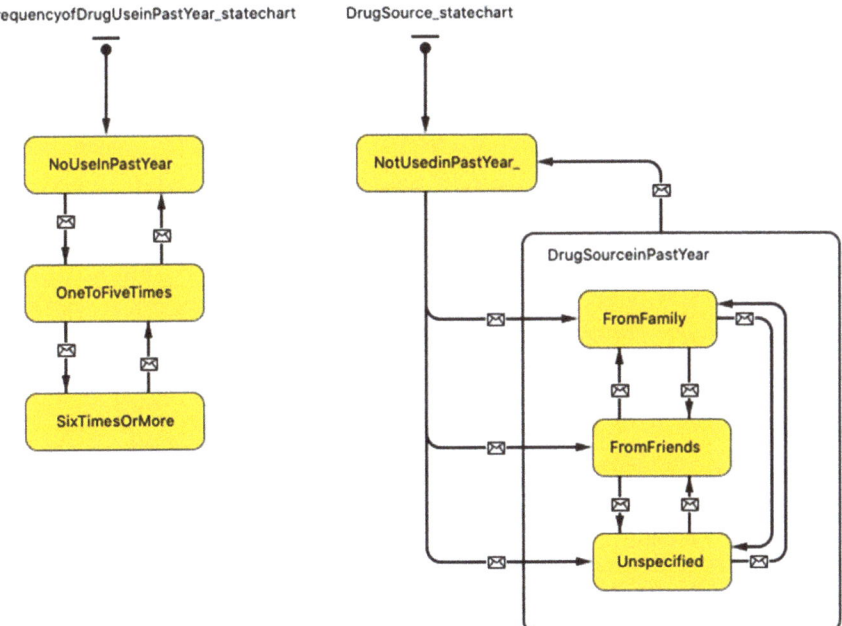

Figure 2. Youth state charts—Youth Drug Use Opinion Evidence state chart at the top middle, Frequency of Drug Use in the past year state chart at the bottom left, and Drug Sources state chart at the bottom right.

The socio-cultural environment for contemporary youth is made up of neighborhoods, recreation areas, social events, and other forces that affect a youth's basic values, perceptions, and preferences. Within the model, a socio-cultural environment agent is implemented to reflect the idea that youth prescription opioid use is particularly high in some specific demographics [68]. Part of the socio-cultural environment within the model is therefore assumed to have some degree of bearing on the valence of a youth's attitude towards drug use.

2.2. Cellular Automata for Spatially Localized Networks

This model uses a three-level spatial grid-based network structure to capture the social context of each youth. All youth are randomly and injectively placed into individual cells (patches) in the cellular automata located in the global environment. The three-level grid containing the youth, family, and socio-cultural environment is a square containing 100 columns and 100 rows. Each patch corresponds to the youth at CA level one (as depicted in Figure 3a), the youth's family at CA level two (as depicted in Figure 3b), and the youth's socio-cultural environment at CA level three (as depicted in Figure 3c).

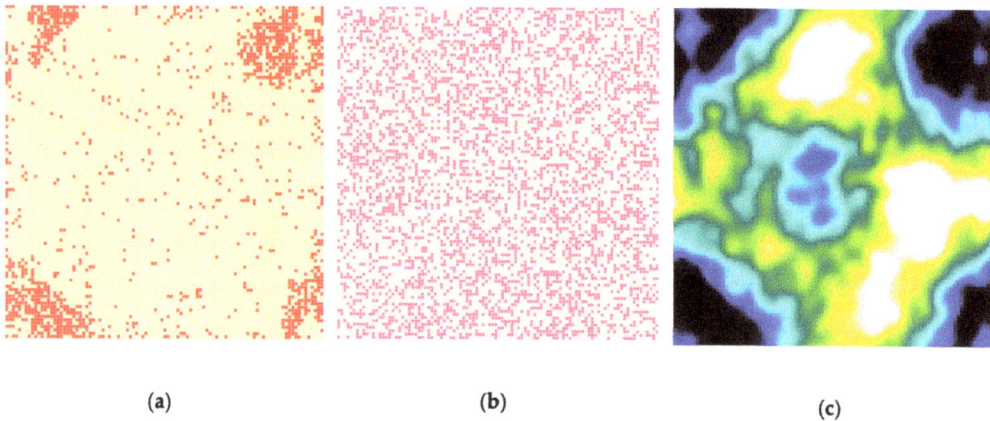

Figure 3. Three-level cellular automata—(**a**) Each patch presents a youth. Colors distinguish youth who are absent nonmedical prescription opioid use experience in the past year (yellow) and with nonmedical prescription opioid use experience in that interval (red). (**b**) Each patch represents family. Corresponding colors for a family with at least one member with current prescribed opioids and family without any prescribed opioids are pink and ivory, respectively. (**c**) Socio-cultural environment, in which the black areas represent a positive perspective toward drug use and gradations towards white represent successively more negative attitudes towards drug use.

This implantation provides a spatially explicit, grid-based network structure for the youth, who remain immobile throughout the simulation. The lack of spatial mobility reflects the fact that many youths exhibited high conservation in their social networks and interaction patterns during and immediately after the pandemic, partly because of the fact that such networks reflect the composition of the family and socio-cultural environment in which the youth is nested [69]. Social network density for youth and their peers at CA level one is operationalized by considering Moore neighborhoods with different diameters (ranges) as shown in Figure 4.

2.3. Social Impact Model of Opinion Formation

The model characterizes how youths' nonmedical use of prescription opioids might be governed by environmental influences, availability of prescription opioids at home, and the actions of their peers following a discrete opinion model based on social impact theory.

The model consists of 10,000 youths and their corresponding family and socio-cultural environment. Each youth is considered to have one of two opposite opinions on nonmedical prescription opioid use, according to whether they currently nonmedically use prescription opioids. The presence or absence of nonmedical prescription drug use is assumed to be dictated entirely by the attitude (opinion) of the youth with respect to drug use.

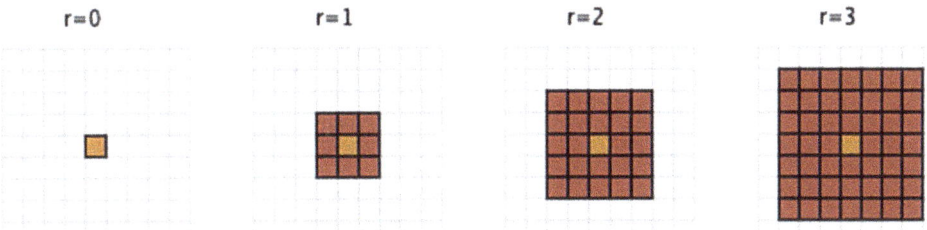

Figure 4. Moore neighborhood with different ranges from left to right: r = 0, r = 1, r = 2, and r = 3.

In accordance with social impact theory, each youth is characterized by two independent parameters called persuasiveness and supportiveness. The strength of persuasiveness is the ability to persuade another youth with a discordant drug use attitude to change their current attitude. The strength of supportiveness characterizes the ability to support another youth with an identical drug use attitude to persist in their current attitude [58].

Following the literature [58,70], the values of the persuasiveness and supportiveness attributes are assigned as random real-number values uniformly drawn between 0 and 100; when youth flip to an alternative attitude and associated behavior, their parameters for persuasiveness and supportiveness are independently drawn from the same distribution.

Youth experience a net impact from interactions with the socio-cultural environment, family, and peers. Employing a formulation drawn from the opinion dynamics literature [58,70], the model characterizes the quantitative value of that impact I_i for an agent i at each drug use occasion with the equation shown in Equation (1).

$$I_i = \left(\left[\sum_{j=1}^{N} \frac{p_j}{d_{ij}^a} (1 - o_i o_j) \right] - \left[\sum_{j=1}^{N} \frac{s_j}{d_{ij}^a} (1 + o_i o_j) \right] \right) - o_i E_i - o_i M_i \quad (1)$$

where j denotes another agent influencing agent i, and o_i and o_j denote the dichotomous (± 1) opinion values of agents i and j, respectively, towards opioid use, where -1 indicates an attitude disfavoring opioid use and $+1$ indicates an attitude in favor of opioid use.

p_j and s_j denote the persuasiveness and supportiveness of agent j, respectively. In accordance with a gravity model formulation, d_{ij} represents the Euclidean distance between youth i and j, and a defines the speed of drop-off of influence with distance. The current model considers peers at Moore neighborhoods with three different levels of influence on nonmedical opioids use for youth; therefore, d is equal to the minimum Moore neighborhood radius with which agents i and j are connected (max = 3). For a given agent i, an agent j lying outside the distance of 3 Moore neighborhoods surrounding agent i is assumed to exert zero influence on agent i (that is, $\frac{p_j}{d_{ij}^a}$ and $\frac{s_j}{d_{ij}^a}$ are considered to be 0). Following the literature [58,70] and consistent with calibrated results of the model, a is considered equal to 2.

The peer impact on youth i is calculated as the difference between the collective impact of the interacting youth exerting influence on youth i to change opinion (characterized by the first bracketed term of Equation (1)) and the collective impact of peers exerting influence to maintain youth i's current opinion (the second bracketed term of Equation (1)).

E_i is a so-called socio-cultural environment pro-drug influence parameter reflecting the level of promotion of drug use by youth i's neighborhoods, recreation areas, social events, and other forces (a value greater than 0 when there is a pro-drug influence and equal to 0 for areas without pro-drug influence). M_i is a child's exposure to opioids at home parameter (family influence), reflecting the level of unsafe opioid storage practices by the youth's family (a value greater than 0 when there is some opioid storage by the youth's family and equal to 0 for youth i in a family without prescription opioids).

If the overall impact from interacting with peers, families, and the socio-cultural environment for a youth who is absent any nonmedical prescription opioids experience as characterized by Equation (1) is greater than 0, then the current youth will immediately initiate nonmedical prescription opioids use. Equation (1) individually governs initiation behavior in youth who are absent nonmedical prescription opioid use experience, as they do not have any acute withdrawal symptoms for opioids prior to any experience.

After initial experience with nonmedical prescription opioid use, the behavior of youth continues to be influenced by peers, families, and the socio-cultural environment; however, another key factor also arises at this point: the severity of acute withdrawal. This factor can serve to either reinforce or discourage youth drug use [29].

Past research has suggested that the temporal evolution of the severity of acute withdrawal symptoms for opioid drugs can be characterized by a lognormal function of days from the last dose [71]. We employed a lognormal function where scale parameter μ ranged between 0 and 1 and shape parameter σ ranged between 1×10^{-3} to 1.5×10^{-3}.

The attitude of youth with nonmedical prescription opioid use experience may change in each drug use situation according to Equation (2).

$$o_i(t+1) = \begin{cases} o_i(t) & \text{with probability } \frac{\exp\left(\frac{-I_i}{T_i}\right)}{\exp\left(\frac{-I_i}{T_i}\right)+\exp\left(\frac{I_i}{T_i}\right)} \\ -o_i(t) & \text{with probability } \frac{\exp\left(\frac{I_i}{T_i}\right)}{\exp\left(\frac{-I_i}{T_i}\right)+\exp\left(\frac{I_i}{T_i}\right)} \end{cases} \qquad (2)$$

The parameter T_i represents the severity of acute withdrawal at the current time, and may be interpreted as a personalized parameter to show randomness in the behavior of youth, who may reject peers, families, and the socio-cultural environment's impact about nonmedical prescription opioid use and elect to quit or relapse. Although the impact (I_i) is a deterministic endogenous parameter that represents a propensity to change—that is, it causes youths who are absent nonmedical prescription opioid experience to initiate opioid use (when the total impact is greater than 0)—any youth with experience of nonmedical prescription opioid use may quit or relapse based on the probability calculated within Equation (2). A higher value of I_i indicates a greater likelihood of changing behavior within Equation (2). Equation (2) is a particular case of the system considered in the literature [72,73].

2.4. In-Person School Closures Implementation Due to the COVID-19 Pandemic

The model characterizes in-person school closures associated with the COVID-19 pandemic as a change in the range of the Moore neighborhood mediating inter-youth interaction starting on 14 March 2020. Specifically, mass in-person school closures are implemented as a Moore neighborhood of range 0 (which has the effect of eliminating the spread of direct—in person—influence between youth) and in the case of the Ontario school closure timeline, the Moore neighborhood range differs for mass closure, partial opening, and phased opening.

2.5. Parametrization, Calibration, and Validation

While the ABM presented in this study is a stylized one, it drew heavily on the Ontario Student Drug Use and Health Survey (OSDUHS) [61,62] to provide data to characterize dynamics of nonmedical prescription opioid use among youth in Canada. The baseline empirically grounded model reflects nonmedical prescription opioids use among students in Grades 7–12 from 2017 to 2021 based on OSDUHS [61,62] and projected until the end of 2025.

Ontario mass in-person school closures were characterized by imposing a Moore neighborhood of range 0 in any phases of the lockdown. The first school closure period was from 14 March 2020 to 8 September 2020, then from 20 December 2020 to 8 January 2021, and finally from 12 April 2021 to 17 January 2022 [12,13]. The period of phased reopening was characterized as imposing a Moore neighborhood of range 2 from 8 September 2020 to 21 September 2020, with partial reopening characterized as a Moore neighborhood of range 1 from 8 January 2021 to 1 February 2021, and as a Moore neighborhood of range 2 from 2 February 2021 to 16 February 2021 to reflect the transition from the mass school closure to full reopening. Finally, the full reopening of Ontario schools was characterized as a Moore neighborhood of range 3.

The model was calibrated so as to match model output against the time-series of the prevalence of youth with nonmedical prescription opioid use, and the time-series of the prevalence of youth using nonmedical prescription opioids frequently (six times or more over the past year) targets from 2017 to 2019 at 2-year intervals and data points of the prevalence of youth using nonmedical prescription opioids obtained from different resources (including families, friends, and unspecified resources) in 2019. During the calibration process, we varied the following set of model parameters by hand until the model outputs approximated empirical data.

Several model parameters were calibrated against the prevalence of youth with nonmedical prescription opioid use and the prevalence of youth using nonmedical prescription opioids obtained from families. Youth exposure to prescription opioids at home was calibrated against the prevalence of youth with nonmedical prescription opioid use and the prevalence of youth using nonmedical prescription opioids obtained from families. The severity of acute withdrawal from nonmedical opioid use was calibrated against the prevalence of youth with nonmedical prescription opioid use. The percentage of the socio-cultural environment with a positive drug use view and the level of drug promotion inside the drug-positive socio-cultural environment were calibrated against the prevalence of youth with nonmedical prescription opioid use. The probability that peers share drugs with peers who request it was calibrated against the prevalence of youth using nonmedical prescription opioids obtained from families. The rate of encountering drug use situations for youth consisted of an initial amount and a coefficient to reflect the current socialization level, and both were calibrated against the prevalence of youth with nonmedical prescription opioid use. The rate of opioid prescription for each family member without prescription opioids and the probability that the duration of the opioid prescription ends for each family member was calibrated to accord with the prevalence of Canadians with an opioid prescription. See Table A1 for more details on parameter values and references.

Finally, to ensure the reliability, validity, and robustness of the current model, a comprehensive validation process was conducted in three phases [74,75]. The first phase, verification, evaluates the correctness of the model by comparing the model's assumptions to the code logic. The second phase, validation, assesses the accuracy of the model's emergent behavior by comparing it to external criteria such as real-world data or expert knowledge. The final phase, sensitivity analysis, examines how variations in model assumptions impact the model's outcomes. The model demonstrates a visually good fit between the observed and model-predicted prevalence of youth with a nonmedical prescription opioid in 2021 during the COVID-19-related in-person school closures.

2.6. Scenarios

To investigate the impact of in-person school closures on nonmedical prescription opioid use among youth, two sets of scenarios were examined. The first set of scenarios examined outcomes from 6, 12, 18, and 24 months of mass in-person school closures followed by partial opening, phased opening, or full opening (i.e., characterizing using different Moore neighborhood ranges) after removing the mass in-person school closures order. For the first set of scenarios, an ensemble of 30 realizations was conducted to secure statistical confidence in results despite stochastic variability.

The second set of scenarios sought to examine the impact of the Ontario school closure timeline and further applied the intervention of reducing youth exposure to prescription opioids at home by 20%, 50%, and 80% at three different time points, considered singly. For the second set of scenarios, an ensemble of 100 realizations was conducted. Furthermore, to generate outcomes of interest that are compatible with the empirical data for the baseline, each simulation employed a 3-year burn-in period for the model. Following the burn-in period, the model was run for a time horizon from 2017 to 2025. Outcomes of interest are plotted daily to see the pattern of changes and recorded yearly to compare with the baseline.

3. Results

This section describes the results of model simulations. The Monte Carlo simulation of the model utilized different realizations to generate a sample of potential outcomes, given a set of inputs and assumptions. Each realization represented a single simulation of the system, utilizing a randomly generated set of inputs. By conducting multiple realizations and introducing randomness in the input parameters, the simulation aimed to gain a deeper understanding of the uncertainty of the results. The results are divided into three subsections, starting with the model-generated prevalence of youth with nonmedical prescription opioid use in the past year for different durations of in-person school closures, followed by a simulation of the model using the Ontario school closure timeline without any intervention. Finally, the impact of safe storage of prescription opioids at home on the prevalence of youth engaged in nonmedical prescription opioid use on the result of the model using the Ontario school closure timeline is explored.

3.1. Results of the Simulation for the Prevalence of Youth with Nonmedical Prescription Opioid Use in the Past Year for Different In-Person School Closure Durations

Figure 5 illustrates the model-generated prevalence of youth with nonmedical prescription opioid use in the past year for the different durations of in-person school closures. There is a small increase in the prevalence of drug use for the first six months of in-person school closures. Following this initial increase in prevalence, scenarios exhibit a decline to a steady level for the next six months of in-person school closures. Following that—for sufficiently long durations of in-person school closures—a plateau persists until the end of the in-person school closures. The prevalence of youth with nonmedical prescription opioid use significantly increases after the lifting of the in-person school closures, regardless of its duration. Nevertheless, the appearance of the increase remained consistent across different levels of in-person socialization following the lifting of in-person school closures, supporting the robustness of this conclusion (See Figures A1 and A2).

3.2. Simulation of the Model Using Ontario School Closure Timeline

Figure 6 represents the model-generated prevalence of youth exhibiting nonmedical prescription opioid use in the past year based on the Ontario school closure timeline. Figure 6 also demonstrates a visually good fit between the observed and model-generated prevalence of youth with nonmedical prescription opioids, persisting even in the middle of in-person school closures in 2021. After the first school closure came into effect on 14 March 2020, the model-generated prevalence of youth exhibiting nonmedical prescription opioid use shows an increasing trend. The increase continues through the year as schooling experiences were more differentiated across Ontario with the different possible levels of socialization for youth. However, as the second mass in-person school closures due to the COVID-19 pandemic lasted for more than six months, the model-generated prevalence of drug use shows a downward shift. The model-generated prevalence of youth exhibiting nonmedical prescription opioid use increases after the lifting of the in-person school closures. Further, we used the model to estimate the overall impact of in-person school closures through the COVID-19 pandemic on youth opioid use by comparing the model-generated prevalence of drug use in 2025, with and without in-person school closures due to the COVID-19 pandemic. The model-generated prevalence of youth exhibiting nonmedical prescription opioid use could show a significant increase (of +195%) in 2025 as a consequence of in-person school closures. Furthermore, the distributions of simulation outputs and the coefficient of variation remain relatively stable under different population sizes (See Figure A3).

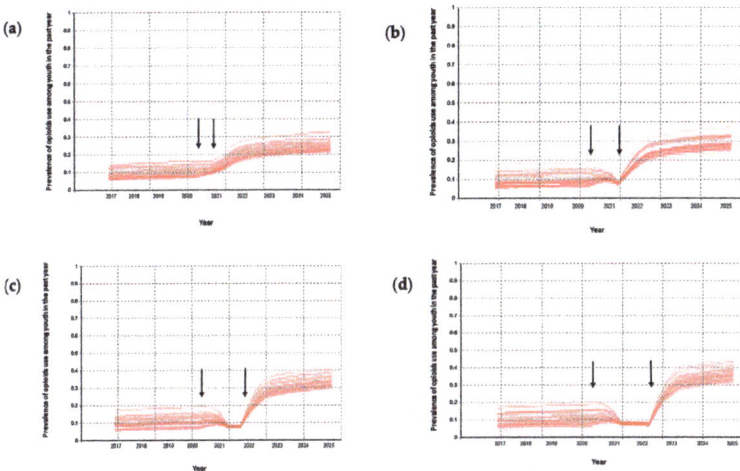

Figure 5. Model-generated prevalence of youth with nonmedical prescription opioid use in the past year for the different durations of in-person school closures (**a–d**). The model predicted the prevalence of youth with nonmedical prescription opioid use in the past year for (**a**) 6-month in-person school closures, (**b**) 12-month in-person school closures, (**c**) 18-month in-person school closures, and (**d**) 24-month in-person school closures. In-person socialization following the lifting of in-person school closures is characterized as a Moore neighborhood of range 3. The two vertical arrows represent the start and end of the in-person school closures for each panel, respectively.

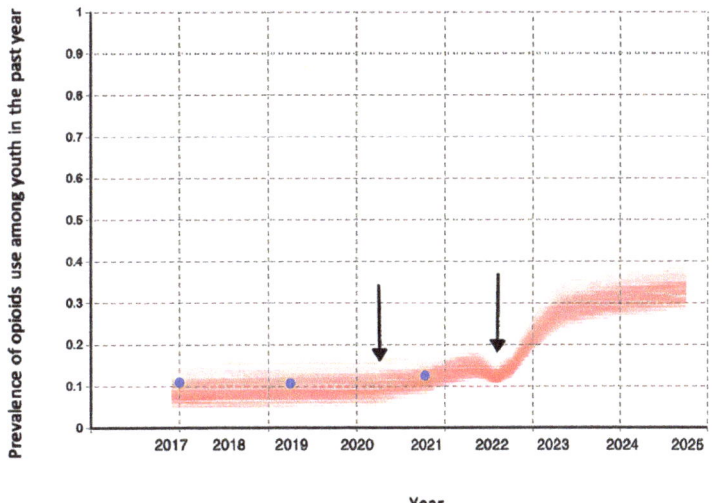

Figure 6. Model-generated prevalence of youth exhibiting nonmedical prescription opioid use in the past year based on Ontario school closure timeline. The blue dots show the empirical data and the two vertical black arrows represent the start and end of the Ontario school closure timeline.

3.3. Impact of Safely Storing Prescription Opioids at Home on the Result of the Model Using the Ontario School Closure Timeline

Figure 7 illustrates the impact of safely storing prescription opioids at home on the prevalence of youth with nonmedical prescription opioid use in the past year. Specifically, it shows the impacts when youth exposure to prescription opioids at home is reduced by 20%. Figure 7b illustrates a scenario in which the intervention of safely storing prescription opioids with a decrease of 20% in youth exposure to prescription opioids at home was implemented in 2017. Figure 7c depicts the effects of this intervention when it was implemented at the start of the COVID-19-related in-person school closures, while Figure 7d depicts the effects of the intervention of securely storing prescription opioids when it was implemented at the start of the 2022–2023 academic year. Cases in which this intervention was implemented before or early in the COVID-19-related in-person school closures slightly mitigate the extent of the increase in prevalence of drug use after the lifting of in-person school closures (Figure 7b,c). However, even a delayed implementation of safely storing prescription opioids—where such precautions are introduced after the lifting of the COVID-19-related in-person school closures—has also achieved a modest reduction in the peak in the prevalence of youth with nonmedical prescription opioid use (Figure 7d).

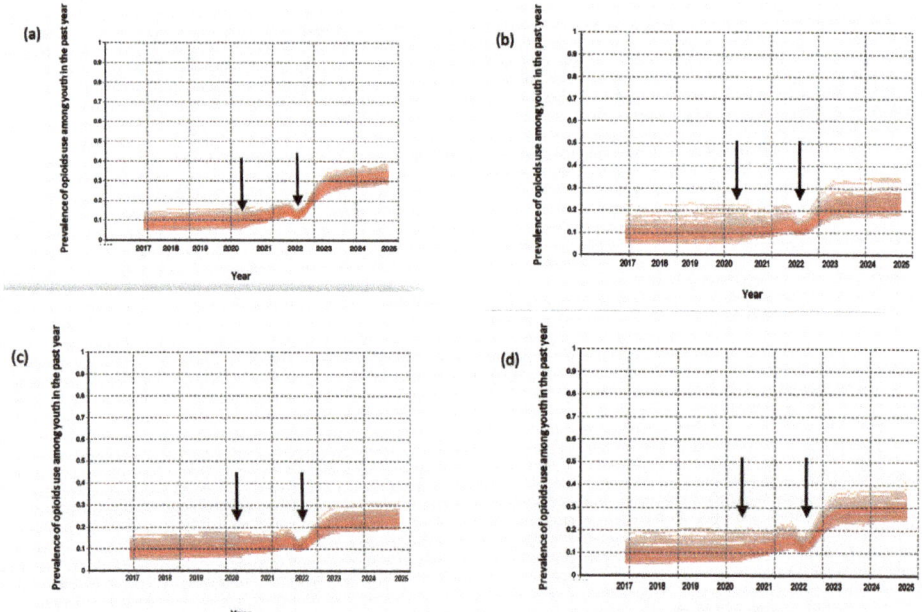

Figure 7. Model-generated prevalence of youth exhibiting nonmedical prescription opioid use in the past year for the baseline scenario (**a**) and after applying safe storage intervention with a decrease of 20% in youth exposure to prescription opioids at home beginning at different time points (**b**–**d**). The two vertical black arrows represent the start and end of the Ontario school closure timeline. (**a**) Model-generated prevalence of youth exhibiting nonmedical prescription opioid use in the past year for the baseline scenario. (**b**) Model-generated prevalence of youth exhibiting nonmedical prescription opioid use in the past year after applying safe storage in 2017. (**c**) Model-generated prevalence of youth exhibiting nonmedical prescription opioid use in the past year after applying safe storage at the beginning of the general COVID-19-related in-person school closures on 14 March 2020. (**d**) Model-generated prevalence of youth exhibiting nonmedical prescription opioid use in the past year after applying safe storage at the start of the 2022–2023 academic year.

Decreasing youth exposure to prescription opioids by 20% would reduce the prevalence of youth with nonmedical prescription opioid use after the lifting of the COVID-19-related in-person school closures by 27% and 28% in 2025 relative to the baseline, depending on whether the intervention was implemented before or at the beginning of the COVID-19-related in-person school closures, respectively. However, late implementation of the intervention at the start of the 2022–2023 academic year would also reduce the prevalence of youth with nonmedical prescription opioid use in 2025 by 9%, relative to the result of the model using the Ontario school closure timeline without any intervention.

The results of the model also indicate that decreasing youth exposure to prescription opioids by 50% can lead to a significant reduction in the prevalence of nonmedical prescription opioid use among youth after the lifting of the COVID-19-related in-person school closures. Specifically, the prevalence of youth with nonmedical prescription opioid use in 2025 would be reduced by 58% and 56%, depending on whether the intervention was implemented before or at the beginning of the COVID-19-related in-person school closures, respectively. With a late implementation at the start of the 2022–2023 academic year, the prevalence of youth with nonmedical prescription opioid use in 2025 would still be reduced by 19% in comparison to the model using the Ontario school closure timeline without any intervention (See Figure A4).

Finally, a significant decrease in youth exposure to prescription opioids by 80% could greatly reduce the prevalence of nonmedical prescription opioid use among youth following the lifting of the COVID-19-related in-person school closures. The prevalence of youth with nonmedical prescription opioid use in 2025 could be lowered by 68% and 66% if the intervention was implemented prior to or at the beginning of the COVID-19-related in-person school closures, respectively. Even with a delayed implementation at the start of the 2022–2023 academic year, the prevalence of youth with nonmedical prescription opioid use in 2025 could still be reduced by 21% compared to the model using the Ontario school closure timeline without any intervention (See Figure A5).

4. Discussion

This simulation demonstrates that public health orders mandating in-person school closures may have had direct and indirect effects on youth opioid use during and after school closure. Limited in-person social interaction changes the circumstances surrounding youth, resulting in unintended consequences on risk factors for opioid use. The simulation illustrates that the pervasiveness of unsafely stored opioids in homes and limited in-person social interaction with anti-drug peers could facilitate the initiation of opioid use among youth. However, decreasing social events for recreational drug use, the absence of peers who might encourage taking certain risks [76], and the negative effect of withdrawal symptoms limit the increase of opioid use further during in-person school closures. The lifting of in-person school closures may lead to a high increase in the prevalence of youth engaged in nonmedical prescription opioid use. The "rebound" effect on the prevalence of nonmedical prescription opioid use after in-person school closures end could occur for several reasons. One possible explanation is that when in-person school closures end, youths may be more likely to come into contact with peers who use drugs. These social networks can play an important role in shaping youth drug use behaviors. The increased socialization that occurs when school is in person can expose young people to a higher risk of peer pressure and influence, which could lead to an increase in drug use. The literature also argues the plausibility that ongoing effects of the COVID-19 pandemic in North America will place youth at a greater risk for nonmedical prescription opioid use [15,77,78]. Factors outside the scope of the model may have influenced such effects in either direction. For example, while family members staying home from work may have restricted youth access to opioids in some households, in some settings, the consequences of concurrent parental unemployment and spending more time at home and witnessing possible elevated levels of family member substance use [19] may put youth at a higher risk for opioid use.

The simulation outcomes demonstrate that interventions that decrease youth exposure to prescription opioids in the home context could constitute an effective intervention pathway to mitigate what could be a significant increase in youth opioid use following the lifting of in-person school closures. Interventions targeting associated risk factors for youth exposure to prescription opioids at home can be beneficial whenever they come into effect, whether before or during in-person school closures; while the benefits secured by intervention at those times are particularly pronounced, later implementations will also help mitigate what could constitute a significant increase in youth opioid use.

The findings from this study should be interpreted within the context of the following limitations. First, the current approach focuses specifically on the in-person peer socialization component of the peer influence process; this work therefore does not consider either peer selection or online peer socialization, which may influence regular substance use among youth [79,80]. Instead, our goal was to identify the extent to which lack of in-person peer socialization as a result of in-person school closures could plausibly influence nonmedical opioid use among youth. Second, research indicates that youth consumption of prescription opioids may be mediated by anxiety and hopelessness [81], as contributed to by the adverse psychological impacts on youth from the pandemic compounded by in-person school closures and isolation from peers. Since this study focused on the sociological aspect of substance use in particular, future research could study psychological factors which may have a reinforcing effect on youth drug use. Third, the current modeling analysis does not explicitly track the effect of opioid tolerance and possible overdoses on later opioid use among youth. Fourth, the current level of model abstraction filtered out some less-essential details for youth within the model, such as youth siblings, youth year in school, and disconnection from peers after school. Finally, exploring alternative network structures and theories of opinion dynamics among youth in future agent-based modeling studies may be worthwhile. Of particular note, more extensive national data on youth opioid use would especially inform the model parameterization and assumptions, support testing the plausibility of model baseline scenario outcomes, and support critical evaluation of the current conclusions.

Despite these limitations, identifying a potential increase in the prevalence of youth with nonmedical prescription opioid use after the lifting of in-person school closures suggests the importance of effective opioid surveillance, and awareness and availability of naloxone and treatment options to prevent serious medical outcomes and death in this vulnerable population. Furthermore, efforts to encourage new opioid packaging, such as personalized pill dispensers, may lower the accessibility of incompletely dispensed prescription opioids. It should be noted that a disruption to the supply of opioids from home should be combined with supporting and promoting awareness of the risks of opioid abuse amongst youth.

Author Contributions: Conceptualization, N.S. and N.D.O.; methodology, N.S. and N.D.O.; software, N.S.; validation, N.S. and N.D.O.; formal analysis, N.S.; writing—original draft preparation, N.S.; writing—review and editing, N.S. and N.D.O.; visualization, N.S.; supervision, N.D.O. All authors have read and agreed to the published version of the manuscript.

Funding: This research received no external funding.

Data Availability Statement: The data presented in this study are openly available at www.camh.ca/osduhs (accessed on 22 January 2023). The implemented model can be found at https://doi.org/10.5281/zenodo.7559419.

Conflicts of Interest: The authors declare no conflict of interest.

Appendix A

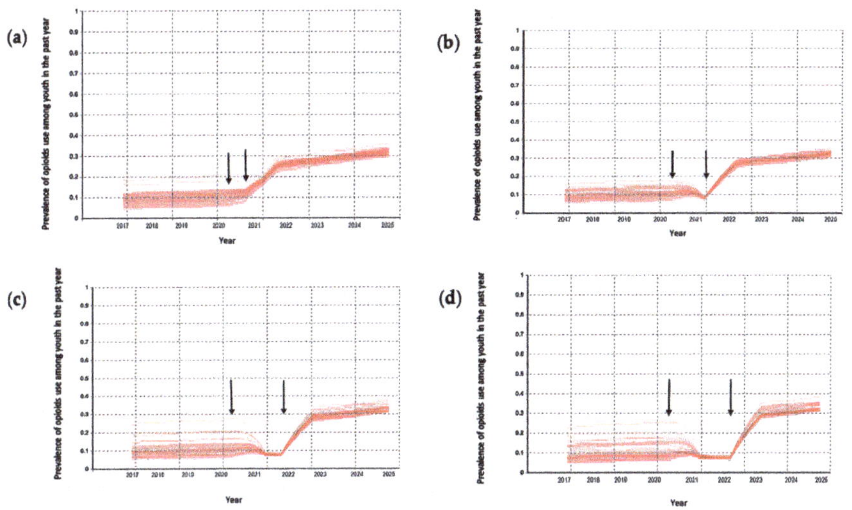

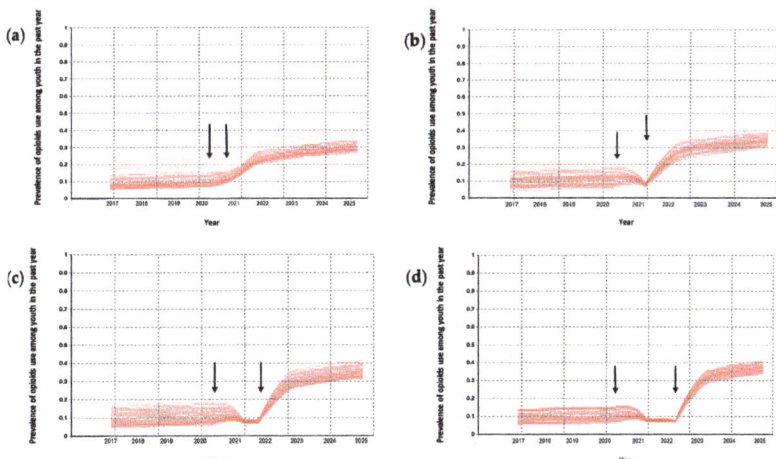

Figure A1. Model-generated prevalence of youth with nonmedical prescription opioid use in the past year for the different durations of in-person school closures (**a–d**). The model predicted the prevalence of youth with nonmedical prescription opioid use in the past year for (**a**) 6-month in-person school closures, (**b**) 12-month in-person school closures, (**c**) 18-month in-person school closures, and (**d**) 24-month in-person school closures. In-person socialization following the lifting of in-person school closures is characterized as a Moore neighborhood of range 1. The two vertical arrows represent the start and end of the in-person school closures for each panel, respectively.

Figure A2. Model-generated prevalence of youth with nonmedical prescription opioid use in the past year for the different durations of in-person school closures (**a–d**). The model predicted the prevalence of youth with nonmedical prescription opioid use in the past year for (**a**) 6-month in-person school closures, (**b**) 12-month in-person school closures, (**c**) 18-month in-person school closures, and (**d**) 24-month in-person school closures. In-person socialization following the lifting of in-person school closures is characterized as a Moore neighborhood of range 2. The two vertical arrows represent the start and end of the in-person school closures for each panel, respectively.

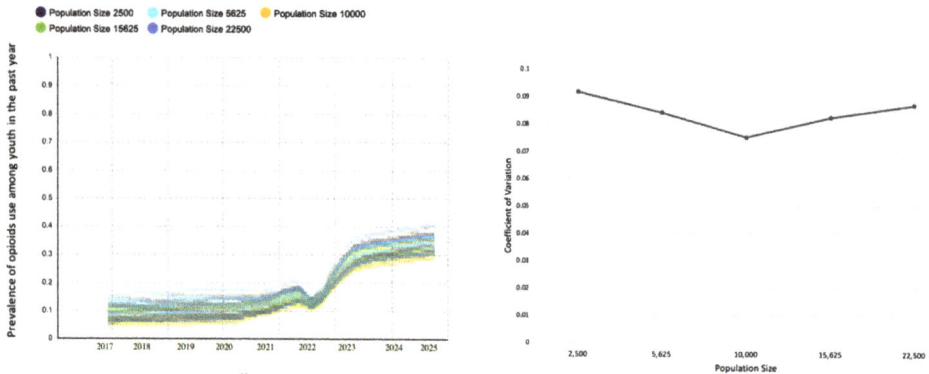

Figure A3. Model-generated prevalence of youth with nonmedical prescription opioid use in the past year (left-hand side) and coefficient of variation for simulation means and standard deviation in 2025 (right-hand side) of the baseline scenario under different population sizes.

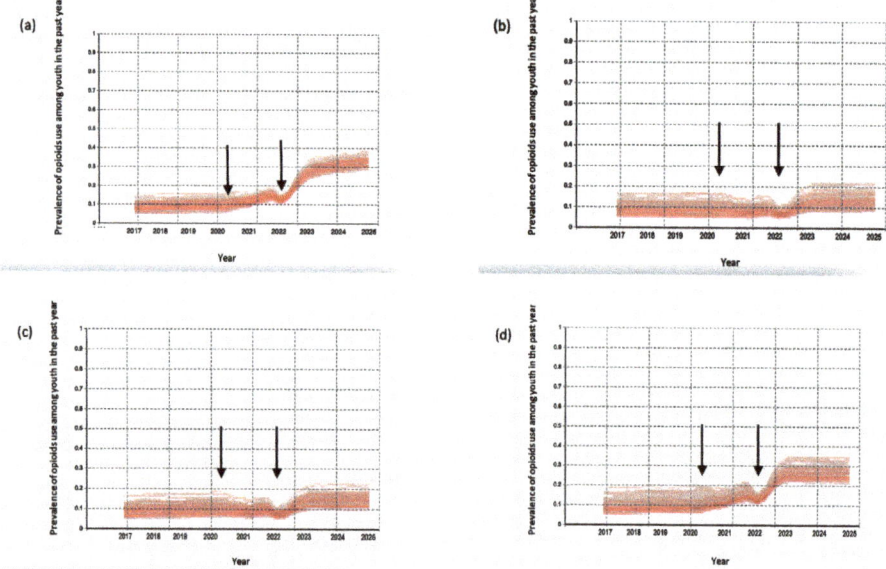

Figure A4. Model-generated prevalence of youth exhibiting nonmedical prescription opioid use in the past year for the baseline scenario (**a**) and after applying safe storage intervention with a decrease of 50% in youth exposure to prescription opioids at home beginning at different time points (**b**–**d**). The two vertical black arrows represent the start and end of the Ontario school closure timeline. (**a**) Model-generated prevalence of youth exhibiting nonmedical prescription opioid use in the past year for the baseline scenario. (**b**) Model-generated prevalence of youth exhibiting nonmedical prescription opioid use in the past year after applying safe storage in 2017. (**c**) Model-generated prevalence of youth exhibiting nonmedical prescription opioid use in the past year after applying safe storage at the beginning of the general COVID-19-related in-person school closures on 14 March 2020. (**d**) Model-generated prevalence of youth exhibiting nonmedical prescription opioid use in the past year after applying safe storage at the start of the 2022–2023 academic year.

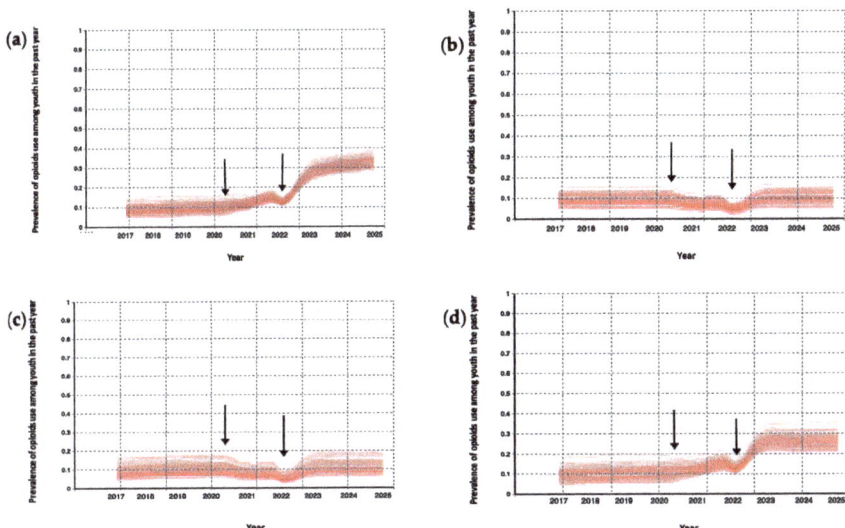

Figure A5. Model-generated prevalence of youth exhibiting nonmedical prescription opioid use in the past year for the baseline scenario (**a**) and after applying safe storage intervention with a decrease of 80% in youth exposure to prescription opioids at home beginning at different time points (**b**–**d**). The two vertical black arrows represent the start and end of the Ontario school closure timeline. (**a**) Model-generated prevalence of youth exhibiting nonmedical prescription opioid use in the past year for the baseline scenario. (**b**) Model-generated prevalence of youth exhibiting nonmedical prescription opioid use in the past year after applying safe storage in 2017. (**c**) Model-generated prevalence of youth exhibiting nonmedical prescription opioid use in the past year after applying safe storage at the beginning of the general COVID-19-related in-person school closures on 14 March 2020. (**d**) Model-generated prevalence of youth exhibiting nonmedical prescription opioid use in the past year after applying safe storage at the start of the 2022–2023 academic year.

Table A1. Parameters, values, and references.

Parameter	Values	References
Youth population size	10,000	Assumed
Total number of family	10,000	Assumed
Family size	Poisson probability distribution	Assumed [66]
Moore neighborhood range	0–3	Assumed
Rate of opioid prescription for each family member without prescription opioids (1/week)	0.003	Calibrated [67]
Probability that the duration of the opioid prescription ends for each family member (1/week)	0.02	Calibrated [67]
Level of youth exposure to prescription opioids at home	Uniform distribution between 450 and 900	Calibrated [61,62]
Percentage of the socio-cultural environment with a positive drug use view	14%	Calibrated [61,62]
Level of drug promotion inside the drug-positive socio-cultural environment	Uniform distribution between 1 and 1500	Calibrated [61,62]
Initial amount of encountering drug use situations for youth	Lognormal distribution	Calibrated [61,62]
Encountering drug use situations coefficient for different level of socialization among youth	Lognormal distribution	Calibrated [61,62]

Table A1. *Cont.*

Parameter	Values	References
Level of supportiveness for peers	Uniform distribution between 0 and 100	Assumed [23,58]
Level of persuasiveness for peers	Uniform distribution between 0 and 100	Assumed [23,58]
Severity of acute withdrawal from nonmedical opioid use	Lognormal distribution	Calibrated [71]
Probability that peers share drugs with peers who request it	0.075	Calibrated [61,62]

References

1. Dash, G.F.; Holt, L.; Kenyon, E.A.; Carter, E.K.; Ho, D.; Hudson, K.A.; Ewing, S.W.F. Detection of Vaping, Cannabis Use, and Hazardous Prescription Opioid Use among Adolescents. *Lancet Child Adolesc. Health* **2022**, *6*, 820–828. [CrossRef] [PubMed]
2. Degenhardt, L.; Stockings, E.; Patton, G.; Hall, W.D.; Lynskey, M. The Increasing Global Health Priority of Substance Use in Young People. *Lancet Psychiatry* **2016**, *3*, 251–264. [CrossRef] [PubMed]
3. Dembo, R.; Blount, W.R.; Schmeidler, J.; Burgos, W. Perceived Environmental Drug Use Risk and the Correlates of Early Drug Use or Nonuse among Inner-City Youths: The Motivated Actor. *Int. J. Addict.* **1986**, *21*, 977–1000. [CrossRef] [PubMed]
4. Rhodes, T.; Lilly, R.; Fernández, C.; Giorgino, E.; Kemmesis, U.E.; Ossebaard, H.C.; Lalam, N.; Faasen, I.; Spannow, K.E. Risk Factors Associated with Drug Use: The Importance of 'Risk Environment'. *Drugs Educ. Prev. Policy* **2003**, *10*, 303–329. [CrossRef]
5. Bauman, K.E.; Ennett, S.T. On the Importance of Peer Influence for Adolescent Drug Use: Commonly Neglected Considerations. *Addiction* **1996**, *91*, 185–198. [CrossRef]
6. Kobus, K. Peers and Adolescent Smoking. *Addiction* **2003**, *98*, 37–55. [CrossRef]
7. Montgomery, S.C.; Donnelly, M.; Bhatnagar, P.; Carlin, A.; Kee, F.; Hunter, R.F. Peer Social Network Processes and Adolescent Health Behaviors: A Systematic Review. *Prev. Med.* **2020**, *130*, 105900. [CrossRef]
8. Salmanzadeh, H.; Ahmadi-Soleimani, S.M.; Pachenari, N.; Azadi, M.; Halliwell, R.F.; Rubino, T.; Azizi, H. Adolescent Drug Exposure: A Review of Evidence for the Development of Persistent Changes in Brain Function. *Brain Res. Bull.* **2020**, *156*, 105–117. [CrossRef]
9. Kandel, D.B.; Yamaguchi, K.; Chen, K. Stages of Progression in Drug Involvement from Adolescence to Adulthood: Further Evidence for the Gateway Theory. *J. Stud. Alcohol* **1992**, *53*, 447–457. [CrossRef]
10. Probst, C.; Elton-Marshall, T.; Imtiaz, S.; Patte, K.A.; Rehm, J.; Sornpaisarn, B.; Leatherdale, S.T. A Supportive School Environment May Reduce the Risk of Non-Medical Prescription Opioid Use Due to Impaired Mental Health among Students. *Eur. Child Adolesc. Psychiatry* **2021**, *30*, 293–301. [CrossRef]
11. Silverman, M.; Sibbald, R.; Stranges, S. Ethics of COVID-19-Related School Closures. *Can. J. Public Health* **2020**, *111*, 462–465. [CrossRef] [PubMed]
12. Gallagher-Mackay, K.; Srivastava, P.; Underwood, K.; Dhuey, E.; McCready, L.; Born, K.; Maltsev, A.; Perkhun, A.; Steiner, R.; Barrett, K. COVID-19 and Education Disruption in Ontario: Emerging Evidence on Impacts. Available online: https://scholars.wlu.ca/laso_faculty/1 (accessed on 22 January 2023).
13. Bialystok, L. Education after COVID. *Philos. Inq. Educ.* **2022**, *29*, 1–4. [CrossRef]
14. Halsall, T.; Mahmoud, K.; Iyer, S.N.; Orpana, H.; Zeni, M.; Matheson, K. Implications of Time and Space Factors Related with Youth Substance Use Prevention: A Conceptual Review and Case Study of the Icelandic Prevention Model Being Implemented in the Context of the COVID-19 Pandemic. *Int. J. Qual. Stud. Health Well-Being* **2023**, *18*, 2149097. [CrossRef]
15. Jayasinha, R.; Nairn, S.; Conrod, P. A Dangerous "Cocktail": The COVID-19 Pandemic and the Youth Opioid Crisis in North America: A Response to Vigo et al.(2020). *Can. J. Psychiatry* **2020**, *65*, 692–694. [CrossRef] [PubMed]
16. de Vaan, M.; Stuart, T. Does Intra-Household Contagion Cause an Increase in Prescription Opioid Use? *Am. Sociol. Rev.* **2019**, *84*, 577–608. [CrossRef]
17. Nguyen, A.P.; Glanz, J.M.; Narwaney, K.J.; Binswanger, I.A. Association of Opioids Prescribed to Family Members with Opioid Overdose among Adolescents and Young Adults. *JAMA Netw. Open* **2020**, *3*, e201018. [CrossRef] [PubMed]
18. Binswanger, I.A.; Glanz, J.M. Pharmaceutical Opioids in the Home and Youth: Implications for Adult Medical Practice. *Subst. Abus.* **2015**, *36*, 141–143. [CrossRef] [PubMed]
19. Griesler, P.C.; Hu, M.-C.; Wall, M.M.; Kandel, D.B. Nonmedical Prescription Opioid Use by Parents and Adolescents in the US. *Pediatrics* **2019**, *143*, e20182354. [CrossRef]
20. Calina, D.; Hartung, T.; Mardare, I.; Mitroi, M.; Poulas, K.; Tsatsakis, A.; Rogoveanu, I.; Docea, A.O. COVID-19 Pandemic and Alcohol Consumption: Impacts and Interconnections. *Toxicol. Rep.* **2021**, *8*, 529–535. [CrossRef]
21. Gohari, M.R.; Varatharajan, T.; MacKillop, J.; Leatherdale, S.T. Examining the Impact of the COVID-19 Pandemic on Youth Alcohol Consumption: Longitudinal Changes from Pre-to Intra-Pandemic Drinking in the COMPASS Study. *J. Adolesc. Health* **2022**, *71*, 665–672. [CrossRef]
22. Osborne, V.; Serdarevic, M.; Crooke, H.; Striley, C.; Cottler, L.B. Non-Medical Opioid Use in Youth: Gender Differences in Risk Factors and Prevalence. *Addict. Behav.* **2017**, *72*, 114–119. [CrossRef] [PubMed]

23. Valente, T.W.; Hoffman, B.R.; Ritt-Olson, A.; Lichtman, K.; Johnson, C.A. Effects of a Social-Network Method for Group Assignment Strategies on Peer-Led Tobacco Prevention Programs in Schools. *Am. J. Public Health* **2003**, *93*, 1837–1843. [CrossRef] [PubMed]
24. Valente, T.W.; Gallaher, P.; Mouttapa, M. Using Social Networks to Understand and Prevent Substance Use: A Transdisciplinary Perspective. *Subst. Use Misuse* **2004**, *39*, 1685–1712. [CrossRef] [PubMed]
25. Ennett, S.T.; Bauman, K.E.; Hussong, A.; Faris, R.; Foshee, V.A.; Cai, L.; DuRant, R.H. The Peer Context of Adolescent Substance Use: Findings from Social Network Analysis. *J. Res. Adolesc.* **2006**, *16*, 159–186. [CrossRef]
26. Michell, M.P. Smoke Rings: Social Network Analysis of Friendship Groups, Smoking and Drug-Taking. *Drugs Educ. Prev. Policy* **2000**, *7*, 21–37. [CrossRef]
27. Jackson, J.C.; Rand, D.; Lewis, K.; Norton, M.I.; Gray, K. Agent-Based Modeling: A Guide for Social Psychologists. *Soc. Psychol. Personal. Sci.* **2017**, *8*, 387–395. [CrossRef]
28. Macy, M.W.; Willer, R. From Factors to Actors: Computational Sociology and Agent-Based Modeling. *Annu. Rev. Sociol.* **2002**, *28*, 143–166. [CrossRef]
29. Agar, M. My Kingdom for a Function: Modeling Misadventures of the Innumerate. *J. Artif. Soc. Soc. Simul.* **2003**, *6*, 1–8.
30. Agar, M. Agents in Living Color: Towards Emic Agent-Based Models. *J. Artif. Soc. Soc. Simul.* **2005**, *8*, 4.
31. Garrison, L.A.; Babcock, D.S. Alcohol Consumption among College Students: An Agent-based Computational Simulation. *Complexity* **2009**, *14*, 35–44. [CrossRef]
32. Lamy, F.; Bossomaier, T.; Perez, P. An Ontologic Agent-Based Model of Recreational Polydrug Use: SimUse. *Int. J. Simul. Process Model.* **2015**, *10*, 207–222. [CrossRef]
33. Agar, M.H.; Wilson, D. Drugmart: Heroin Epidemics as Complex Adaptive Systems. *Complexity* **2002**, *7*, 44–52. [CrossRef]
34. Perez, P.; Dray, A.; Moore, D.; Dietze, P.; Bammer, G.; Jenkinson, R.; Siokou, C.; Green, R.; Hudson, S.L.; Maher, L. SimAmph: An Agent-Based Simulation Model for Exploring the Use of Psychostimulants and Related Harm amongst Young Australians. *Int. J. Drug Policy* **2012**, *23*, 62–71. [CrossRef]
35. Agar, M.; Reisinger, H.S. Using Trend Theory to Explain Heroin Use Trends. *J. Psychoact. Drugs* **2001**, *33*, 203–211. [CrossRef]
36. Di Clemente, R.; Pietronero, L. Statistical Agent Based Modelization of the Phenomenon of Drug Abuse. *Sci. Rep.* **2012**, *2*, 532. [CrossRef]
37. Coates, A.; Han, L.; Kleerekoper, A. A Unified Framework for Opinion Dynamics. In Proceedings of the 17th International Conference on Autonomous Agents and Multiagent Systems, International Foundation for Autonomous Agents and Multiagent Systems, Stockholm, Sweden, 10–15 July 2018.
38. Grabisch, M.; Rusinowska, A. A Survey on Nonstrategic Models of Opinion Dynamics. *Games* **2020**, *11*, 65. [CrossRef]
39. Anderson, B.D.; Ye, M. Recent Advances in the Modelling and Analysis of Opinion Dynamics on Influence Networks. *Int. J. Autom. Comput.* **2019**, *16*, 129–149. [CrossRef]
40. Sun, R.; Mendez, D. An Application of the Continuous Opinions and Discrete Actions (CODA) Model to Adolescent Smoking Initiation. *PLoS ONE* **2017**, *12*, e0186163. [CrossRef]
41. Moore, T.W.; Finley, P.D.; Apelberg, B.J.; Ambrose, B.K.; Brodsky, N.S.; Brown, T.J.; Husten, C.; Glass, R.J. An Opinion-Driven Behavioral Dynamics Model for Addictive Behaviors. *Eur. Phys. J. B* **2015**, *88*, 1–28. [CrossRef]
42. Clifford, P.; Sudbury, A. A Model for Spatial Conflict. *Biometrika* **1973**, *60*, 581. [CrossRef]
43. Castellano, C.; Muñoz, M.A.; Pastor-Satorras, R. Nonlinear Q-Voter Model. *Phys. Rev. E* **2009**, *80*, 041129. [CrossRef] [PubMed]
44. Castellano, C.; Loreto, V.; Barrat, A.; Cecconi, F.; Parisi, D. Comparison of Voter and Glauber Ordering Dynamics on Networks. *Phys. Rev. E* **2005**, *71*, 066107. [CrossRef] [PubMed]
45. Mobilia, M. Does a Single Zealot Affect an Infinite Group of Voters? *Phys. Rev. Lett.* **2003**, *91*, 028701. [CrossRef]
46. Malik, N.; Mucha, P.J. Role of Social Environment and Social Clustering in Spread of Opinions in Coevolving Networks. *Chaos Interdiscip. J. Nonlinear Sci.* **2013**, *23*, 043123. [CrossRef] [PubMed]
47. Krapivsky, P.L.; Redner, S. Dynamics of Majority Rule in Two-State Interacting Spin Systems. *Phys. Rev. Lett.* **2003**, *90*, 238701. [CrossRef]
48. Galam, S. Minority Opinion Spreading in Random Geometry. *Eur. Phys. J. B-Condens. Matter Complex Syst.* **2002**, *25*, 403–406. [CrossRef]
49. Sznajd-Weron, K.; Sznajd, J. Opinion Evolution in Closed Community. *Int. J. Mod. Phys. C* **2000**, *11*, 1157–1165. [CrossRef]
50. Sznajd-Weron, K.; Sznajd, J.; Weron, T. A Review on the Sznajd Model—20 Years After. *Phys. A: Stat. Mech. Its Appl.* **2021**, *565*, 125537. [CrossRef]
51. Sznajd-Weron, K. Sznajd Model and Its Applications. *arXiv* **2005**, arXiv:physics/0503239.
52. Deffuant, G.; Amblard, F.; Weisbuch, G.; Faure, T. How Can Extremism Prevail? A Study Based on the Relative Agreement Interaction Model. *J. Artif. Soc. Soc. Simul.* **2002**, *5*, 4.
53. Deffuant, G.; Neau, D.; Amblard, F.; Weisbuch, G. Mixing Beliefs among Interacting Agents. *Adv. Complex Syst.* **2001**, *3*, 87–98. [CrossRef]
54. Martins, A.C. Continuous Opinions and Discrete Actions in Opinion Dynamics Problems. *Int. J. Mod. Phys. C* **2008**, *19*, 617–624. [CrossRef]
55. Fan, K.; Pedrycz, W. Emergence and Spread of Extremist Opinions. *Phys. A Stat. Mech. Its Appl.* **2015**, *436*, 87–97. [CrossRef]

56. Martins, A.C.; Kuba, C.D. The Importance of Disagreeing: Contrarians and Extremism in the Coda Model. *Adv. Complex Syst.* **2010**, *13*, 621–634. [CrossRef]
57. Latané, B. The Psychology of Social Impact. *Am. Psychol.* **1981**, *36*, 343. [CrossRef]
58. Nowak, A.; Szamrej, J.; Latané, B. From Private Attitude to Public Opinion: A Dynamic Theory of Social Impact. *Psychol. Rev.* **1990**, *97*, 362. [CrossRef]
59. Castellano, C.; Fortunato, S.; Loreto, V. Statistical Physics of Social Dynamics. *Rev. Mod. Phys.* **2009**, *81*, 591. [CrossRef]
60. Hołyst, J.A.; Kacperski, K.; Schweitzer, F. Social Impact Models of Opinion Dynamics. *Annu. Rev. Comput. Phys.* **2001**, 253–273. [CrossRef]
61. Boak, A.; Elton-Marshall, T.; Mann, R.E.; Hamilton, H.A. *Drug Use among Ontario Students, 1977–2019: Detailed Findings from the Ontario Student Drug Use and Health Survey (OSDUHS)*; Centre for Addiction and Mental Health: Toronto, ON, Canada, 2020.
62. Boak, A.; Elton-Marshall, T.; Hamilton, H.A. *The Well-Being of Ontario Students: Findings from the 2021 Ontario Student Drug Use and Health Survey (OSDUHS)*; Centre for Addiction and Mental Health: Toronto, ON, Canada, 2022.
63. Berryman, M. Review of Software Platforms for Agent Based Models. Available online: https://citeseerx.ist.psu.edu/document?repid=rep1&type=pdf&doi=f3acb55df14e3e83f60bb14f067f5fcb5afc97d1 (accessed on 22 January 2023).
64. Nikolai, C.; Madey, G. Tools of the Trade: A Survey of Various Agent Based Modeling Platforms. *J. Artif. Soc. Soc. Simul.* **2009**, *12*, 2.
65. Borshchev, A. *The Big Book of Simulation Modeling: Multimethod Modeling with AnyLogic 6*; AnyLogic: New York, NY, USA, 2013; ISBN 0-9895731-7-6.
66. Average Number of People per Family in Canada in 2019, by Province. Available online: https://www.statista.com/statistics/478954/average-family-size-in-canada-by-province/ (accessed on 22 January 2023).
67. Carrière, G.; Garner, R.; Sanmartin, C. Significant Factors Associated with Problematic Use of Opioid Pain Relief Medications among the Household Population, Canada, 2018. *Health Rep.* **2021**, *32*, 11–26.
68. Sharma, B.; Bruner, A.; Barnett, G.; Fishman, M. Opioid Use Disorders. *Child Adolesc. Psychiatr. Clin.* **2016**, *25*, 473–487. [CrossRef] [PubMed]
69. Branstetter, S.A.; Low, S.; Furman, W. The Influence of Parents and Friends on Adolescent Substance Use: A Multidimensional Approach. *J. Subst. Use* **2011**, *16*, 150–160. [CrossRef] [PubMed]
70. Mansouri, A.; Taghiyareh, F. Effect of Segregation on the Dynamics of Noise-Free Social Impact Model of Opinion Formation through Agent-Based Modeling. *Int. J. Web Res.* **2019**, *2*, 36–44.
71. Lerner, A.; Klein, M. Dependence, Withdrawal and Rebound of CNS Drugs: An Update and Regulatory Considerations for New Drugs Development. *Brain Commun.* **2019**, *1*, fcz025. [CrossRef] [PubMed]
72. Bordogna, C.M.; Albano, E.V. Dynamic Behavior of a Social Model for Opinion Formation. *Phys. Rev. E* **2007**, *76*, 061125. [CrossRef]
73. Hołyst, J.A.; Kacperski, K.; Schweitzer, F. Phase Transitions in Social Impact Models of Opinion Formation. *Phys. A Stat. Mech. Its Appl.* **2000**, *285*, 199–210. [CrossRef]
74. Cooley, P.; Solano, E. Agent-Based Model (ABM) Validation Considerations. In Proceedings of the Third International Conference on Advances in System Simulation (SIMUL 2011), Barcelona, Spain, 23–29 October 2011; pp. 134–139.
75. Sayama, H. *Introduction to the Modeling and Analysis of Complex Systems*; Open SUNY Textbooks: Albany, NY, USA, 2015.
76. Andrews, J.L.; Foulkes, L.; Blakemore, S.-J. Peer Influence in Adolescence: Public-Health Implications for COVID-19. *Trends Cogn. Sci.* **2020**, *24*, 585–587. [CrossRef]
77. Cho, J.; Bello, M.S.; Christie, N.C.; Monterosso, J.R.; Leventhal, A.M. Adolescent Emotional Disorder Symptoms and Transdiagnostic Vulnerabilities as Predictors of Young Adult Substance Use during the COVID-19 Pandemic: Mediation by Substance-Related Coping Behaviors. *Cogn. Behav. Ther.* **2021**, *50*, 276–294. [CrossRef]
78. Pelham III, W.E.; Tapert, S.F.; Gonzalez, M.R.; McCabe, C.J.; Lisdahl, K.M.; Alzueta, E.; Baker, F.C.; Breslin, F.J.; Dick, A.S.; Dowling, G.J. Early Adolescent Substance Use before and during the COVID-19 Pandemic: A Longitudinal Survey in the ABCD Study Cohort. *J. Adolesc. Health* **2021**, *69*, 390–397. [CrossRef]
79. Miller, B.L.; Lowe, C.C.; Kaakinen, M.; Savolainen, I.; Sirola, A.; Stogner, J.; Ellonen, N.; Oksanen, A. Online Peers and Offline Highs: An Examination of Online Peer Groups, Social Media Homophily, and Substance Use. *J. Psychoact. Drugs* **2021**, *53*, 345–354. [CrossRef]
80. Huang, G.C.; Unger, J.B.; Soto, D.; Fujimoto, K.; Pentz, M.A.; Jordan-Marsh, M.; Valente, T.W. Peer Influences: The Impact of Online and Offline Friendship Networks on Adolescent Smoking and Alcohol Use. *J. Adolesc. Health* **2014**, *54*, 508–514. [CrossRef] [PubMed]
81. Nairn, S.A.; Audet, M.; Stewart, S.H.; Hawke, L.D.; Isaacs, J.Y.; Henderson, J.; Saah, R.; Knight, R.; Fast, D.; Khan, F. Interventions to Reduce Opioid Use in Youth At-Risk and in Treatment for Substance Use Disorders: A Scoping Review. *Can. J. Psychiatry* **2022**, 07067437221089810. [CrossRef] [PubMed]

Disclaimer/Publisher's Note: The statements, opinions and data contained in all publications are solely those of the individual author(s) and contributor(s) and not of MDPI and/or the editor(s). MDPI and/or the editor(s) disclaim responsibility for any injury to people or property resulting from any ideas, methods, instructions or products referred to in the content.

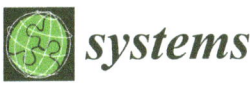 systems

Article

Simulation-Based Assessment of Cholera Epidemic Response: A Case Study of Al-Hudaydah, Yemen

Pei Shan Loo [1,2], Anaely Aguiar [1] and Birgit Kopainsky [1,*]

1 System Dynamics Group, University of Bergen, NO-5020 Bergen, Norway
2 Health Systems and Policies Group, Swiss Tropical and Public Health Institute, 4123 Allschwil, Switzerland
* Correspondence: birgit.kopainsky@uib.no

Abstract: Cholera kills between 21,000 and 143,000 people globally each year. It is often fatal, killing up to 50% of the severely symptomatic patients; but death by cholera is preventable with timely treatment, so that the fatality rate can drop to less than 1%. Due to cholera's multi-pathway transmission, a multifaceted and multi-sectoral approach to combat this disease is needed. Such complexity gives rise to uncertainty about where it is best to intervene, as stakeholders have to balance prevention and treatment under highly constrained resources. Using Al-Hudaydah, Yemen as a case study, this paper demonstrates how a system dynamics model can be built using a classic infection structure with empirically grounded operational structures: health treatment, water, sanitation, and hygiene (WASH), vaccination, and a data surveillance system. The model explores the implications of the joint interventions with different start times. The model analysis revealed that the historical interventions likely prevented 55% more deaths in 2017 as compared to a counterfactual business-as-usual scenario with no interventions in the past. At the same time, some 40% of deaths could potentially have been prevented if interventions (with the same resources as historical data) had been initiated earlier in April 2017. Further research will explore each intervention impact for more detailed policy analysis and simulations into the future.

Keywords: cholera response; system dynamics; computational modeling; cholera epidemics; policy testing; humanitarian response

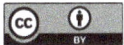

Citation: Loo, P.S.; Aguiar, A.; Kopainsky, B. Simulation-Based Assessment of Cholera Epidemic Response: A Case Study of Al-Hudaydah, Yemen. *Systems* **2023**, *11*, 3. https://doi.org/10.3390/systems11010003

Academic Editor: William T. Scherer

Received: 30 October 2022
Revised: 4 December 2022
Accepted: 6 December 2022
Published: 21 December 2022

Copyright: © 2022 by the authors. Licensee MDPI, Basel, Switzerland. This article is an open access article distributed under the terms and conditions of the Creative Commons Attribution (CC BY) license (https://creativecommons.org/licenses/by/4.0/).

1. Introduction

Cholera is an acute diarrheal infection caused by consuming food or water contaminated with the bacterium *Vibrio cholerae* [1,2]. *Vibrio cholerae* causes profuse watery diarrhea and vomiting that can quickly progress to dehydration and hypovolemic shock, killing up to 50% of patients who do not receive adequate rehydration [1]. Even healthy people can die within hours if they develop severe cholera symptoms. Conversely, if symptomatic individuals receive healthcare treatment in time, the case fatality rate can be less than 1%.

Cholera treatment, control, and prevention are the responsibility of national government health ministries and non-governmental organizations (NGOs) [3–5]. Once cases are identified, interventions to control and prevent cholera include surveillance and case management (treatment), water, sanitation, and hygiene (WASH) interventions, provision of oral cholera vaccinations, and strengthening education programs [1,6,7].

While universal access to clean water and sanitation is the long-term solution to cholera, this is typically linked with the country's economic and political development; and is therefore vulnerable to environmental and humanitarian crises [5]. WHO [7] reported 2.5 million suspected cholera cases and nearly 4000 deaths in Yemen as of November 2020. Figure 1 illustrates the cholera epidemic prevalence from 2017 to 2018 and first oral cholera vaccination campaign in Al-Hudaydah, Yemen. The literature identifies two groups of problems that allowed an epidemic of this magnitude to occur: Yemen's precarious conditions and the humanitarian response.

Yemen has been devastated by a complex civil war [5,8]. It was classified as a level 3 emergency by the United Nations (UN) in 2015, triggering the highest level of resource mobilization across the humanitarian system [5]. By 2016, only 46% of all healthcare facilities remained operational. In addition to severely damaged water and sewage infrastructure, the dire situation has been exacerbated by a lack of energy—mainly electricity and fuel, spare parts, operating and maintenance funds, and three years of unpaid civil servants [3,5,8,9].

Furthermore, most civilians' movements are confined by the ongoing conflicts; and food insecurity has put more than half of the population at risk of famine. Yemen has the highest number of people in need of humanitarian assistance of any country. On 28 September 2016, a large-scale cholera epidemic began and the number of people in need of humanitarian assistance and protection reached as high as 20 million in 2017 [10].

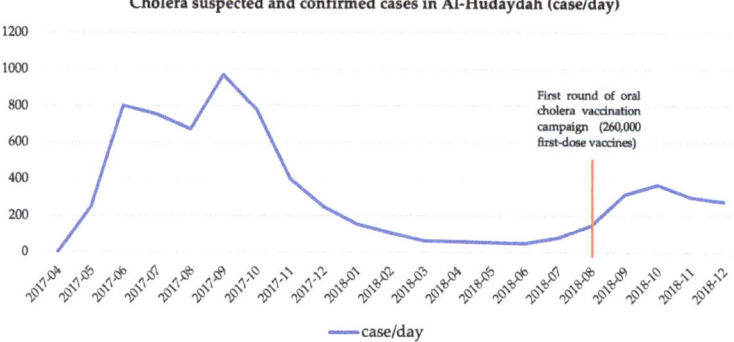

Figure 1. Timeline of key events in Al-Hudaydah Yemen cholera epidemic from 2016 to 2018, daily number of cases [5,11,12].

Lessons learned from Yemen's cholera response are well documented, reporting that Yemen lacked an adequate cholera preparedness and response plan, despite previous outbreaks, regional endemicity, and active conflict [3,5,9,13,14]. The key questions revolve around: How can the recommendation be implemented? How does one actualize what ought to be done into how and when it can be done? Previous studies concluded that the delayed response was due to two factors.

First, multi-sector coordination structures were confused, with the roles of the clusters, cholera task force, and incident management system either overlapping or incompletely developed. Lack of coordination across these areas hampered management, technical output, and agency trust [3–5,8,14].

Second, a lack of a functioning surveillance system, hence, a lack of data. Despite that, policy decisions must be made, frequently under high uncertainty and pressure conditions, especially when the fatality rate is high. Where a lack of data makes precise predictions impossible, simulation models may still provide valuable insights to aid decision-making under unknown circumstances. Such scientifically informed exploration can add clarity to decisions, allowing for more effective policy choices.

From the simulation model literature review, Barciela et al. [15] developed a Cholera Risk Model (CRM) for cholera control in Yemen, specifically on WASH interventions. It is a predictive tool that integrates data on rainfall, temperature, and water security to determine the risk of cholera trigger and transmission. Harpring et al. [4] use a causal loop diagram to visualize the compounding factors influencing the cholera outbreak in Yemen. Along with the susceptible, infected, and recovered (SIR) dynamics, they discovered a strong connection between humanitarian response and the existing infrastructure development to the cholera epidemic. Pruyt [16] developed a cholera epidemic System Dynamics (SD) model for Zimbabwe that tested two policies: sanitary infrastructure and health services.

The model uses percentage change on these two policy parameters instead of detailed operational policy structures.

On the other hand, ordinary differential equation (ODE) cholera models were reviewed and half of them contain only SIR model structure [17]. The other half of cholera transmission models included a maximum of three interventions focusing mainly on vaccination, antibiotics, and water provision. None of the reviewed models include structures of both asymptomatic and symptomatic individuals as well as sanitation intervention (sewage system) and health services.

With the dynamic complexity of cholera control and death reduction, a multifaceted approach is crucial. To address the identified research gaps above, this paper aims to demonstrate how operational policy structures are built upon a system dynamics classic infection model to explore the impact of the interventions. In other words, the present model bridges the endogenous feedback mechanisms that drive both symptomatic and asymptomatic cholera infectious dynamics, with the empirically grounded operational structures: oral rehydration corner, diarrhea treatment center, water, sanitation and hygiene (WASH), vaccination, and data surveillance system.

2. Materials and Methods

System Dynamics (SD) uses computer simulation for policy analysis and design. Its origins are in servomechanisms engineering and management, and the approach uses a perspective based on information feedback and circular causality to understand the dynamics of complex social systems. Mathematically, SD models can be described as a system of coupled, nonlinear, first-order differential equations [18] that are solved using numerical methods. SD is a useful modeling approach for piloting complex systems modeling in the humanitarian sector, because it enables humanitarian response simulation even in contexts with limited data [19].

The data collected during the model's development and validation can be classified into three categories:

Structural data: variables and interrelationships in the model were extracted from literature review, see Supplementary Materials for further information.

Epidemiological data: information on the characteristics of *Vibrio cholerae* infections (e.g., duration of infection, severity proportions), as well as their prevalence in Al-Hudaydah governorate (e.g., number of suspected and confirmed cases, deaths).

Cholera response (interventions) data: information and data on the implemented interventions between 2017 to 2018 was collected from WASH sector [11] and health sector [12,20] (see Supplementary Materials for further detail).

Data quality issues have been regarded as a significant obstacle to an effective humanitarian response to the cholera epidemic. Inadequate access to health facilities may have resulted in underestimating the cholera burden, most notably mortality [5]. For example, infected individuals who choose traditional medicine or private clinics over these specialized treatment centers are not captured by the surveillance system. Even mortality statistics are subject to reporting errors when deaths occur beyond the treatment facilities. On the other hand, Camacho et al. [21] stated that overreporting of other acute watery diarrhea (AWD) cases was likely to contribute to underestimates of the epidemic's case fatality rate.

2.1. Cholera Susceptible-Infected-Recovered/Susceptible

Building on the Yemen cholera response—causal loop diagram of Harpring et al. [4], and Pruyt's model [22] that simulates the 2008 cholera outbreak in Zimbabwe, the cholera response model is an extended SIR model that integrates the epidemic response's operational dynamics.

Al-Hudaydah governorate had a population of 3,238,199 in 2017 [11]. In an SIR model, the population is divided into several compartments called stocks, depending on their status of being susceptible to the infection (S), being infected and infectious (I), and having recovered from the infection (R) [22]. In the case of cholera, the recovered population becomes susceptible again after a delay, which makes the model an SIS model. Figure 2 is a high-level and simplified view of the main stocks and flows in the model. Table 1 summarizes the feedback loops in Figure 2.

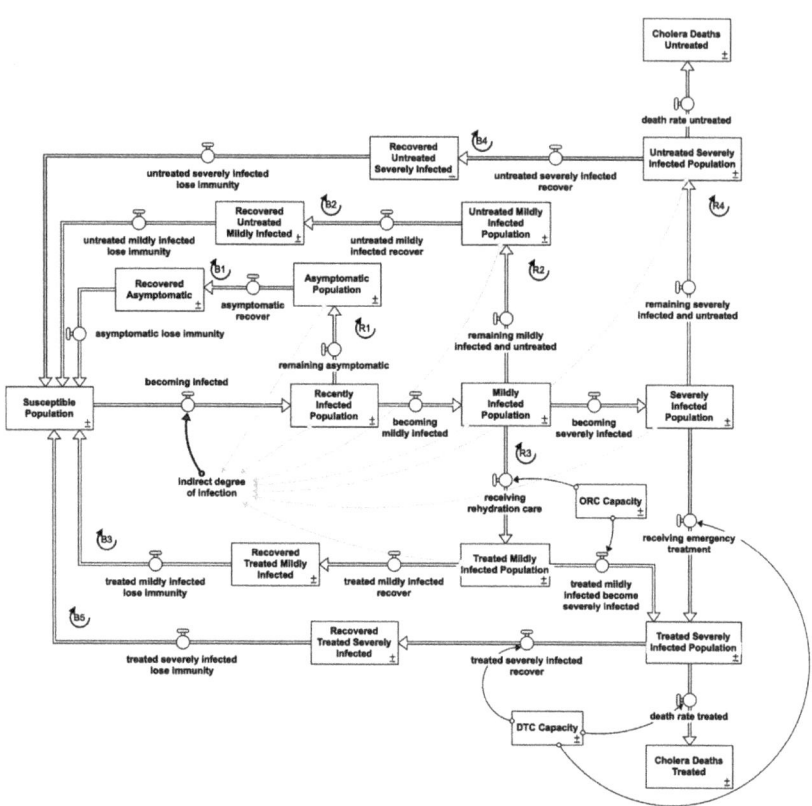

Figure 2. Core cholera infection stock and flow diagram providing an overview of the key pop-ulation groups and the transitions among them.

Table 1. Summary of feedback loops.

Infectious State	Treatment	Loop	Shown
Asymptomatic (75%)	No	Asymptomatic infected loop	R1
		Asymptomatic recovered loop	B1
Mild symptoms (15%)	No	Untreated mildly infected loop	R2
	No	Untreated mildly recovered loop	B2
	Yes	Treated mildly infected loop	R3
	Yes	Treated mildly recovered loop	B3
Severe symptoms (10%)	No	Untreated severely infected loop	R4
	No	Untreated severely recovered loop	B4
	Yes	Treated severely recovered loop	B5

2.1.1. Indirect Infection

This model only incorporates indirect infection through contaminated water by infected individuals. When susceptible individuals become infected with cholera, they shift to the recently infected population after one day. The rate of cholera infection is a product of the indirect degree of infection and the size of the susceptible population (S). In turn, the indirect degree of infection depends on the connectedness of aquifers and smoothed fraction of contaminated water.

Although sporadic cholera cases may occur as a result from ingestion of insufficiently cooked seafood contaminated with *Vibrio cholerae*, humans are the primary reservoir for the pathogen during periods of active transmission (epidemic) via fecal contamination of drinking water or food [1,6,23,24]. A meta-analysis of the role of water, sanitation, and hygiene exposures in 51 case–control cholera studies found that cases were significantly more likely than controls to report the use of untreated drinking water, open defecation, unimproved sanitation, and poor hand hygiene [25]. Hence, the smoothed fraction of contaminated water is water contaminated by bacteria shedding from the infected individuals [23].

The smoothed fraction of contaminated water uses the water contamination from total bacteria shedding from the fraction of infected with a delay of two and a half days. *Vibrio cholerae* survival in the aquatic environment is highly dependent on the chemical, biological, and physical conditions of the aquatic environment: *Vibrio cholerae* survives in surface water for periods ranging from one hour to thirteen days [26].

Three days is used for the time period to affect water in aquifers in this model. A third-order delay is used to account for the fact that there are different stages in the process [23] between bacteria shedding by the infected individuals to contaminating the water.

Connectedness of aquifers is the "contact rate" between the susceptible population with contaminated water. More than 19 million Yemenis are believed to be without access to safe drinking water and sanitation [8,21,27]. According to WHO-UNICEF statistics, only 55% of the population had access to drinking water from improved water sources in 2014 [9]. Grad et al. [28] explained that the "contact rate" is largely unknown in most contexts, and there are no simple methods for converting experimental study results into a "contact rate" between susceptible individuals and bacteria in water. Since various factors determine the rate at which susceptible individuals become infected, the connectedness of aquifers is calibrated to the historical data. 0.02 is used in this model.

2.1.2. Asymptomatic Reinforcing Feedback Loop (R)

Individuals in the recently infected population leave the stock after an average incubation time of one day and flow in two directions: as asymptomatic infected to the asymptomatic population if they show no symptoms, or as mildly infected to the mildly infected population if they show mild symptoms. Pruyt's model [23] makes no distinction between asymptomatic and symptomatic infections. Other works highlighted that these are essential elements and incorporated an asymptomatic feedback loop into their model [1,26,29–31].

First, most infected individuals (75% of infections) remain clinically unapparent, while the remaining 25% develop mild to severe symptoms (depending on the strain involved) [1]. Only symptomatic infections from treatment centers are captured in surveillance data [1,17]. When calibrating modeling outputs to historical data, Fung [17] concluded that underreporting of cases, including asymptomatic cases, should be considered. Chao et al. [29] found their model sensitive to the fraction of infected people who became symptomatic: The higher the symptomatic proportion, the higher the incidence of reported cases.

Second, the bacterial shedding rate is lower in asymptomatic individuals than in symptomatic individuals (60–90 percent of infected individuals are asymptomatic). Studies [1,26,30] have reported that some individuals can be infected with *Vibrio cholerae* and yet show no symptoms but then tend to shed the organism into the environment, even for only a few days. In a non-cholera epidemic area, *Vibrio cholerae* can be isolated from wastewater effluents [26].

Third, research emphasizes the distinction between immunity from asymptomatic infection and protection from disease (symptomatic) following recovery [30,31].

2.1.3. Bacteria Shedding

The model includes bacteria shedding as part of the indirect infection pathway. According to Kaper, Morris, and Levine [30], doses of 10^11 Colony Forming Units (CFU) of *Vibrio cholerae* were needed to trigger diarrhea in healthy North American volunteers. For example, ingestion of 10^6 *Vibrio cholerae* with fish and rice resulted in a high attack rate (100%). On the other hand, a symptomatic mildly infected individual can shed *Vibrio cholerae* in the stool in low but potentially infectious concentrations, up to 10^8 *Vibrio cholerae* organisms per g of stool [32]. An individual with acute cholera, severely diseased, excretes 10^7 to 10^8 *Vibrio cholerae* organisms per gram of stool. For patients who have 5 to 10 L of diarrheal stool, the total output of *Vibrio cholerae* can be in the range of 10^11 to 10^13 CFU [30].

This model uses 10^6 *Vibrio cholerae* as the amount to infect an individual.
The value of:

1. bacteria shedding from symptomatic is 10^4, hence, normalized to $10^4/10^6 = 0.01$
2. bacteria shedding from a mildly infected individual is 10^8, hence, normalized to $10^8/10^6 = 100$
3. bacteria shedding from a severely infected individual is 10^12, hence, normalized to $10^{12}/10^6 = 1{,}000{,}000$

2.1.4. Symptomatic Reinforcing Feedback Loops (R)

The mildly infected population consists of mild cases of *Vibrio cholerae* infection that may be clinically indistinguishable from other causes of diarrheal illness [33]. Hence, not all seek healthcare services [1]. Depending on access to healthcare services, this model disaggregates mildly infected individuals into two different stocks: treated and untreated mildly infected individuals. Mildly infected individuals leave the stock after the time period to progress to the next stage (one day) and flow to three directions: treated mildly infected population, untreated mildly infected population, or intone of the severe disease population stocks.

The severely infected population consists of severe cases of *Vibrio cholerae* infection that are characterized by a sudden onset of acute voluminous watery diarrhea, described as 'rice water stools' and vomiting leading to rapid dehydration (fluid losses of up to one liter per hour), and death if left untreated [1,30]. Among individuals developing symptoms, 60 to 80% of episodes are of mild or moderate severity [1,23]. In other words, only 5 to 10% of the recently infected population in the base model becomes very ill. Mildly infected individuals move to the severely infected population after an average time to progress to the next stage. Severely infected individuals then move into two different stocks based on access to healthcare services: treated and untreated. The treated severely infected population stock does not contribute to the infectious reinforcing feedback loop as the excreted wastewater is disinfected at the healthcare sewage treatment facilities [1].

2.1.5. Recovered Balancing Feedback Loops (B)

All individuals belonging to the asymptomatic population, treated and untreated mildly infected population, recover after an average illness duration (asymptomatic for five days and symptomatic for nine days) [32,33]. On the other hand, individuals in the treated and untreated severely infected population either die (cholera deaths) or recover and become immune (recovered from severe infection) after the same average duration of the illness of nine days.

The proportion of the treated severely infected population that die or recover is determined by the capacity of healthcare services, as overloading in the health services results in lower care quality. Hence, an increase in fatality fraction. In 2017, the case fatality rate in Al-Hudaydah governorate was 0.0019 [11]. For severely infected individuals who are not accessing healthcare services, the untreated fatality fraction uses 0.004, assuming that the fatality fraction is double the case fatality rate with treated death fraction of 0.0021.

2.1.6. Immunity Waning

Studies have shown a difference between protection from asymptomatic infection and protection from disease (symptomatic) after recovery [30,31]. Pruyt's model [22] aggregates both mildly and severely infected population into one stock of recovered temporarily immune population where they flow back to the susceptible population after an average immunity period of six years. Studies reported that clinical cholera (symptomatic) conferred protection against subsequent cholera for at least three years [30] while a study by Leung and Matrajt [31] identified that the asymptomatic protection period lasts between 3 to 12 months. The model uses six months for the average asymptomatic infection acquired immunity period and three years for the average symptomatic infection acquired immunity period [30,31].

2.2. Cholera Response-Intervention Structure

In the event of a cholera epidemic, the focus must be on limiting mortality and stopping the disease from spreading. It should be comprehensive and multi-sectoral, encompassing epidemiology (surveillance), case management, water, sanitation, hygiene, logistics, community engagement, and risk communication [34]. Figure 3 illustrates the stock and flow diagrams of each intervention. Further description is listed in the Supplementary Materials.

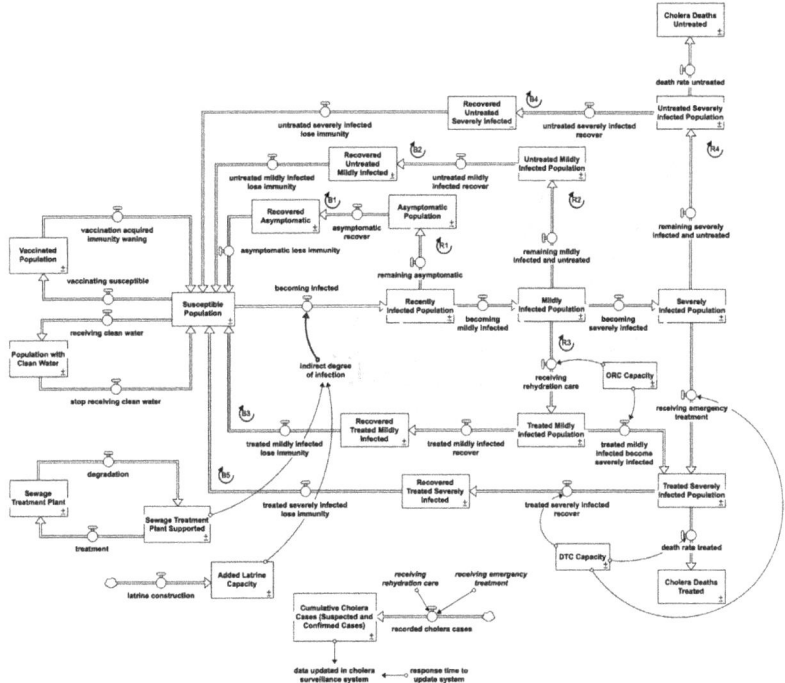

Figure 3. Stock and flow diagram of the overall cholera response model.

2.2.1. Water, Sanitation and Hygiene Interventions (WASH)

Water, sanitation, and hygiene (WASH) interventions are commonly used to prevent and control cholera by reducing exposure to risk factors for disease transmission [25]. In

Yemen, water trucking, latrine construction, chlorine tablet distribution, filter distribution, and hygiene kit distribution are the primary focuses of WASH [5].

Clean Water Provision

Water interventions improve the quantity of water (water trucking), the quality of water (chlorinating water), or the management of water (safe storage). Figure 4 shows that susceptible individuals who receive clean water shift to population with clean water stock after one day.

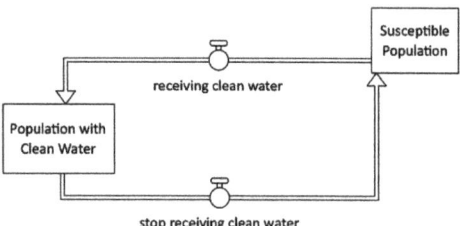

Figure 4. Clean water provision intervention stock and flow diagram.

Sewage Treatment Plant

Figure 5 illustrates that the sewage treatment helps remove contaminants from sewage to produce effluent suitable for discharge to the surrounding environment or reuse and therefore prevent contamination of water sources [1,26,35].

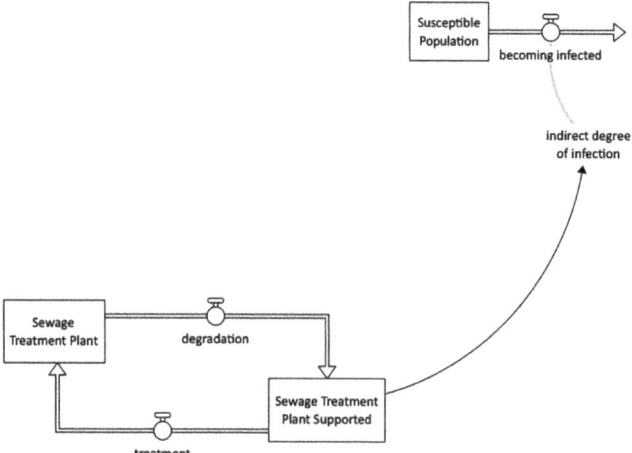

Figure 5. Sewage treatment intervention stock and flow diagram.

Latrine Construction

This model latrine construction intervention is based on the need for latrine capacity: the 1% of the population openly defecating (Figure 6). While the Médecins Sans Frontières' cholera response manual [1] recommends prioritizing public latrine placement in areas with a high risk of transmission (markets, train stations, and bus stations).

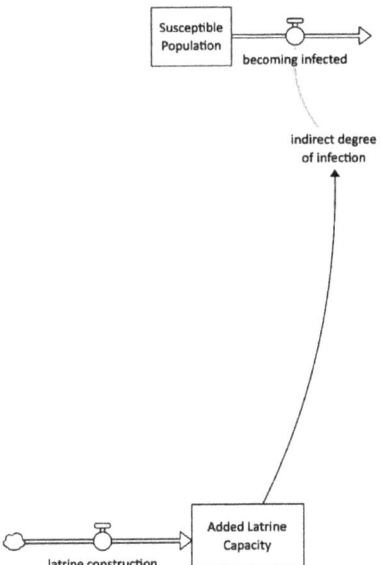

Figure 6. Latrine construction intervention stock and flow diagram.

2.2.2. Healthcare Interventions

Diarrhea Treatment Centre (DTC)

A DTC is a specialized inpatient healthcare facility dedicated to managing severe cholera cases. A DTC is located outside the main hospital to prevent disease spread and is completely self-sufficient in general services (toilets, showers, kitchen, laundry, morgue, and waste area), stocks, and resources (medical and logistics, water, and electricity). Severity affects the intensity of shedding, and so the average contribution of an infectious person to transmission may change systematically with time as the distribution of infectious doses changes [30,32]. The "severely infected not in DTC" excludes treated severely infected population because at DTC, the sewage system is in place with disinfection. Hence, Figure 7 shows that all patients at DTC do not attribute their bacteria shedding back into the environment.

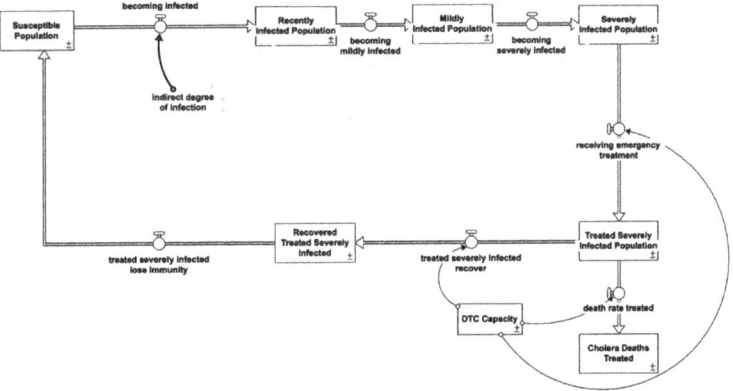

Figure 7. Diarrhea treatment centre intervention stock and flow diagram.

Oral Rehydration Corner (ORC)

ORCs are small, decentralized outpatient care facilities that operate only during daylight hours (8 to 12 h per day). They are primarily used to administer oral rehydration therapy. Figure 8 illustrates that early oral therapy can help prevent the onset or aggravation of severe dehydration, which requires hospitalization [1,24,36].

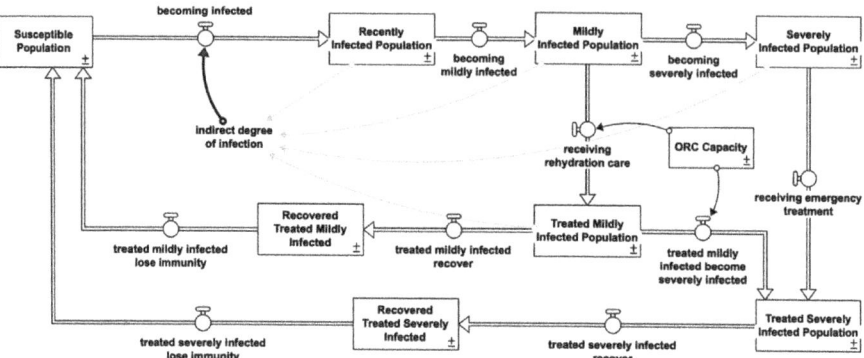

Figure 8. Oral rehydration corner intervention stock and flow diagram.

Vaccination

Figure 9 shows that vaccination decreases the number of fully susceptible individuals, decreases infectiousness (the rate of water contamination), and decreases the likelihood of becoming symptomatic when infected [21,28]. Oral cholera vaccine (OCV) has been shown to be safe, logistically feasible, and acceptable by recipients. OCV is also inexpensive in a variety of settings, with total costs including procurement and delivery per fully vaccinated individual being less than USD 10 [3,37,38].

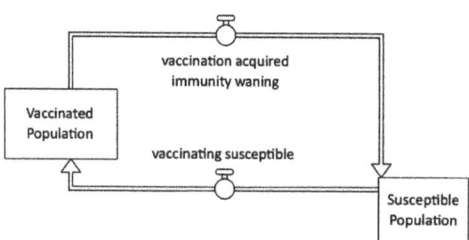

Figure 9. Vaccination intervention stock and flow diagram.

2.2.3. Surveillance System

According to Camacho et al. [21], Yemen's health authorities established a national cholera surveillance system to collect data on suspected cholera cases presenting to health facilities (no mass screening, the data depends on the availability of ORCs, DTCs, and health seeking ratio). Only symptomatic infections are likely to seek treatment and be reported. Figure 10 shows that simulated suspected and confirmed cases that replicate the historical data are a product of individuals seeking rehydration care and emergency treatment with suspected cholera infection.

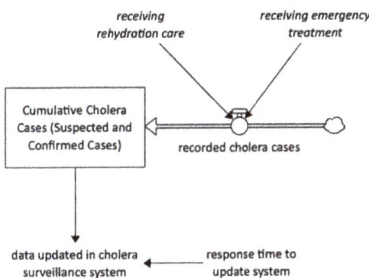

Figure 10. Surveillance system intervention stock and flow diagram.

2.3. Other Model Settings

The model conceptual framework and structure has now been discussed and a detailed description of key assumptions, model equations, and numeric inputs are provided in the Supplementary Materials. The simulation of the model was conducted using Stella Architect version 3.0. This model has a relatively short time horizon, as its purpose is to explore the implications of cholera response interventions during the 2017 and 2018 epidemics. As such, the model commences on 1 January 2017 and continues for 730 days, ending on 31 December 2018. A retrospective analysis and policy testing were conducted rather than the more conventional future timeline projection for epidemic preparedness. A DT of 1/4 with Euler's integration method is used to run this model.

Table 2 below outlines key parameters used in the model. For more information and a complete list of parameters, refer to the Supplementary Materials.

Table 2. Literature sources for key parameters in the model.

No	Parameters	Sensitivity Test (Numerical)	Values	Unit	Sources
1	connectedness of aquifers		0.02	1/day	Calibrated; [14,38]
2	time to affect water in aquifers		3.5	day	Calibrated; [14]
3	ratio of asymptomatic		0.75	dmnl	[1,30]
4	average incubation time		1	day	[1,30,32]
5	average duration of illness asymptomatic		5	day	[1,29,30]
6	susceptible population		3,238,199	person	[18]
7	recently infected population		500	person	[18]
8	normal ratio of severe disease		0.3	dmnl	[1,30]
9	average duration of illness symptomatic		9	day	[32,39]
10	average asymptomatic infection acquired immunity period		180	day	[31]
11	average symptomatic infection acquired immunity period		1095	day	[30,31]
12	fraction mildly infected seeking care		0.3	dmnl	Estimation from Camacho et al. [21]
13	fraction severely infected seeking care		0.4	dmnl	[1,21]
14	treated fatality fraction		0.0021	dmnl	[18]
15	bacteria shedding from asymptomatic		0.67	dmnl	[30] (normalized value)
16	bacteria shedding from mildly infected		1.33	dmnl	[32] (normalized value)
17	bacteria shedding from severely infected		2	dmnl	[30] (normalized value)

Indicators: ▢ Sensitive ▢ Highly sensitive.

2.4. Model Validation

A system dynamics model is generally validated in two ways. A structural validation of the model seeks to determine whether it accurately corresponds to the real world. Behavioral validation focuses on model behavior during simulation and evaluates the level of confidence that can be placed in the results [22,40,41]. Adhering to the guidelines, formal model analysis and validation procedures were conducted to support model development and testing throughout the research process. The procedures involved iterative cycles of data collection, model building, simulation, analysis, validation, and documentation. They are described in detail in the Supplementary Materials.

2.4.1. Comparison to Historical Data

Three uncertain parameter values: connectedness to aquifer, initial value of recently infected population, and time (of bacteria shed by infected individuals) to affect water in aquifer, were estimated through full-model calibration. Figure 11 compares simulated behavior with historical data (from 2017 to 2018) for fitted variables, using estimated parameter values from the full-model calibration. First, the model incorporates the dynamic of an asymptomatic feedback loop, as the collected data are the suspected and confirmed cases in Al-Hudaydah. In other words, infected individuals who are sick enough to seek healthcare services (symptomatic). Second, the model takes account of the data source; suspected and confirmed cases were collected from the DTC. Hence, the capacity structure of the DTC is built as part of the intervention structures.

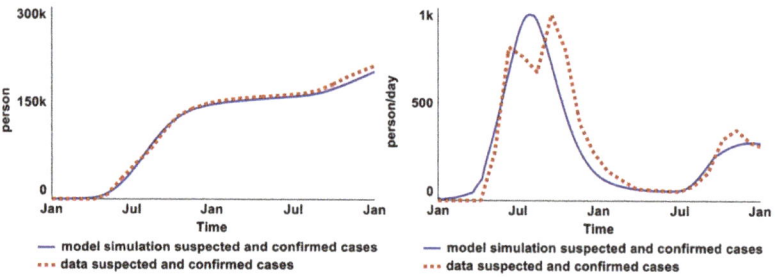

Figure 11. Comparison between model behaviors and historical data in total suspected and confirmed cases graph (**left**) and in the infection rate of suspected and confirmed cases graph (**right**).

On the other hand, the infection rate of suspected and confirmed cases graph (right) illustrates the marginal difference in infection rates between suspected and confirmed cases (right). The plausible explanation is that DTCs and ORCs lacked capacity at the start of the epidemic due to a delay in capacity development (constructing new DTCs and ORCs).

Camacho et al. [21] explained that scarcity of adequate treatment is more common during the initial phase of unexpected outbreaks and in crisis settings. The absence of DTCs and ORCs indicates a data collection gap (according to Yemen's surveillance system). When infected individuals have access to a DTC and ORC, there is an over-reporting problem because other patients with acute watery diarrhea (AWD) seek care at the ORC and DTC [3,5]. It is reasonable for the simulated infection rate to be slightly higher than the data at the start and slightly lower than the data following the establishment of DTCs and ORCs.

No explanation regarding the two peaks in the data is available from the literature. One plausible reason is that the healthcare system was over-stretched by the drastic increase in infected patients; healthcare and the data surveillance system could not perform as usual under such an overloaded condition. Once the system capacity increased (after a delay), the data collection function also increased, resulting in a second peak. Another reason could be that the rainfall intensified the infection rate [15].

2.4.2. Sensitivity Test

A multivariate Monte-Carlo sensitivity analysis was conducted on all exogenous parameters and initial values using a Sobol Sequence. A base case run was given initially, and each sensitivity run utilized these values and changed one of the values in uniform distribution within a preset range (see Supplementary Materials). The following Figures 12 and 13 present the sensitive parameters that indicate the potential leverage points for policy tests.

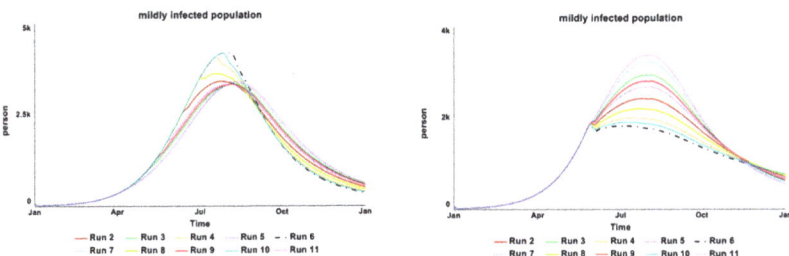

Figure 12. The (**left**) behavior-over-time graphs show the result from the vaccination start time parameter test, while the (**right**) over-time graph shows the result of the desired number of vaccines pa-rameter test.

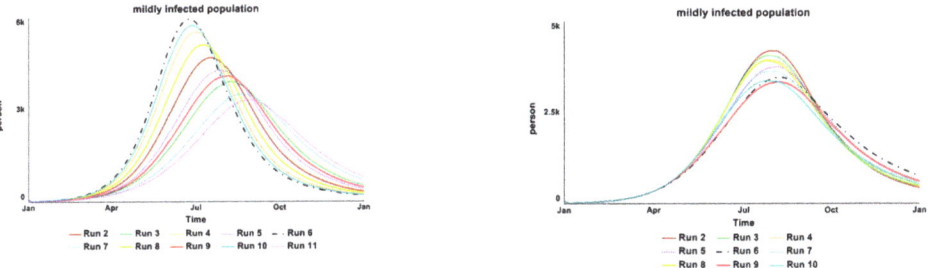

Figure 13. The (**left**) over-time graph shows the results from the 'bacteria shedding from asymptomatic cases' parameter test while the (**right**) over-time graph shows the result of the desired sewage plant treatment parameter test.

Figure 12 shows the result from the parameter "vaccination start time" (left behavior-over-time graph). The model is numerically sensitive to changes in the tested value from day 90 to 365, with the same amount of vaccine provision in Al-Hudaydah (260,000 vaccines—intervention historical data), as expected. An earlier vaccine campaign shows a significant reduction in the infected population. With the model setting the vaccination start time as day 120 (April 2017), the sensitivity test continued with another parameter of "desired vaccine number". The model shows a high numerical sensitivity to the tested range of vaccines number, between 200,000 to 1,000,000.

The left over-time graph in Figure 13 shows that the model is strongly (numerically) sensitive to changes in the value of "bacteria shedding from asymptomatic cases" as expected. Although the tested values are the lowest among the three infectious levels of bacteria shedding (asymptomatic, mildly, and severely symptomatic individuals), asymptomatic individuals have the highest ratio (75%) among the total infected population. Hence, contributing to the high sensitivity of this parameter value.

The right over-time graph in Figure 13 shows that the model is strongly (numerically) sensitive to changes in the values of "desired sewage plant treatment", as expected. The tested range included start time and the capacity of the sewage plant treatment intervention. The infection reinforcing feedback loop is affected by the water source contamination by the infected individuals. If the current sewage plant treatment is well supported, there is less water contamination by the Vibrio cholera bacteria.

3. Scenario Analysis and Discussion

BAU-BASE-Early Response

The model was run under the following three different conditions to understand the interventions' impact on the cholera epidemic dynamics. Figure 14 presents the results from each scenario simulation.

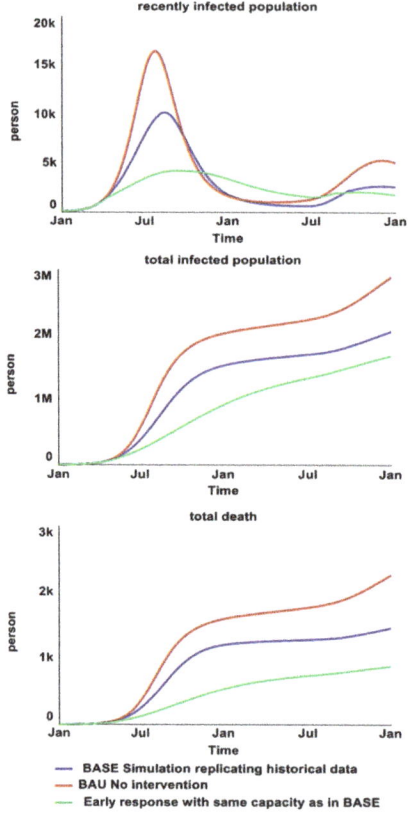

Figure 14. Behavior over time graphs that present the results for recently infected populations (**top**), rec-orded suspected and confirmed cases (**middle**), and treated and untreated death rate (**bottom**) of BAU-BASE-Early response simulations.

BASE. BASE is the simulation scenario that replicates the historical data. This scenario included interventions implemented in 2017. A detailed intervention timeline simulated in "BASE" with the capacity of treatment centers over time and vaccine distribution can be found in Supplementary Materials (variables with "data" in their name).

Business as Usual (BAU). BAU is the scenario where all interventions are deconstructed from BASE to explore a counterfactual worst-case scenario for the cholera epidemic.

Early Response. An early response explores the impact of all interventions if the starting day were in April 2017, using the same capacity from the BASE. In addition, similar interventions were added in as responses to the second wave from June 2018. Using capacity of interventions similar to historical data aims to avoid overly unrealistic policy recommendations, particularly in a conflict-affected context where intervention implementation faces immense challenges. Further policy analysis of each intervention will be explored in future research.

Cholera epidemic control is highly complex in a conflict-affected context such as Yemen. While the epidemic lessons learned were widely discussed in the literature (mostly qualitatively), it is still not fully understood what the best strategies for cholera response are. Existing cholera related simulation models mainly study vaccination, antibiotics, and water provision. None of the reviewed models include structures of both asymptomatic and symptomatic individuals as well as sanitation intervention (sewage system) and health services. In this paper, the cholera response model explores the dynamic interplay between the classic infection SIR/SIS structure and the empirically grounded operational structures: oral rehydration corners, diarrhea treatment centers, water, sanitation and hygiene (WASH), vaccination, and the data surveillance system. The following insights emerge from the sensitivity and the three scenario policy tests.

First, deconstructing the interventions from BASE to BAU has shown significant impacts from the humanitarian cholera response in 2017. The results from Table 3 show that there would have been 55% more deaths if nothing had been done in Al-Hudaydah. In the BAU scenario, the cholera infection reinforcing feedback loops (R1, 2, 3, and 4) continue to dominate the SIR/SIS dynamics without attenuation from exogenous interventions; more infected individuals lead to more susceptible persons being infected, and the epidemic curve increases exponentially. In addition to the decline in the susceptible population (over time), more infected individuals recover or die; the balancing feedback loops (B1, 2, 3, 4, and 5) gain strength. The epidemic curve peaks and eventually falls.

Table 3. Results of BASE, BAU, and Early Response simulations.

Scenario	Total Infected Population	Total Death
BASE	2,055,712	1,468
BAU	2,888,484	2,268
	+41%	+55%
Early Response	1,681,105	891
	−18%	−39%

This endogenous SIR/SIS dynamic of reinforcing and balancing feedback loops shed lights on some of the questions asked in the reviewed literature. For instance, an epidemiologist who was interviewed in a study by Spiegel et al. [5] asked why the second wave was so massive. After the mild first wave, the susceptible population is still very large. Such a condition enables the infection reinforcing feedback loops to dominate in the second wave if there is no exogenous intervention to counter the strength of the reinforcing feedback loops (or to strengthen the balancing feedback loops).

Second, the simulation results also reveal that a potential 40% of deaths could have been prevented if interventions, especially vaccination, had been initiated earlier. Studies have reported that concern was raised by the Yemeni government and some humanitarian actors that mass immunization would be logistically difficult with ongoing security problems [3,9,13]. Another reason is that vaccination would have a minimal effect given the magnitude of the outbreak: it may be too late for vaccination, and the benefits would not outweigh the risks of initiating a campaign.

Yemen's government, the United Nations, and the WHO stated that the decision was made on a technical basis to ensure that efforts would be concentrated on WASH intervention targeting approximately 16 million people [13]. Vaccines were finally distributed to 540,000 people by the WHO and UNICEF in August 2018, nearly 16 months after the outbreak began. Al-Hudaydah vaccinated 260,000 people with two-dose oral cholera vaccines (OCVs).

Indeed, the conflict situation posed significant logistical challenges for mass vaccination. Burki [8], on the other hand, reported that coverage of the pentavalent vaccine is estimated to be around 88% in 2015—the same as in 2014. The past pentavalent vaccine campaign indicates that a mass vaccination campaign is feasible if well-planned and supported. Moreover, Médecins Sans Frontières' [1] cholera response manual stated that OCVs are administered orally (not via injection) and rarely cause serious adverse effects, and mass cholera vaccination campaigns do not require a large number of medical personnel. Hence, an earlier vaccination campaign would not have been impossible in Yemen.

Third, the sensitivity test findings show that the model is not sensitive to the water provision intervention. This is an unexpected result as one might anticipate a greater impact from water provision on cholera epidemic control, given that WASH intervention is considered to be one of the most critical components of such an emergency response [1].

In Al-Hudaydah, clean water provision activities comprise chlorination of wells, communal water tanks, distribution of chlorine tablets, and the daily chlorination of water trucks at water filling stations. In this cholera response model, susceptible individuals who receive clean water shift to the population with clean water stock after one day. Compared to the model of Tuite et al. [42] with 100% reduction of "contact" rate if covered by clean water provision, this model assumes only 70% of individuals who receive clean water shift into the population with clean water stock. Having clean water does not ensure a 100% reduction in susceptibility [25]. It is unrealistic to assume that those who receive clean water are 100% protected from cholera infection, as cholera is transmitted via multiple pathways (as illustrated in Figure 15). With other words, removing a single source of infection through water provision may not effectively prevent the disease.

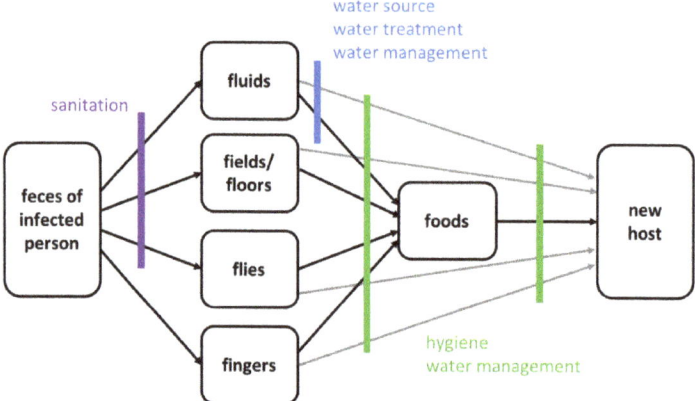

Figure 15. Pathways of fecal–oral cholera transmission and opportunities to interrupt transmission from Water 1st International (cited in Wolfe et al. [25]).

Water can also still be viewed as a source of cholera outbreaks. Even when routine water treatments are carried out, cholera can still be transmitted when: dosing errors are made, treatment is forgotten, or the piped water supply is contaminated [25]. In fact, John Snow made history in public health by tracing and discovering that the source of the London cholera epidemic in 1854 was contaminated water from a water pump.

This discussion does not intend to discredit the crucial role of clean water provision. Having access to safe drinking water is central to living a life in dignity and upholding human rights [38]. However, it is problematic when resources are overly focused on WASH interventions. During the major wave of the epidemic, when stakeholders chose not to vaccinate the public but instead prioritized WASH [13]; and after the epidemic, when humanitarian actors utilized the water-fighting system, Cholera Risk Model predictive tool [15] without considering the endogenous feedback loops of cholera transmission. Such policy is likely to result in the "Shifting the Burden" system archetype; relying on reactive quick fixes that lead to unintended consequences of lower priorities and fewer resources for other interventions. For instance, vaccination provides three-year protection compared to one-day protection from water provision.

One might argue that the water provision should eventually transition from emergency water trucking or chlorine tablets to building water treatment plants. Nevertheless, such a long-term WASH development strategy is not part of the emergency cholera response model boundary. Additionally, such policy is not suitable in a conflict-affected context where the infrastructures are intentionally being obliterated.

Fourth, sewage plant treatment can potentially be the leverage point for the silent spreaders who make the cholera transmission harder to fight. The sensitivity test findings highlight that the model is strongly (numerically) sensitive to changes in the value of "bacteria shedding from asymptomatic cases" due to asymptomatic individuals having the highest ratio (75%) among the total infected population. It is rather challenging to intervene in this population at the individual level as they are asymptomatic. However, it is still crucial to have intervention(s) targeting or controlling the impact from the silent spreaders. One of the potential interventions is sanitation, such as sewage plant treatment.

The sensitivity test results also show that the model is strongly sensitive towards sewage system treatment. Sewage management and food safety are two critical areas for preparedness and response to the cholera outbreak. However, because these fields are not mandated by the health care system or the WASH cluster, they are frequently overlooked or dealt with ad hoc during the response [14,25]. This problem is also indicated by the lack of cholera modeling literature on sewage treatment.

The highest numbers of cholera cases have been reported in areas with non-functional sewage treatment plants [43]. Without functional sewage treatment plants, sewage effluents are frequently diverted to impoverished neighborhoods and agricultural lands, contaminating shallow aquifers and wells used by local civilians and private tankers [1,26]. The reuse of sewage effluents for irrigation is an essential alternative water source for Yemen.

Sewage treatment helps remove contaminants from sewage to produce effluent suitable for discharge to the surrounding environment or reuse [1,26,35]. For instance, farmers in Yemen collect sewage effluent directly from stabilization ponds to irrigate various crops [44]. A study by Al-Sharabee in 2009 (cited in Al-gheeti et al. [35]) reports that the zone area near the Sana'a wastewater treatment plant depends upon the sewage effluents for 95% of crop irrigation. However, Yemen's current sewage effluent quality is generally poor, since none of the existing sewage treatment plants produce effluents that comply with the effluent quality regulations [44].

Although reports specifying project impact evaluation are uncommon in the published literature [17], a well-maintained sewage treatment plant is assumed to produce effluents that meet quality regulations, thereby improving sanitary conditions and reducing *Vibrio cholerae* contamination in drinking water sources [1,26].

While this cholera response model is useful for clarifying policy problems and reshaping mental models, it is just as important to be transparent regarding the model's limitations, assumptions, and boundary conditions. The cholera response model has several limitations, many of which stem from data quality or availability problems when approximating or estimating more detailed quantified representations of important dynamics. For instance, a lack of information regarding the weight of various WASH intervention impacts on the overall sanitary conditions in Al-Hudaydah. Sensitivity analysis has been used to provide some insurance against such uncertainties. The model's limitations nonetheless restrict the quantitative precision of the model's projections, which should be borne in mind when interpreting its results. In other words, this cholera response model is not intended for high-precision quantitative forecasting or prediction.

Regardless of the outlined limitations, this cholera response model has shown both the compounding factors that exacerbate the epidemic and the operational dynamics in controlling the epidemics. The model stresses the importance of distinct asymptomatic and symptomatic reinforcing feedback loops, where interventions must target both. Most importantly, the intervention starting time plays the essential role in controlling the epidemic.

Lastly, the model identifies the unknown unintended consequences, such as 'shifting the burden' from overly focused water provision intervention. To conclude, the model paves the way for a more robust cholera response policy analysis in the future. The next steps include further analysis of how each intervention impacts the epidemic control, building a use-friendly model interface, and adapting the model to reflect cholera outbreaks in other countries.

Supplementary Materials: The following supporting information can be downloaded at: https://www.mdpi.com/article/10.3390/systems11010003/s1, Table S1 (Documentation) and Table S2 (Sensitivity Analysis). References [45–57] list in Supplementary Materials file.

Author Contributions: Conceptualization, P.S.L.; methodology, P.S.L.; software, P.S.L.; validation, P.S.L., A.A. and B.K.; formal analysis, P.S.L.; investigation, P.S.L.; resources, P.S.L.; data curation, P.S.L.; writing—original draft preparation, P.S.L.; writing—review and editing, A.A. and B.K.; visualization, P.S.L.; supervision, A.A. and B.K.; project administration, A.A. and B.K. All authors have read and agreed to the published version of the manuscript.

Funding: This research received no external funding.

Institutional Review Board Statement: Not applicable.

Informed Consent Statement: Not applicable.

Data Availability Statement: Not applicable.

Acknowledgments: The model is built upon the findings from Rocca [19]. The authors are grateful for early guidance from humanitarian experts Leonardo Milano and data fellow Roberta Rocca. The authors would also like to thank Billy Schoenberg and Wang Zhao for their feedback on the model.

Conflicts of Interest: The authors declare no conflict of interest.

References

1. Médecins Sans Frontières. Management of a Cholera Epidemic. 2018th ed. 2018. Available online: https://medicalguidelines.msf.org/viewport/CHOL/english/management-of-a-cholera-epidemic-23444438.html (accessed on 20 September 2022).
2. World Health Organization. *Guidelines for Cholera Control*; World Health Organization: Geneva, Switzerland, 1993; Available online: https://apps.who.int/iris/handle/10665/36837 (accessed on 20 September 2022).
3. Federspiel, F.; Ali, M. The Cholera Outbreak in Yemen: Lessons Learned and Way Forward. *BMC Public Health* **2018**, *18*, 1338. [CrossRef] [PubMed]
4. Harpring, R.; Maghsoudi, A.; Fikar, C.; Piotrowicz, W.D.; Heaslip, G. An Analysis of Compounding Factors of Epidemics in Complex Emergencies: A System Dynamics Approach. *J. Humanit. Logist. Supply Chain Manag.* **2021**, *11*, 198–226.
5. Spiegel, P.; Ratnayake, R.; Hellman, N.; Lantagne, D.S.; Ververs, M.; Ngwa, M.; Wise, P.H. *Cholera in Yemen: A Case Study of Epidemic Preparedness and Response*; Johns Hopkins Center for Humanitarian Health: Baltimore, MD, USA, 2018.
6. Davis, W.; Narra, R.; Mintz, E.D. Cholera. *Curr. Epidemiol. Rep.* **2018**, *5*, 303–315. [CrossRef]
7. World Health Organization. Cholera Situation in Yemen December 2020 [Infographic]. Available online: https://applications.emro.who.int/docs/WHOEMCSR314E-eng.pdf?ua=1 (accessed on 20 September 2022).
8. Burki, T. Yemen's Neglected Health and Humanitarian Crisis. *Lancet* **2016**, *387*, 734–735. [CrossRef]
9. Qadri, F.; Islam, T.; Clemens, J.D. Cholera in Yemen—An Old Foe Rearing Its Ugly Head. *N. Engl. J. Med.* **2017**, *377*, 2005–2007. [CrossRef]
10. Emergency Operation Center. Cholera Response Health Actors and Partner Activities. 2021. Available online: https://app.powerbi.com/view?r=eyJrIjoiNTY3YmU0NTItMmFjYy00OTUxLWI2NzEtOTU5N2Q0MDBjMjE5IiwidCI6ImI3ZTNlYmJjLTE2ZTctNGVmMi05NmE5LTVkODc4ZDg3MDM5ZCIsImMiOjl9 (accessed on 20 September 2022).
11. United Nations Office for the Coordination of Humanitarian Affairs. Yemen: Cholera Outbreak Tracker Governorate Profiles. Available online: https://public.tableau.com/views/001CholeraYemenTracker/FacilityBaseline?%3Aembed=y&%3AshowVizHome=no&%3Adisplay_count=y&%3Adisplay_static_image=y#!%2Fpublish-confirm (accessed on 20 September 2022).
12. UNICEF. UNICEF Yemen Humanitarian Situation Report. Available online: https://reliefweb.int/sites/reliefweb.int/files/resources/UNICEFYemenHumanitarianSituationReport-August2018.pdf (accessed on 20 September 2022).
13. Al-Mekhlafi, H.M. Yemen in a Time of Cholera: Current Situation and Challenges. *Am. J. Trop. Med. Hyg.* **2018**, *98*, 1558–1562. [CrossRef] [PubMed]
14. Bellizzi, S.; Pichierri, G.; Cegolon, L.; Panu Napodano, C.M.; Ali Maher, O. Coordination during Cholera Outbreak Response: Critical Insights from Yemen. *Am. J. Trop. Med. Hyg.* **2021**, *105*, 1155–1156. [CrossRef]

15. Barciela, R.; Bilge, T.; Brown, K.; Champion Christophe, A.S.; Shields, M.; Ticehurst, H.; Jutla, A.; Usmani, M.; Colwell, R. *Early Action for Cholera Project. Yemen Case Study*; Met Office: Exeter, UK, 2021.
16. Pruyt, E. *Small System Dynamics Models for Big Issues: Triple Jump towards Real-World Complexity*; TU Delft Library: Delft, The Netherlands, 2013.
17. Fung, I.C.-H. Cholera Transmission Dynamic Models for Public Health Practitioners. *Emerg. Themes Epidemiol.* **2014**, *11*, 1. [CrossRef]
18. Richardson, G.P. System Dynamics: Simulation for Policy Analysis from a Feedback Perspective. In *Qualitative Simulation Modeling and Analysis*; Springer: Berlin/Heidelberg, Germany, 1991; pp. 144–169.
19. Rocca, R. *Complex Systems Modeling for Humanitarian Action: Methods and Opportunities*; United Nations Office for the Coordination of Humanitarian Affairs: Geneva, Switzerland, 2021.
20. Diphtheria & Cholera Response. Available online: https://www.humanitarianresponse.info/sites/www.humanitarianresponse.info/files/documents/files/eoc_sitrep_25_yemen.pdf (accessed on 20 September 2022).
21. Camacho, A.; Bouhenia, M.; Alyusfi, R.; Alkohlani, A.; Naji, M.A.M.; de Radiguès, X.; Abubakar, A.M.; Almoalmi, A.; Seguin, C.; Sagrado, M.J.; et al. Cholera Epidemic in Yemen, 2016–2018: An Analysis of Surveillance Data. *Lancet Glob. Health* **2018**, *6*, e680–e690. [CrossRef]
22. Sterman, J. *Business Dynamics. Systems Thinking and Modeling for a Complex World*; McGraw Hill Higher Education: Boston, MA, USA, 2000.
23. Pruyt, E. Making System Dynamics Cool? Using Hot Testing & Teaching Cases. In Proceedings of the 27th International Conference of the System Dynamics Society. System Dynamics Society, Albuquerque, New Mexico, 26 July 2009.
24. Mwasa, A.; Tchuenche, J.M. Mathematical Analysis of a Cholera Model with Public Health Interventions. *Biosystems* **2011**, *105*, 190–200. [CrossRef]
25. Wolfe, M.; Kaur, M.; Yates, T.; Woodin, M.; Lantagne, D. A Systematic Review and Meta-Analysis of the Association between Water, Sanitation, and Hygiene Exposures and Cholera in Case-Control Studies. *Am. J. Trop. Med. Hyg.* **2018**, *99*, 534–545. [CrossRef] [PubMed]
26. Okoh, A.I.; Sibanda, T.; Nongogo, V.; Adefisoye, M.; Olayemi, O.O.; Nontongana, N. Prevalence and Characterisation of Non-Cholerae Vibrio Spp. in Final Effluents of Wastewater Treatment Facilities in Two Districts of the Eastern Cape Province of South Africa: Implications for Public Health. *Environ. Sci. Pollut. Res.* **2015**, *22*, 2008–2017. [CrossRef] [PubMed]
27. Ng, Q.X.; De Deyn, M.L.Z.Q.; Loke, W.; Yeo, W.S. Yemen's Cholera Epidemic Is a One Health Issue. *J. Prev. Med. Public Health* **2020**, *53*, 289. [CrossRef] [PubMed]
28. Grad, Y.H.; Miller, J.C.; Lipsitch, M. Cholera Modeling: Challenges to Quantitative Analysis and Predicting the Impact of Interventions. *Epidemiology* **2012**, *23*, 523–530. [CrossRef]
29. Chao, D.L.; Longini, I.M., Jr.; Morris, J.G., Jr. Modeling Cholera Outbreaks. *Curr. Top. Microbiol. Immunol.* **2014**, *379*, 195–209. [CrossRef]
30. Kaper, J.B.; Morris, J.G., Jr.; Levine, M.M. Cholera. *Clin. Microbiol. Rev.* **1995**, *8*, 48–86. [CrossRef]
31. Leung, T.; Matrajt, L. Protection Afforded by Previous Vibrio Cholerae Infection against Subsequent Disease and Infection: A Review. *PLoS Negl. Trop. Dis.* **2021**, *15*, e0009383. [CrossRef]
32. Nelson, E.J.; Harris, J.B.; Morris, J.G., Jr.; Calderwood, S.B.; Camilli, A. Cholera Transmission: The Host, Pathogen and Bacteriophage Dynamic. *Nat. Rev. Microbiol.* **2009**, *7*, 693–702. [CrossRef]
33. Chao, D.L.; Halloran, M.E.; Longini, I.M. Vaccination Strategies for Epidemic Cholera in Haiti with Implications for the Developing World. *Proc. Natl. Acad. Sci. USA* **2011**, *108*, 7081–7085. [CrossRef]
34. Global Task Force on Cholera Control. Roadmap 2030. Available online: https://www.gtfcc.org/about-gtfcc/roadmap-2030/ (accessed on 20 September 2022).
35. Al-Gheethi, A.A.S.; Abdul-Monem, M.O.; Al-Zubeiry, A.H.S.; Efaq, A.N.; Shamar, A.M.; Al-Amery, R.M.A. Effectiveness of Selected Wastewater Treatment Plants in Yemen for Reduction of Faecal Indicators and Pathogenic Bacteria in Secondary Effluents and Sludge. *Water Pract. Technol.* **2014**, *9*, 293–306. [CrossRef]
36. Miller Neilan, R.L.; Schaefer, E.; Gaff, H.; Fister, K.R.; Lenhart, S. Modeling Optimal Intervention Strategies for Cholera. *Bull. Math. Biol.* **2010**, *72*, 2004–2018. [CrossRef] [PubMed]
37. Parker, L.A.; Rumunu, J.; Jamet, C.; Kenyi, Y.; Lino, R.L.; Wamala, J.F.; Mpairwe, A.M.; Ciglenecki, I.; Luquero, F.J.; Azman, A.S.; et al. Adapting to the Global Shortage of Cholera Vaccines: Targeted Single Dose Cholera Vaccine in Response to an Outbreak in South Sudan. *Lancet Infect. Dis.* **2017**, *17*, e123–e127. [CrossRef] [PubMed]
38. World Health Organization. Ending Cholera a Global Roadmap to 2030. In *Ending Cholera a Global Roadmap to 2030*; UNICEF: Yemen, Yemen, 2017; p. 32.
39. LaRocque, R.; Harris, J.B. Cholera: Clinical Features, Diagnosis, Treatment, and Prevention. This Top. Available online: https://www.uptodate.com/contents/cholera-clinical-features-diagnosis-treatment-and-prevention (accessed on 20 September 2022).
40. Barlas, Y. Formal Aspects of Model Validity and Validation in System Dynamics. *Syst. Dyn. Rev.* **1996**, *12*, 183–210. [CrossRef]
41. Turner, B.L. Model Laboratories: A Quick-Start Guide for Design of Simulation Experiments for Dynamic Systems Models. *Ecol. Modell.* **2020**, *434*, 109246. [CrossRef]
42. Tuite, A.R.; Tien, J.; Eisenberg, M.; Earn, D.J.; Ma, J.; Fisman, D.N. Cholera Epidemic in Haiti, 2010: Using a Transmission Model to Explain Spatial Spread of Disease and Identify Optimal Control Interventions. *Ann. Intern. Med.* **2011**, *154*, 593–601. [CrossRef]

43. Abu-Lohom, N.; Muzenda, D.; Mumssen, Y.U. A WASH Response to Yemen's Cholera Outbreak. World Bank Blogs 2018. Available online: https://blogs.worldbank.org/water/wash-response-yemen-s-cholera-outbreak (accessed on 20 September 2022).
44. Al-Gheethi, A.; Noman, E.; Jeremiah David, B.; Mohamed, R.; Abdullah, A.; Nagapan, S.; Hashim Mohd, A. A Review of Potential Factors Contributing to Epidemic Cholera in Yemen. *J. Water Health* **2018**, *16*, 667–680. [CrossRef]
45. Centers for Disease Control and Prevention. Antibiotic Treatment. Available online: https://www.cdc.gov/cholera/treatment/antibiotic-treatment.html (accessed on 20 September 2022).
46. International Organization for Migration. Task Force for Population Movement Yemen August 2018. 2021. Available online: https://displacement.iom.int/yemen (accessed on 20 September 2022).
47. Ali, A. IDPs in Hudaydah: Where Aid, Protection Don't Always Reach; 2021. Available online: https://sanaacenter.org/ypf/idps-in-hudaydah/ (accessed on 20 September 2022).
48. McCrickard, L.; Massay, A.E.; Narra, R.; Mghamba, J.; Mohamed, A.A.; Kishimba, R.S.; Urio, L.J.; Rusibayamila, N.; Magembe, G.; Bakari, M.; et al. Cholera Mortality during Urban Epidemic, Dar Es Salaam, Tanzania, August 16, 2015–January 16, 2016. *Emerg. Infect. Dis. J.* **2017**, *23*, 13. [CrossRef]
49. UNICEF. UNCEF Cholera Tookit 2013. Available online: https://sites.unicef.org/cholera/Cholera-Toolkit-2013.pdf (accessed on 20 September 2022).
50. Ochoa, B.; Surawicz, C.M. Diarrheal Diseases–Acute and Chronic. Available online: https://gi.org/topics/diarrhea-acute-and-chronic/ (accessed on 20 September 2022).
51. Michas, F. Number of Patients That Physicians in the U.S. Saw per Day from 2012 to 2018. 2020. Available online: https://www.statista.com/statistics/613959/us-physicians-patients-seen-per-day/ (accessed on 20 September 2022).
52. Günther, I.; Niwagaba, C.B.; Lüthi, C.; Horst, A.; Mosler, H.-J.; Tumwebaze, I.K. When Is Shared Sanitation Improved Sanitation?- The Correlation between Number of Users and Toilet Hygiene. 2012. Available online: https://www.ircwash.org/resources/when-shared-sanitation-improved-sanitation-correlation-between-number-users-and-toilet (accessed on 22 September 2022).
53. Worldbank. People Practicing Open Defecation, Urban (% of urban population)-Yemen, Rep. Available online: https://data.worldbank.org/indicator/SH.STA.ODFC.UR.ZS?locations=YE (accessed on 20 September 2022).
54. Ministry of Electricity and Water. Environmental Impact Assessment. Available online: Chrome-extension://efaidnbmnnnibpcajpcglclefindmkaj/https://documents1.worldbank.org/curated/en/279131468335060537/pdf/E4940V60P0576020Box353756B01PUBLIC1.pdf (accessed on 20 September 2022).
55. Pezzoli, L. Global Oral Cholera Vaccine Use, 2013–2018. *Vaccine* **2020**, *38*, A132–A140. [CrossRef]
56. Durham, L.K.; Longini, I.M., Jr.; Halloran, M.E.; Clemens, J.D.; Azhar, N.; Rao, M. Estimation of Vaccine Efficacy in the Presence of Waning: Application to Cholera Vaccines. *Am. J. Epidemiol.* **1998**, *147*, 948–959. [CrossRef]
57. Shim, E.; Galvani, A.P. Distinguishing Vaccine Efficacy and Effectiveness. *Vaccine* **2012**, *30*, 6700–6705. [CrossRef]

Disclaimer/Publisher's Note: The statements, opinions and data contained in all publications are solely those of the individual author(s) and contributor(s) and not of MDPI and/or the editor(s). MDPI and/or the editor(s) disclaim responsibility for any injury to people or property resulting from any ideas, methods, instructions or products referred to in the content.

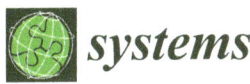

Hypothesis

Identifying Policy Gaps in a COVID-19 Online Tool Using the Five-Factor Framework

Janet Michel [1,*], David Evans [2], Marcel Tanner [3,4] and Thomas C. Sauter [1]

1. Department of Emergency Medicine, Inselspital, University Hospital, University of Bern, 3010 Bern, Switzerland
2. World Bank Health Economist, 7 Bis Avenue de la Paix, 1202 Geneva, Switzerland
3. Department of Epidemiology and Public Health, Swiss Tropical and Public Health Institute, 4002 Basel, Switzerland
4. Faculty of Science, University of Basel, 4001 Basel, Switzerland
* Correspondence: janetmichel71@gmail.com

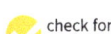

Citation: Michel, J.; Evans, D.; Tanner, M.; Sauter, T.C. Identifying Policy Gaps in a COVID-19 Online Tool Using the Five-Factor Framework. *Systems* **2022**, *10*, 257. https://doi.org/10.3390/systems10060257

Academic Editors: Philippe J. Giabbanelli and Andrew Page

Received: 20 September 2022
Accepted: 12 December 2022
Published: 15 December 2022

Publisher's Note: MDPI stays neutral with regard to jurisdictional claims in published maps and institutional affiliations.

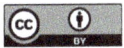

Copyright: © 2022 by the authors. Licensee MDPI, Basel, Switzerland. This article is an open access article distributed under the terms and conditions of the Creative Commons Attribution (CC BY) license (https://creativecommons.org/licenses/by/4.0/).

Abstract: Introduction: Worldwide health systems are being faced with unprecedented COVID-19-related challenges, ranging from the problems of a novel condition and a shortage of personal protective equipment to frequently changing medical guidelines. Many institutions were forced to innovate and many hospitals, as well as telehealth providers, set up online forward triage tools (OFTTs). Using an OFTT before visiting the emergency department or a doctor's practice became common practice. A policy can be defined as what an institution or government chooses to do or not to do. An OFTT, in this case, has become both a policy and a practice. Methods: The study was part of a broader multiphase sequential explanatory design. First, an online survey was carried out using a questionnaire to $n = 176$ patients who consented during OFTT usage. Descriptive analysis was carried out to identify who used the tool, for what purpose, and if the participant followed the recommendations. The quantitative results shaped the interview guide's development. Second, in-depth interviews were held with a purposeful sample of $n = 19$, selected from the OFTT users who had consented to a further qualitative study. The qualitative findings were meant to explain the quantitative results. Third, in-depth interviews were held with healthcare providers and authorities ($n = 5$) that were privy to the tool. Framework analysis was adopted using the five-factor framework as a lens with which to analyze the qualitative data only. Results: The five-factor framework proved useful in identifying gaps that affected the utility of the COVID-19 OFTT. The identified gaps could fit and be represented by five factors: primary, secondary, tertiary, and extraneous factors, along with a lack of systems thinking. Conclusion: A theory or framework provides a road map to systematically identify those factors affecting policy implementation. Knowing how and why policy practice gaps come about in a COVID-19 OFFT context facilitates better future OFTTs. The framework in this study, although developed in a universal health coverage (UHC) context in South Africa, proved useful in a telehealth context in Switzerland, in Europe. The importance of systems thinking in developing digital tools cannot be overemphasized.

Keywords: utility; five-factor framework; policy gaps; COVID-19 OFTT; systems thinking

1. Introduction

Worldwide health systems are being faced with unprecedented COVID-19-related challenges ranging from the problems of a novel condition and a shortage of personal protective equipment to frequently changing medical guidelines [1]. Online forward triage tools (OFTTs) facilitate the interaction between a user/human and a computer system and gives a recommendation on what to do based on the input received [1–3]. Many institutions were forced to innovate and many hospitals as well as telehealth providers set up online forward triage tools (OFTTs) [1]. Using an OFTT before visiting the emergency department or a doctor's practice, therefore, became common practice.

A policy is defined as what an institution or government chooses to do or not to do [4]. The policy process is widely conceptualized as six stages: (1) problem emergence; (2) agenda setting; (3) consideration of policy options; (4) decision-making; (5) implementation; (6) evaluation [5]. The policy cycle is also described as policy development, policy communication, policy implementation, and policy evaluation [6]. In light of the above, the COVID-19 OFTT is both a policy and a practice.

The SARS-CoV-2 pandemic accelerated the adoption of telehealth services, particularly OFTTs [1,7,8]. OFTTs have been reported to reduce the health system burden, to inform and direct patients toward the appropriate level of care, e.g., to test or not to test, how to conduct self-care, as well as how to relieve anxiety [1,9]. The Inselspital, University Hospital Bern, set up an OFTT, coronatest.ch, on 2 March 2020, to cope with the influx of SARS-CoV-2 patients. The tool was updated regularly, based on the changing testing criteria issued by the Swiss Federal Office of Public Health [1].

Due to the urgency of the situation, patients or potential tool users could not be consulted during tool development but the tool was pilot-tested by ER physicians. With no active advertisement, the tool was offered by the Inselspital hospital. It is noteworthy that involving end users, policy implementers, and beneficiaries facilitates successful policy implementation [10–12].

Evaluating policy implementation facilitates learning which in turn leads to success and positive outcomes. Many OFTTs have however not been evaluated. Identifying frameworks that work is the first step in that direction. A theory or framework provides a road map for systematic evaluation, identifying factors that actors perceive as affecting implementation. We utilized the five-factor framework as our analytic tool [11]. The purpose of this manuscript is to assess the utility of the five-factor framework in identifying how and why policy–practice gaps come about in a COVID-19 OFTT implementation context.

2. Methods

2.1. Context

The Emergency Department, Inselspital University Hospital Bern decided to set up coronatest.ch, an OFTT, in March 2020. The assessment tool, coronatest.ch, was designed to deal with an influx of patients during the SARS-CoV-2 pandemic.

2.2. Study Aim

The aim of the study was to assess the utility of the five-factor framework in identifying how and why policy–practice gaps came about within the context of a COVID-19 online forward triage tool.

2.3. Study Design

This study was part of a broader multiphase sequential explanatory study.

Participants included OFTT users aged 18 and above who used the Insel COVID-19 OFTT between 2 March and 12 May 2020. A total of 6272 users consulted the COVID-19 OFTT and quantitative data was collected from 560 participants, who consented to a follow-up survey and provided valid email addresses. A total of $n = 176$ out of the 560 participants completed the online survey. First, a descriptive analysis was carried out to identify who used the online tool and for what purpose, and if, indeed, they followed the recommendations (see Table 1, below). The quantitative results guided the interview guide development. Second, in-depth interviews were held with a purposeful sample, $n = 19$, selected from the OFTT users who had consented to a further qualitative study. The qualitative findings were meant to explain the quantitative results. Third, in-depth interviews were held with healthcare providers and authorities ($n = 5$) who were privy to the analytical tool due to their professional roles. Framework analysis was adopted, using the five-factor framework as a lens, to analyze the qualitative data only.

Table 1. The socio-demographic characteristics of the survey participants (quantitative data) [13].

	Total	(n = 176)	Female	(n = 101)	Male	(n = 75)	p-Value *
Age [mean, SD]	50.1	[±15.4]	45.9	[±14.1]	55.7	[±15.4]	<0.001
Education							
Did not want to answer	6	[3.4]	3	[3.0]	3	[4.0]	
University	120	[68.2]	67	[66.3]	53	[70.7]	
Higher secondary school	27	[15.3]	17	[16.8]	10	[13.3]	
Lower secondary school	23	[13.1]	14	[13.9]	9	[12.0]	0.871
Income per month							
Did not want to answer	29	[16.5]	17	[16.8]	12	[16.0]	
<4000 CHF	26	[14.8]	20	[19.8]	6	[8.0]	
4000–6000	42	[23.9]	27	[26.7]	15	[20.0]	
>6000	79	[44.9]	37	[36.6]	42	[56.0]	0.037
Work							
Did not want to answer	33	[18.8]	14	[13.9]	19	[25.3]	
Employed	106	[60.2]	64	[63.4]	42	[56.0]	
Self-employed	24	[13.6]	13	[12.9]	11	[14.7]	
Unemployed	3	[1.7]	3	[3.0]	0	[0.0]	
Lost work (COVID-19)	1	[0.6]	1	[1.0]	0	[0.0]	
Student/trainee	9	[5.1]	6	[5.9]	3	[4.0]	0.236
Insurance							
Do not know	5	[2.8]	3	[3.0]	2	[2.7]	
General	68	[38.6]	39	[38.6]	29	[38.7]	
Telemedicine	12	[6.8]	6	[5.9]	6	[8.0]	
GP	83	[47.2]	47	[46.5]	36	[48.0]	
Other	8	[4.5]	6	[5.9]	2	[2.7]	0.859
Nationality							
Did not want to answer	1	[0.6]	1	[1.0]	0	[0.0]	
Switzerland	147	[83.5]	80	[79.2]	67	[89.3]	
Germany	13	[7.4]	8	[7.9]	5	[6.7]	
French	1	[0.6]	0	[0.0]	1	[1.3]	
Italy	3	[1.7]	2	[2.0]	1	[1.3]	
Other Europe	4	[2.3]	3	[3.0]	1	[1.3]	
Other	7	[4.0]	7	[6.9]	0	[0.0]	0.202

* Chi-squared for categorical variables and Wilcoxon rank sum test for continuous variables; data are total number and percentage if not mentioned otherwise

3. Qualitative Data Collection

The qualitative interviews were conducted with purposefully selected key informants who gave their consent during the survey (see Table 2 below).

Table 2. Key informants (patients, healthcare providers, and authorities).

Key Informants	Male	Female	Total
OFTT users—patients	10	9	19
Healthcare providers and authorities	1	4	5
Total	11	13	24

Video rather than face-to-face interviews were held with most participants in September 2020, due to social-distancing rules. A combination of video and telephonic interviews was conducted with three participants who encountered technical difficulties and a telephone-only interview was held with one lady, aged over 65, who had no computer access. Three face-to-face interviews were held with three key informants: one was a hospital healthcare worker and two other key informants worked close to Bern University Hospital. A semi-structured interview guide, informed by the quantitative results, was used (see Supplementary Materials Figures S1–S3). This guide was adapted iteratively throughout the data collection period. Two qualitative researchers sat in each session, fielding questions in turn. All interviews were conducted in German by two researchers who were fluent in both English and German. The interviews lasted between 45 min to one and a half hours. Two audio recorders were used in each session. All participants gave individual written consent as well as oral consent to their being recorded at the beginning of each session (see Table 2 for a summary of the key informants).

Qualitative Data Analysis

All audio recordings were transcribed verbatim, analyzed, and triangulated with the results from the quantitative data. Qualitative narratives were explored for their fit with the five factors of the analytic framework [11]. Two qualitative researchers analyzed the transcripts independently and developed and agreed on a code book. All the concepts fitted into the five factor themes.

4. Measures to Ensure the Trustworthiness of the Data

To ensure dependability, the data collection process and analysis were performed iteratively, continuously adjusting our interview guide to capture newly emerging themes. Two qualitative researchers kept reflexive journals and debriefed at the end of each interview throughout the data collection phase. A comprehensive description of the participants, context, and data collection process has been outlined here to ensure transferability. Data were managed and analyzed with the aid of MAXQDA2020.

4.1. Ethics Approval

Our study is embedded in an online forward triage tool set up by the Insel University Hospital within a pandemic setting, primarily to prevent health-system overload. The evaluation of the usefulness of this tool to the health stakeholders, patients, healthcare providers, and health authorities was deemed to be a quality evaluation; hence, the ethics committee of the province (canton) of Bern, Switzerland, waived the need for a full ethical review (Req-2020-00289) on the 23 March 2020 and granted us permission to carry out the study.

4.2. Central Questions

How well do the identified themes fit into the five-factor framework?
How well does the five-factor framework explain why and how the policy–practice gaps came about?

4.3. The Five-Factor Framework [11]

A theory or framework provides a road map for systematically identifying those factors perceived by all stakeholders as affecting implementation. With the aid of the five-factor framework, we identified COVID-19 OFTT (coronatest.ch) policy gaps. This framework, developed in a universal health coverage (UHC) context [11], goes beyond identifying barriers and facilitators of policy to explain how and why these policy–practice gaps came about.

4.4. Five Groups of Factors Identified as Bringing about Policy–Practice Gaps

(1) Primary factors stem from a direct lack of a critical component for policy implementation, whether tangible or intangible—resources, the policy itself, information, motivation, power, and context;
(2) Secondary factors stem from a lack of efficient processes or systems, e.g., budget processes, financial delegations, communication channels, top-down directives, supply chains, supervision, and performance management processes;
(3) Tertiary factors stem from human factors—perception, cognition, and calculated human responses to a lack of primary, secondary, and or extraneous factors as coping mechanisms (ideal reporting and audit driven compliance);

(4) Extraneous factors stem from beyond the health system—economy, weather, climate, and drought;
(5) An overall lack of systems thinking also brings about this type of gap. See Figure 1 below.

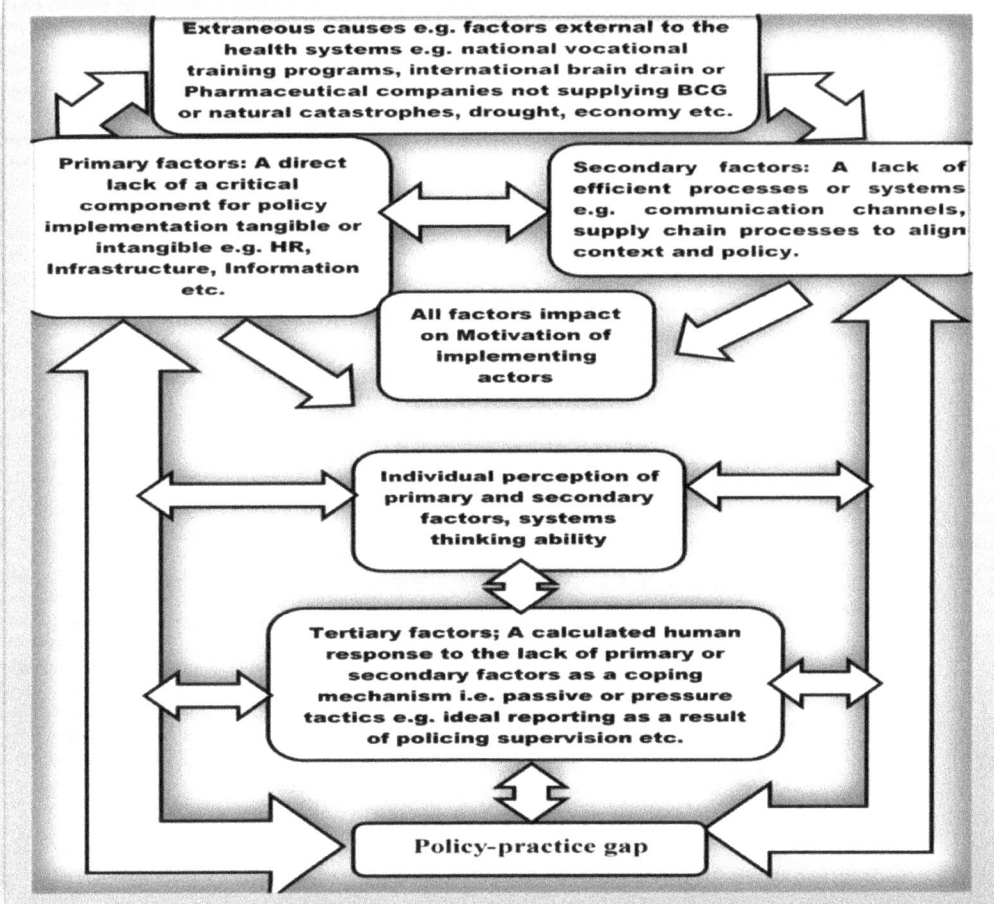

Figure 1. The five-factor framework [11].

5. Findings

5.1. Primary Factors Stemming from the Direct Lack of a Critical Component for Policy Implementation, Whether Tangible or Intangible—Resources, Information, Motivation, and Power

The policy itself, regarding the use of OFTT to reduce the health-system burden, was shown to be good in itself. Most of the participants, however, discovered the tool by chance, as the tool itself was not advertised. There was no coordinated way of communicating the tool's availability to other healthcare providers either.

> "The tool is meant for adults. A similar tool that is child-specific would be very helpful."
>
> Key informant 2 (healthcare provider)

The first OFTT, coronatest.ch, was adult-oriented and so child-specific information was missing. The first interviews revealed this lack, which led to the birth of another initiative, the launch of coronabambini, a child-specific OFTT [14].

5.2. Secondary Factors Stemming from a Lack of Efficient Processes or Systems—Budget Processes, Limited Financial Delegation, Top-Down Directives, Communication Channels, Supply-Chain Processes, Ineffective Supervision, and Performance Management Systems

The availability of the OFTTs was not communicated widely; neither were they advertised. Notwithstanding the communication challenge, many participants reported using the tool and receiving the recommendation to be tested, only to be met with test-kit shortages. Others reported that their GPs and pediatricians were not aware of the tool and so refused to give them the test. Other healthcare providers reported that shortages in terms of test availability prevented them from doing so.

> "We did not have sufficient test kits at the beginning; we ran out and could not test."
>
> Key informant (healthcare provider)

5.3. Tertiary Factors Stemming from Human Factors—Perception and Cognition, and the Calculated Human Responses to a Lack of Primary, Secondary, and/or Extraneous Factors as Coping Mechanisms (Ideal Reporting and Audit-Driven Compliance with Core Standards)

The system is only as good as the people within the system. The GPs responded in different ways when patients suspected that they had COVID-19, as revealed below:

> "When I asked for a test, my GP told me that this is [a] hysterical [response], everyone now thinks that they have COVID-19."
>
> Key informant (patient)

> "What is interesting is that the GPs were open to testing children, while the pediatricians refused [to test] the children."
>
> Key informant (patient)

5.4. Extraneous Factors Stemming from Beyond the Health System (National Vocational Training, Leading to a National Shortage of Plumbers)

COVID-19, a novel infection, took the world by surprise. There was a lack of knowledge of the disease signs and symptoms, progression, and even management. This made the guidelines change frequently as a result, with sometimes conflicting information being given, including those concerning mask mandates.

> "The whole pandemic took us all by surprise."
>
> Key informant (health authority)

5.5. An Overall Lack of Systems Thinking

An OFTT is dependent upon other parts of the system, for example, the supply chain, testing centers, and the readiness of the patients to follow recommendations. Fear, social media, rumors, and disinformation, although not primarily health system factors, also affected attitudes to OFTT testing recommendations. Some participants revealed the following:

> "Many people did not test for fear of a positive test result. They would rather not know."
>
> Key informant (patient)

6. Discussion

We assessed the utility of the five-factor framework in identifying how and why policy–practice gaps came about within a COVID-19 online forward triage tool. The themes that emerged from the qualitative data could fit into the five factors: primary, secondary, tertiary, and extraneous factors, along with a lack of systems thinking, and helped explain how and why policy–practice gaps come about in the context of a COVID-19 OFTT. See Table 3 and Figure 1 above.

Table 3. Summary of the emergent themes.

Theme	Category	Unit Meaning
1. Primary factors stemming from a direct lack of a critical component for policy implementation, tangible or intangible—resources, information, motivation, power	Policy communication	- Often, it was not advertised
2. Secondary factors stemming from a lack of efficient processes or systems—budget processes, limited financial delegations, top-down directives, communication channels, supply chain processes, ineffective supervision, and performance management systems	Supply chain challenges Infrastructural challenges	- Test kit shortages - Laboratory testing capacity
3. Tertiary factors stemming from human factors—perception and cognition and calculated human responses to a lack of primary, secondary, and or extraneous factors, as coping mechanisms (ideal reporting and audit-driven compliance with core standards)	Human factors	- GPs told patients that they are being hysterical, they cannot have COVID-19
4. Extraneous factors stemming from beyond the health system (national vocational training, leading to a national shortage of plumbers)	Factors beyond the health system	- A novel condition; therefore, no one knew what to expect with COVID-19 - Economic factors
5. An overall lack of systems thinking	The utility of the tool in testing is affected by so many factors	- Test kit shortages, psychological readiness to test, the healthcare provider's trust in the tool

6.1. Primary Factors Stemming from the Direct Lack of a Critical Component for Policy Implementation, Whether Tangible or Intangible—Resources, Information, Motivation, and Power

The Inselspital Emergency Department responded to the high volumes of calls by setting up an OFTT, so as to reduce the burden on the health system. Neither the healthcare providers nor the patients were involved in tool development. The tool itself was not advertised and those that used the tool discovered it by chance, revealing an information gap. This five-factor framework recommends the involvement of both policymakers and policy implementers and their beneficiaries, where appropriate, as a way of achieving the buy-in and uptake of future tools. This shortcoming is also highlighted by Greenhalgh et al. [15]. The communication of this policy, although closely related to policy development, is, in itself, very important for successful policy implementation [15]. This identified gap might have resulted in a low buy-in from healthcare providers and in some patient groups who are not technology-aware being excluded.

6.2. Secondary Factors Stemming from a Lack of Efficient Processes or Systems-Budget Processes, Limited Financial Delegations, Top-Down Directives, Communication Channels, Supply Chain Processes, Ineffective Supervision, and Performance Management Systems

The five-factor framework revealed that healthcare providers were not involved, and patients reported being refused a test by some doctors who were not aware of the tool and, hence, did not trust the recommendations affecting policy implementation (OFFT). Shortages of test kits were reported at the beginning of the pandemic. This points toward supply-chain issues, a secondary factor in the five-factor framework. The shortage of test kits represents a supply-chain issue that affected the usefulness of the OFTT on testing, since those who needed a test could not access one. In line with our findings, supply-chain issues can impact policy implementation, either positively or negatively [16].

6.3. Tertiary Factors Stemming from Human Factors—Perception and Cognition and Calculated Human Responses to a Lack of Primary, Secondary, and or Extraneous Factors as Coping Mechanisms (Ideal Reporting and Audit-Driven Compliance with Core Standards)

The utility of the assessment tool in reducing the health-system burden was acknowledged by patients, providers, and authorities. Some aspects, such as the utility of the tool in relieving fear and anxiety, were acknowledged by patients but were disputed by healthcare providers. Human factors play a role in implementation; being a patient or healthcare provider changes how one perceives the utility of a tool [11,17]. The importance of human factors in policy implementation cannot be overemphasized [18].

6.4. Extraneous Factors Stemming from beyond the Health System (National Vocational Training, Leading to a National Shortage of Plumbers)

COVID-19 is a novel condition. Neither the authorities nor the clinicians had knowledge of its pathology at the beginning of the outbreak, leading to ever-changing guidelines and conflicting messages since there was no prior knowledge to fall back on. This underlies the fact that some issues affecting implementation go far beyond the health system. In addition, a number of OFTT users who received the recommendation to be tested for COVID-19 did not go on to do so. Many cited the fear of losing income and possibly their jobs, revealing how factors beyond the health system, such as economic factors, affected OFTT implementation, concurring with the findings reported elsewhere [18]. Contrary to our findings, OFTTs have been associated with risk aversion, resulting in increased healthcare service use rather than the reduction of the healthcare system burden [19,20]. It is worth highlighting that while as OFTTs can educate clients and provide information on symptoms, they cannot talk to the patient, touch, feel, or look the patient in the eye, a vital shortcoming that underlies the importance of the human factor in health care [20].

6.5. An Overall Lack of Systems Thinking

A proportion of people who received a recommendation to test did not do so. This finding was associated with the psychological readiness of patients to test, which, in turn, was influenced by the fear of receiving a positive test result. Even after resolving the supply-chain issues, having the test kits alone did not resolve this issue, highlighting the interconnectedness of things and the importance of systems thinking. Senge also emphasizes the importance of systems thinking in policy implementation [21].

6.6. Strengths and Limitations

1. Our study tested the utility of a five-factor framework, thereby contributing to the body of OFTT evaluation frameworks.
2. Knowing how and why policy practice gaps come about in a COVID-19 OFFT context facilitates success in future and better OFTTs.
3. Our study demonstrated the importance of systems thinking in developing digital tools and this importance cannot be overemphasized.
4. The key informants were sampled from online OFTT users. The perspectives of key informants that do not have access to or do not use OFTTs are not represented.

Few OFTTs have been evaluated; one of the major stumbling blocks is a lack of OFTT evaluation frameworks. Our study tested the utility of a five-factor framework, thereby contributing to the body of OFTT evaluation frameworks. Identifying frameworks that work is the first step. A theory or framework provides a road map for systematic evaluation, identifying those factors that actors perceive as affecting implementation. Knowing how and why policy practice gaps come about in a COVID-19 OFFT context facilitates success in future and better OFTTs. The five-factor framework, although developed in a universal health coverage (UHC) context in South Africa, proved useful in identifying policy–practice gaps in a COVID-19 OFTT used in Switzerland, in Europe. Our study demonstrated the importance of systems thinking in developing digital tools and this cannot be overemphasized. The key informants in this study were sampled from online OFTT users. The perspectives of key informants that do not have access to or do not use OFTTs are, thus, not represented. To the best of our knowledge, this selection bias could not be prevented due to data protection regulations, which impose voluntary participation and prohibit the technically possible automatic tracking of participants.

7. Conclusions

The five-factor framework proved useful in identifying gaps that affected the utility of the COVID-19 OFTT. The identified gaps could fit and be represented by the five factors: primary, secondary, tertiary, and extraneous factors, along with a lack of systems thinking. The framework, although developed in a universal health coverage (UHC) context in South Africa, proved useful in a telehealth context in Switzerland, in Europe. A theory or framework provides a road map to systematically identify those factors affecting policy implementation [22]. Knowing how and why policy practice gaps came about in a COVID-19 OFFT context facilitates success in future and better OFTTs. These findings are encouraging, and we recommend that others should test this framework in other settings and contexts to assess its utility in identifying how and why policy–practice gaps come about. This is particularly important to address, as evidence repeatedly points out that policies are rarely translated into practice [11,23–26].

Supplementary Materials: The following supporting information can be downloaded at: https://www.mdpi.com/article/10.3390/systems10060257/s1, Figure S1: Interview Guide: Key Informants—Patients; Figure S2: Interview Guide: Key Informants—Healthcare Providers; Figure S3: Interview Guide: Key Informants—Health Authorities.

Author Contributions: Study design and ideas: J.M., D.E., M.T. and T.C.S.; qualitative data analysis, J.M., D.E., M.T. and T.C.S.; writing of the first draft: J.M., D.E., M.T. and T.C.S.; revision of final draft and approval, J.M., D.E., M.T. and T.C.S.; project administrator, T.C.S. All authors have read and agreed to the published version of the manuscript.

Funding: Swiss National Science Foundation (Project ID: 196615).

Data Availability Statement: Due to the nature of the study (OFTT), participants did not agree that their data should be shared publicly. The data that support the findings are available on reasonable request. Please contact the corresponding author, J.M.

Conflicts of Interest: The authors declare no conflict of interest. The present manuscript is partially funded by the Swiss National Foundation (Project ID: 196615). The funder has no influence on the content of the manuscript or the decision to publish it. T.C.S. holds the endowed professorship for emergency telemedicine at the University of Bern, Switzerland. The funder, Touring Club Switzerland, has no influence on the research performed, the content of any manuscript, or any decision to publish. All other authors have nothing to disclose.

References

1. Hautz, W.E.; Exadaktylos, A.; Sauter, T.C. Online forward triage during the COVID-19 outbreak. *Emerg. Med. J.* **2020**, *38*, 106–108. [CrossRef] [PubMed]
2. Shingte, K.; Chaudhari, A.; Patil, A.; Chaudhari, A.; Desai, S. Chatbot Development for Educational Institute. *SSRN Electron. J.* **2021**. [CrossRef]
3. Nudging, Remote Monitoring and Chatbots: How Virtual Care Is Being Brought to the Patient. Available online: https://vator.tv/news/2020-07-03-nudging-remote-monitoring-and-chatbots-how-virtual-care-is-being-brought-to-the-patient (accessed on 29 September 2022).

4. Burke, K.; Morris, K.; McGarrigle, L.; Centre for Effective Services. *An Introductory Guide to Implementation: Terms, Concepts and Frameworks*; Centre for Effective Services: Dublin, Ireland, 2012; ISBN 978-0-9568037-2-6.
5. Policy Process—An Overview. Available online: https://www.sciencedirect.com/topics/social-sciences/policy-process (accessed on 23 March 2021).
6. Michel, J.; Mohlakoana, N.; Bärnighausen, T.; Tediosi, F.; McIntyre, D.; Bressers, H.T.A.; Tanner, M.; Evans, D. Varying universal health coverage policy implementation states: Exploring the process and lessons learned from a national health insurance pilot site. *J. Glob. Health Rep.* **2020**, *4*, e2020036. [CrossRef]
7. Nittas, V.; von Wyl, V. COVID-19 and telehealth: A window of opportunity and its challenges. *Swiss Med. Wkly.* **2020**, *150*, w20284. [CrossRef] [PubMed]
8. Michel, J.; Hautz, W.; Sauter, T. Telemedicine and Online Platforms as an Opportunity to Optimise Qualitative Data Collection, Explore and Understand Disease Pathways in a Novel Pandemic Like COVID-19. *J. Int. Soc. Telemed. EHealth* **2020**, *8*, e9. [CrossRef]
9. Effects and Utility of an Online Forward Triage Tool during the SARS-CoV-2 Pandemic: Patient Perspectives. Available online: https://preprints.jmir.org/preprint/26553 (accessed on 4 January 2021).
10. van Deen, W.K.; Cho, E.S.; Pustolski, K.; Wixon, D.; Lamb, S.; Valente, T.W.; Menchine, M. Involving end-users in the design of an audit and feedback intervention in the emergency department setting—A mixed methods study. *BMC Health Serv. Res.* **2019**, *19*, 270. [CrossRef] [PubMed]
11. Michel, J.; Chimbindi, N.; Mohlakoana, N.; Orgill, M.; Bärnighausen, T.; Obrist, B.; Tediosi, F.; Evans, D.; McIntyre, D.; Bressers, H.T.; et al. How and why policy-practice gaps come about: A South African Universal Health Coverage context. *J. Glob. Health Rep.* **2019**, *3*, e2019069. [CrossRef]
12. Mohlakoana, N. *Implementing the South African Free Basic Alternative Energy Policy: A Dynamic Actor Interaction*; University of Twente: Enschede, The Netherlands, 2014.
13. Michel, J.; Mettler, A.; Stuber, R.; Müller, M.; Ricklin, M.; Jent, P.; Hautz, W.E.; Sauter, T.C. Effects and utility of an online forward triage tool during the SARS-CoV-2 pandemic: A mixed method study and patient perspectives, Switzerland. *BMJ Open* **2022**, *12*, e059765. [CrossRef] [PubMed]
14. Coronabambini. Available online: https://www.coronabambini.ch/login/main_sprachvar.cfm?typ=o&sprachprepo=&startpos=0&frage=0&danke=0&v=1&setinitial= (accessed on 24 August 2021).
15. Greenhalgh, T.; Wherton, J.; Papoutsi, C.; Lynch, J.; Hughes, G.; A'Court, C.; Hinder, S.; Fahy, N.; Procter, R.; Shaw, S. Beyond Adoption: A New Framework for Theorizing and Evaluating Nonadoption, Abandonment, and Challenges to the Scale-Up, Spread, and Sustainability of Health and Care Technologies. *J. Med. Internet Res.* **2017**, *19*, e8775. [CrossRef] [PubMed]
16. Hoeyi, P.K.; Makgari, K.R. The impact and challenges of a public policy implemented in the South African Police Service, Northern Cape. *Afr. Public Serv. Deliv. Perform. Rev.* **2021**, *9*, 374. [CrossRef]
17. Adams-Jack, U.L. Implementation gaps, policy change and health system transformation in the Western Cape Province, South Africa. *Politeia* **2016**, *35*, 1–18. [CrossRef] [PubMed]
18. Tezera, D. Factors for the Successful Implementation of Policies. *Merit Res. J. Educ. Rev.* **2019**, *7*, 092–095. Available online: https://core.ac.uk/download/pdf/228209627.pdf (accessed on 24 August 2022).
19. Cerami, C.; Galandra, C.; Santi, G.C.; Dodich, A.; Cappa, S.F.; Vecchi, T.; Crespi, C. Risk-Aversion for Negative Health Outcomes May Promote Individual Compliance to Containment Measures in Covid-19 Pandemic. *Front. Psychol.* **2021**, *12*, 666454. [CrossRef] [PubMed]
20. Bauman, D. Online Symptom Checkers—What Do They Really Do for Consumers? Available online: https://info.isabelhealthcare.com/blog/online-symptom-checkers-what-should-they-really-do-for-consumers (accessed on 21 February 2022).
21. Senge, P.M. *The Fifth Discipline: The Art and Practice of the Learning Organization*; Random House Business Books: London, UK, 1999; ISBN 978-0-7126-5687-0.
22. Bressers Hans. *Implementing Sustainable Development: How to Know What Works, Where, When and How*; Edward Elgar: Cheltenham, UK, 2004; pp. 284–318.
23. Robinson, T.; Bailey, C.; Morris, H.; Burns, P.; Melder, A.; Croft, C.; Spyridonidis, D.; Bismantara, H.; Skouteris, H.; Teede, H. Bridging the research–practice gap in healthcare: A rapid review of research translation centres in England and Australia. *Health Res. Policy Syst.* **2020**, *18*, 117. [CrossRef] [PubMed]
24. Translating Research into Practice (TRIP)-II. Available online: https://archive.ahrq.gov/research/findings/factsheets/translating/tripfac/trip2fac.html (accessed on 13 August 2021).
25. Tomm-Bonde, L.; Schreiber, R.S.; Allan, D.E.; MacDonald, M.; Pauly, B.; Hancock, T. Fading vision: Knowledge translation in the implementation of a public health policy intervention. *Implement. Sci.* **2013**, *8*, 59. [CrossRef] [PubMed]
26. Michel, J.; Obrist, B.; Bärnighausen, T.; Tediosi, F.; McIntyre, D.; Evans, D.; Tanner, M. What we need is health system transformation and not health system strengthening for universal health coverage to work: Perspectives from a National Health Insurance pilot site in South Africa. *S. Afr. Fam. Pract.* **2020**, *62*, 15. [CrossRef] [PubMed]

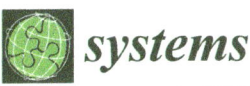

Article

On the Relationships among Nurse Staffing, Inpatient Care Quality, and Hospital Competition under the Global Budget Payment Scheme of Taiwan's National Health Insurance System: Mixed Frequency VAR Analyses

Wen-Yi Chen

Department of Senior Citizen Service Management, National Taichung University of Science and Technology, Taichung 403301, Taiwan; chenwen@nutc.edu.tw; Tel.: +886-422196932

Abstract: Background: Time series analyses on the relationship between nurse staffing and inpatient care quality are rare due to inconsistent frequencies of data between common observations of nurse-staffing (e.g., monthly) and inpatient care quality indicators (e.g., quarterly). Methods: In order to deal with the issue of mixed frequency data, this research adopted the MF-VAR model to explore causal relationships among nurse staffing, inpatient care quality, and hospital competition under the global budget payment scheme of Taiwan's healthcare system. Results: Our results identified bi-directional causation between nurse staffing and patient outcomes and one-way Granger causality running between nurse staffing and reimbursement payments for inpatient care services. Impulse-response analyses found positive (negative) effects of the patient-to-nurse ratio on adverse patient outcomes (reimbursement payments) in all types of hospitals and detrimental effects of adverse patient outcomes on the patient-to-nurse ratio in medical centers and regional hospitals across a 12-month period. Conclusions: These findings suggest that nurse staffing is an essential determinant of both patient outcomes and reimbursement payments. Strategic policies such as direct subsidy and hospital accreditation for appropriate nurse staffing levels should be implemented for medical centers and regional hospitals to mitigate the harmful effects of adverse patient outcomes on nurse staffing.

Keywords: nurse staffing; inpatient care quality; hospital competition; Mixed Frequency VAR; global budget payment scheme; National Health Insurance

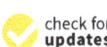

Citation: Chen, W.-Y. On the Relationships among Nurse Staffing, Inpatient Care Quality, and Hospital Competition under the Global Budget Payment Scheme of Taiwan's National Health Insurance System: Mixed Frequency VAR Analyses. *Systems* **2022**, *10*, 187. https://doi.org/10.3390/systems10050187

Academic Editors: Philippe J. Giabbanelli and Andrew Page

Received: 31 August 2022
Accepted: 11 October 2022
Published: 14 October 2022

Publisher's Note: MDPI stays neutral with regard to jurisdictional claims in published maps and institutional affiliations.

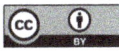

Copyright: © 2022 by the author. Licensee MDPI, Basel, Switzerland. This article is an open access article distributed under the terms and conditions of the Creative Commons Attribution (CC BY) license (https://creativecommons.org/licenses/by/4.0/).

1. Introduction

In their pioneering work on the relationship between hospital nurse staffing and patient outcomes and factors influencing nurse retention, Aiken and her colleagues identified the patient-to-nurse ratio (PNR, hereafter) as an essential determinant of patient outcomes and nurse retention [1]. A crucial conclusion of their study is that each additional patient per nurse is associated with higher patient mortality in the US. Continuing this line of research, one strand of studies provided evidence of the positive effect of hospital nurse staffing levels on patient mortality worldwide, such as in Australia [2,3], Belgium [4], Canada [5], Chile [6], England [7], Finland [8], Korea [9], Norway [10], Taiwan [11–13], and a group of European and OECD countries [14–18]. Another strand of the literature investigated the relationships between nurse staffing levels and various nursing-sensitive patient outcomes such as fall, pressure ulcer, medication error, various infections, physical restraint, missed observation, failure to respond to patients, length of stay, readmission to hospitals, emergency department attendance, etc. [2,19–25].

It is important to address that hospital competition under a publicly financed healthcare system may create a vicious cycle. In general, the cycle starts with quantity competition in inpatient care services leading to a high PNR and then further worsens patient outcomes or inpatient care quality (ICQ, hereafter). For example, Taiwan's National Health Insurance (NHI, hereafter) system is a publicly financed healthcare system delivering universal coverage of healthcare services with moderate cost-sharing for all Taiwanese residents. The beneficiaries of Taiwan's NHI pay 5.17% of the payroll income for the regular insurance premium rate and 2.11% of the non-payroll income (such as bonuses, part-time income, professional service income, dividend income, interest income, and rental income) for a supplementary premium rate [26]. Additionally, the covered benefits of Taiwan's NHI system include outpatient care, inpatient care, emergence department (ED, hereafter) care, dental care, eye care, maternity delivery, physiotherapy and rehabilitation services, home health care, chronic mental illness, prescription drugs, and traditional Chinese medicine [26]. Nevertheless, the copayment for the outpatient care (ED care) per visit varies from USD 1.67 (USD 5.00) to USD 14.00 (USD 18.33), and the co-insurance rate for inpatient care per diem varied from 5% to 30% depending on various healthcare providers and the length of stay, respectively [26].

As with other publicly financed healthcare systems such as the National Health Services (NHS, hereafter) and Social Health Insurance systems (SHI, hereafter), it is expected that financial difficulty will be the most challenging issue under Taiwan's NHI system [26–29]. In order to constrain the upward trend in healthcare expenditure, the Taiwan National Health Insurance Administration (NHIA, hereafter) applied the Global Budget Payment Scheme (GBPS, hereafter) to reimburse for healthcare services in the hospital sector since 2002 [26,30–32]. In general, the GBPS assigns a fixed total budget for inpatient care services with hospitals being reimbursed on a fee-for-service basis, and it follows that hospitals have strong incentives to compete with quantity rather than quality of inpatient care services in order to obtain target revenues under a fixed total budget of healthcare expenditure [26,30–32].

It is also important to point out that the hospital sector of Taiwan's NHI system consists of three different types of hospitals, these being district hospitals (delivering secondary care), regional hospitals (providing tertiary care), and medical centers (handling the most complicated illnesses and supporting teaching and research in clinical practices) [29,30]. In order to prevent the negative effects of hospital (quantity) competition on patient outcomes under the GBPS of Taiwan's NHI system, Taiwan's NHIA imposed a PNR mandate such that the PNR of the day-shift should be below 7 for hospital wards in the three different types of hospitals. Nonetheless, the mean PNR of the three shifts (i.e., day, afternoon, and night shifts) within a daily cycle can legally vary from 9, 12, and 15 for hospital wards in medical centers, regional hospitals, and district hospitals, respectively [33]. This mandated PNR policy, in fact, is not restrictive, but flexible, for hospitals to adjust their nurse labor force to cope with severe quantity competition of inpatient care services in the hospital sector of Taiwan's NHI system. Therefore, the most likely response of hospitals to market (quantity) competition under the GBPS of Taiwan's NHI system is to shift their PNRs upward in order to maintain their own share of a fixed total budget [34]. It follows that a heavier workload imposed on incumbent nurses would not only increase the likelihood of nurses' burnout but also worsen patient outcomes [1,35]. Therefore, a vicious cycle originating from hospital (quantity) competition under the GBPS should be anticipated which will deteriorate ICQ through inappropriate nurse staffing levels under Taiwan's NHI system.

From the perspective of preventing the vicious cycle triggered by hospital (quantity) competition under the GBPS, the surveillance of PNR time series at hospital wards is an important managerial strategy for the healthcare administration to use to maintain high ICQ, better nursing work environments, and a reasonable inpatient care expenditure (ICE, hereafter) to reimburse hospitals for their inpatient care services. Nevertheless, time series analyses on the relationship between nurse staffing and patient outcomes are limited in the literature. Some studies relating to the nurse staffing and patient outcomes nexus focused on identifying potential structural changes in ICQ indicators due to initiating new nurse staffing regulations [19,36], and other research applied conventional time series methodologies (such as the trend and seasonality decomposition method and the latent growth model) to investigate the determinant of patient outcomes and trajectory of ICQ indicators [37,38]. Although these time series studies provide some justification for nurse staffing as an important determinant of patient outcomes, these studies were not grounded in a time series theoretical foundation with regards to three aspects: First, the causal linkage between nurse staffing and patient outcomes cannot be established in these studies, especially for the existence of bidirectional causality between these two variables. Second, these studies fail to provide precautionary information in terms of the propagation mechanism of a nurse staffing policy shock across a period of time. Third, a recent study proposed by Winter and his colleagues cautioned against a potential data aggregation effect on estimations of the nurse staffing and patient outcomes relationship [39]. Moreover, nurse staffing and patient outcomes can be reported in different time frequencies. For example, variables for nurse staffing and patient outcomes may be reported either monthly or quarterly. In order to perform time series analyses with all variables being single frequency, these studies aggregated high frequency data (e.g., monthly data) into low frequency data (e.g., quarterly data). Such temporal aggregation was proven to have some adverse impacts on statistical inferences of time series analyses [40,41].

In this study, we specifically investigate the interdependences between nurse staffing, patient outcomes, and hospital competition under the GBPS of Taiwan's NHI system. The motivation of this study is three-fold: First, Taiwan has experienced a fast demographic transition from an aging society to an aged society within 25 years (from the period of 1993~2018), and it is projected to become a hyper-aged country in 2025 [42]. The growth of the aging population will burden Taiwan's NHI system in terms of rising healthcare expenditures. It can be expected that more stringent cost-containment policies will be enforced to suppress an upward trend of healthcare expenditures, and it is predictable that such policies would create an even more competitive market for hospitals. Second, although Taiwan's NHI system has been successful in providing comprehensive healthcare services for all Taiwanese residents, the quality of healthcare services has been challenged regarding various dimensions of the OECD Health Care Quality Indicator Project [43]. Third, the nurse labor participation rate (defined as the total number of incumbent nurses divided by the total number of licensed nurses) has been around 60% since 2005, meaning that approximately 40% of total licensed nurses are reluctant to engage in nursing works [44]. It was reported that 89.76% of local hospitals had difficulty recruiting nurses in Taiwan, and the shortage of nurses and the poor environment at nursing workplaces are overwhelming problems negatively influencing the appropriate deployment of nursing staffs in the hospital sector of Taiwan's NHI system [34,45,46].

In order to incorporate mixed frequency data into the investigation of the causal relationship between nurse staffing and patient outcomes under the GBPS of Taiwan's NHI system, we first adopted the Mixed Frequency Vector Auto-regressive (MF-VAR, hereafter) model proposed by Ghysel and his colleagues [47,48] to test the causal linkages among nurse staffing (measured by monthly PNR), patient outcomes (measured by two quarterly ICQ indicators defined in the next section), and hospital (quantity) competition (measured by quarterly real ICE per admission) based on three pairs of causal relationships: (1) PNR leading ICQ versus ICQ leading PNR, (2) PNR leading ICE versus ICE leading PNR, and (3) ICQ leading ICE versus ICE leading ICQ. The identification of these three pairs of causal relationships allows us to establish potential mechanisms triggering the vicious cycle of hospital competition under the GBPS of Taiwan's NHI system.

In this study, the conventional VAR model based on the temporal aggregation of mixed frequency data into single frequency data is referred to as the Low Frequency Vector Auto-regressive (LF-VAR, hereafter) model. The MF-VAR model has several advantages against the LF-VAR model from four aspects. First, the MF-VAR model incorporates a high-frequency nurse staffing variable (i.e., monthly PNR used in this study) into the time series analyses. This allows us to demonstrate heterogeneous effects on low frequency variables reflecting patient outcomes (i.e., quarterly ICQ indicators) across the high frequency timescale (three months) within each low frequency time-span (say, one quarter timespan) [40,47–49]. Second, the impulse-response functions (IRFs, hereafter) for the mixed frequency data were estimated in order to capture the propagation mechanism of a nurse-staffing policy (or patient outcomes) shock across a period of time, which can then be used to evaluate the responses of ICQ indicators (PNR) on the change in PNR (ICQ indicators). Third, forecast error variance decomposition analyses for the mixed frequency data were conducted to show that an aggregation of monthly nurse staffing data into quarterly data is likely to underestimate the influence of nurse staffing on patient outcomes. Fourth, all statistical inferences from the MF-VAR model are based on the bootstrap method, which is capable of accommodating the small sample size of data used in this study [40,49]. Therefore, the results obtained from the MF-VAR model provide new insights into the linkages among nurse staffing, patient outcomes, and hospital competition under the GBPS of Taiwan's NHI system.

2. Materials and Methods

2.1. Data and Variables

The main purpose of this study is to explore the interdependences between nurse staffing, patient outcomes, and hospital competition under the GBPS of Taiwan's NHI system. The average PNR of the three shifts (i.e., day, afternoon, and night shifts) of the daily cycle at hospital wards was used to indicate the nurse staffing level. Taiwan's NHIA reports PNR monthly for the three different types of hospitals (i.e., medical centers, regional hospitals, and district hospitals). The re-emergency-department-visit rate in the same hospital within 3 days after discharge (hereafter, 3-day EDV rate) and the unplanned readmission rate within 14 days after discharge (hereafter, 14-day readmission rate) were suggested by Taiwan's NHIA to measure ICQ under the GBPS of Taiwan's NHI system [50]. In order to avoid inconsistencies in monetary values across different periods of time, the real ICE per admission (adjusted by the medical price index based on the 2016 price level) was used to measure reimbursement payments for inpatient care services provided by the three different types of hospitals. Since the GBPS was applied to reimburse inpatient care services, the real ICE per admission also serves as a measure of hospital (quantity) competition in the hospital sector of Taiwan's NHI system. Note that Taiwan's NHIA reported the two ICQ indicators and reimbursed healthcare services quarterly for the three different types of hospitals. Hence, the quarterly data of ICQ indicators and the real ICE per admission and monthly data of PNR were used for our empirical analyses.

Since all data used in this study belong to time series data, we need to deal with the unit root property involved in time-series data in order to avoid spurious correlations among nurse staffing, patient outcomes, and hospital (quantity) competition [27,30]. Previous studies utilized cyclical components extracted from time series data to obtain the stationarity of time series [27]. Accordingly, we extracted the cyclic components of these time series data through the Hodrick and Prescott filter method to assure the stationarity of the time series [51]. Note that cyclic components of these time series data have two important features: First, the long-run trend of times series was removed, so cyclic components of these time series data have a zero mean without a time trend. Second, these cyclic components are interpreted as the percentage deviating from the long-run trend of the original time series. The aggregate cyclic component of PNR (used to estimate the LF-VAR model) was computed as an average of the three individual cyclic components of PNR across a 3-month cycle of a quarter timespan. All the data used in this study were obtained from the Open Database of National Health Insurance administrated by Taiwan's NHIA. The data collection process was approved by the Research Ethics Committee of Taichung Tzu Chi Hospital with the Certificate of Exempt Review ID: REC REC110-23. The quarterly and monthly sample periods start from 2015: Q1 to 2021: Q4 and 2015: M1 to 2021: M12, resulting in a total of 28 and 84 quarterly and monthly observations, respectively.

2.2. VAR Models

The relationship between nurse staffing and patient outcomes can be represented by the hospital production function below:

$$Q_t = f(L_t, K_t, E_t) \tag{1}$$

where the ICQ indicator (Q_t) is the output of a hospital production function. L_t and K_t represent labor and capital inputs of a hospital production function, respectively. E_t measures the environmental factors such as hospital competition under the GBPS. The labor (L_t) and capital (K_t) inputs of a hospital production function were measured by PNR, and three different types of hospitals (such as district hospitals for secondary care, regional hospitals for tertiary care, and medical centers for the most complicated sicknesses and research and development for clinic practices) were used to control different levels of capital inputs in a hospital production function. Hospital competition is signified by the real ICE per admission under the GBPS of Taiwan's NHI system. The same specification of hospital production was used in previous studies on the association between nurse staffing and patient outcomes [11–13]. Since the output and inputs of a hospital production function are all endogenous in clinical practices, Equation (1) could be established as the MF-VAR model as follows:

$$\begin{bmatrix} L_{1t} \\ L_{2t} \\ L_{3t} \\ Q_t \\ E_t \end{bmatrix} = \sum_{k=1}^{\ell} \begin{bmatrix} a_{11,k} & a_{12,k} & a_{13,k} & a_{14,k} & a_{15,k} \\ a_{21,k} & a_{22,k} & a_{23,k} & a_{24,k} & a_{25,k} \\ a_{31,k} & a_{32,k} & a_{33,k} & a_{34,k} & a_{35,k} \\ a_{41,k} & a_{42,k} & a_{43,k} & a_{44,k} & a_{45,k} \\ a_{51,k} & a_{52,k} & a_{53,k} & a_{54,k} & a_{55,k} \end{bmatrix} \begin{bmatrix} L_{1t-1} \\ L_{2t-1} \\ L_{3t-1} \\ Q_{t-1} \\ E_{t-1} \end{bmatrix} + \begin{bmatrix} \varepsilon_{1t} \\ \varepsilon_{2t} \\ \varepsilon_{3t} \\ \varepsilon_{4t} \\ \varepsilon_{5t} \end{bmatrix} \tag{2}$$

where, given a fixed capital input of hospital production (e.g., medical centers, regional hospitals, or district hospitals), L_{it} ($i = 1,2,3$) represents the PNR in the ith month of a quarter timespan. Q_t and E_t signify the ICQ indicator and real ICE per admission, respectively. $t \in \{1, 2, \ldots, T\}$ denotes each quarter during our study period. The lag length (ℓ) was selected based on the method proposed by Newey and West with the maximal lag set at 3 in order to capture the potential seasonal (or monthly) effect [52]. $a_{ij,k}$ ($i, j \in \{1,2,3,4,5\}$ and $k \in \{1,2,3\}$) are the elements of the parameter matrix in the VAR system. ε_{it} ($i = 1,2,\ldots,5$) denote error terms. Since the cyclic components of these time series data were used for the estimation of the MF-VAR model, the estimated parameters of constant terms in the parameter matrix were skipped due to the zero mean property of the Hodrick and Prescott filter method. The way we established our model specification in Equation (2) is the same as for prior studies applying the MF-VAR model for time series analyses in the field of social sciences [40,49]. The technical details of the notations in the parsimonious specification of the MF-VAR model can be found in Ghysel's study [47].

For the sake of model specification comparison between the MF-VAR and LF-VAR models, it should be noted that the individual monthly PNRs (L_{1t}, L_{2t}, and L_{3t}) are stacked in a vector, and one of the possible relationships among PNR, ICQ, and real ICE per admission can be expressed as the 4th low of Equation (2) as follows:

$$Q_t = \sum_{k=1}^{\ell} \left[\sum_{j=1}^{3} a_{4j,k} L_{j,t-k} + a_{44,k} Q_{t-k} + a_{45,k} E_{t-k} \right] + \varepsilon_{4t} \tag{3}$$

As indicated in Equation (3), nurse staffing from each month (L_{it}, $i = 1,2,3$) has heterogeneous effects ($a_{4j,k}$, $j = 1,2,3$) on ICQ. In contrast to the MF-VAR model, the model specification of the LF-VAR model is given by Equation (4):

$$\begin{bmatrix} L_t \\ Q_t \\ E_t \end{bmatrix} = \sum_{k=1}^{3} \begin{bmatrix} a_{11,k} & a_{12,k} & a_{13,k} \\ a_{21,k} & a_{22,k} & a_{23,k} \\ a_{31,k} & a_{32,k} & a_{33,k} \end{bmatrix} \begin{bmatrix} L_{t-k} \\ Q_{t-k} \\ E_{t-k} \end{bmatrix} + \begin{bmatrix} \varepsilon_{1t} \\ \varepsilon_{2t} \\ \varepsilon_{3t} \end{bmatrix} \tag{4}$$

where, L_t represents the quarterly PNR calculated as the average of monthly PNR (i.e., $L_t = (L_{1t} + L_{2t} + L_{3t})/3$). Other notations used in Equation (4) share the same definitions as those used in Equations (2) and (3). Analogous to Equations (2) and (3), one of the possible linkages among PNR, ICQ, and real ICE per admission can be written as the 2nd low of Equation (4) as follows:

$$Q_t = \sum_{k=1}^{3} \left[a_{21,k} \left(\frac{1}{3} \sum_{i=1}^{3} L_{i,t-k} \right) + a_{22,k} E_{t-k} + a_{23,k} L_{t-k} \right] + \varepsilon_{2t} \qquad (5)$$

The specification in Equation (5) implies that L_{1t}, L_{2t}, and L_{3t} have a homogeneous impact ($a_{21,k}/3$) on ICQ (Q_t), and, in turn, the possibilities of monthly effects and lagged information transmission within each quarter are excluded from the LF-VAR model. Finally, the MF-VAR model can be estimated in the same way as the LF-VAR model because these two models share the same asymptotic theory. Nevertheless, the p values for testing the causal (lead-lag) relationships among PNR, ICQ, and real ICE per admission and confidence intervals of IRFs were generated by the bootstrap method due to a small size of samples used in this study.

2.3. Granger Causality Tests

Since all variables establishing a hospital production function are endogenous in clinical practices, the assumption of the interdependence of variables is fulfilled to specify our MF-VAR model and apply the mixed frequency Granger causality tests to investigate the lead-lag relationships among nurse staffing, patient outcomes, and hospital competition. In order to introduce mixed frequency Granger causality tests, we rewrote Equation (2) in the following matrix form:

$$\mathbf{X_t} = \sum_{k=1}^{\ell} \mathbf{A}_k \mathbf{X}_{t-k} + \varepsilon_t \qquad (6)$$

where, $\mathbf{X_t} = (L_{1t}, L_{2t}, L_{3t}, Q_t, E_t)'$, $\varepsilon_t = (\varepsilon_{1t}, \varepsilon_{2t}, \varepsilon_{3t}, \varepsilon_{4t}, \varepsilon_{5t})'$, and $\mathbf{A}_t$ is the parameter matrix comprised of elements $a_{ij,k} = A_k(i,j), i,j \in \{1,2,3,4,5\}$, and $k \in \{1,2,3\}$. The joint zero hypothesis specified by $A_k(i,j) = 0, i \neq j$ postulates a non-causal linkage running from variable j to variable i. The Wald test statistic derived from Ghysel and his colleagues [48] was used to test for this hypothesis. Nonetheless, previous studies [48,49] indicated that the asymptotic distribution of the Wald statistic under the null hypothesis of non-causality from the MF-VAR model suffers from a severe size distortion with a small sample size. Therefore, the heteroscedasticity-robust parametric bootstrap method with 10,000 repetitions proposed by Gonçalves and Kilian [53] was used for calculating p values in order to accommodate size distortion and potential heteroscedasticity under the MF-VAR model, as suggested by Ghysel and his colleagues [48]. Six causal linkages among PNR, ICQ, and real ICE per admission (these being PNR leading ICQ, ICQ leading PNR, PNR leading ICE, ICE leading PNR, ICQ leading ICE, and ICE leading ICQ) were examined using the Granger causality tests. The investigation of these six causal relationships allows us to understand potential mechanisms activating the vicious cycle of hospital competition under the GBPS of Taiwan's NHI system.

2.4. Impulse-Response and Variance Decomposition

Once the causal relationships among nurse staffing, patient outcomes, and hospital competition were justified using the Granger causality tests, then the impulse response effect of a standard error shock in the jth element of $\mathbf{X}_t$ at time t on $\mathbf{X}_{t+h}$ could be expressed as follows:

$$IRF(h) = \sigma_{jj}^{-0.5} A_h \Omega e_j \text{ for } h = 1, 2, 3, \ldots, 12 \qquad (7)$$

where Ω is the variance-covariance matrix in the MF-VAR system, and σ_{jj} is the variance elements in the Ω matrix. e_j is an indicator vector where its jth element equals one. We plotted the impulse-response relationships among PNR, ICQ, and real ICE per admission based on the Granger causality tests, and the 90% confidence intervals of the IRFs were constructed using the Monte Carlo simulation method with 10,000 repetitions in order to investigate whether or not the estimated impulses are statistically significant at the 10% significance level. The forecast error variance decompositions for both LF-VAR and MF-VAR models were conducted following the estimation of the IRFs in Equation (6). Note that the estimation of Equation (7) involves a selection of the Cholesky order. The Cholesky orders for the LF-VAR and MF-VAR models were established as $L_t \rightarrow Q_t \rightarrow E_t$ and $L_{1t} \rightarrow L_{2t} \rightarrow L_{3t} \rightarrow Q_t \rightarrow E_t$, respectively. These settings comply with the process of reimbursement paid for inpatient care services in the hospital sector under the GPBS of Taiwan's NHI system.

3. Results

3.1. Descriptive Statistics

Table 1 summarizes the descriptive statistics for the monthly PNR and quarterly real ICE per admission, 3-day EDV rate, and 14-day readmission rate for medical centers, regional hospitals, and district hospitals over the period of 2015:Q1–2021:Q4. As indicated in Table 1, means of the 3-day EDV rate (14-day readmission rate) for medical centers, regional hospitals, and district hospitals were 2.489% (6.428%), 2.814% (7.259%), and 2.599% (7.460%), respectively. The real ICE per admission on average varied from USD 2629.971, USD 1826.339, and USD 1679.079, corresponding to payments reimbursed for inpatient care services per admission for medical centers, regional hospitals, and district hospitals, respectively. In addition, the average PNR at hospital wards ranging from the lowest to highest were 7.436 at medical centers, 7.573 at district hospitals, and 9.261 at regional hospitals, and variations of average PNR at hospital wards were found within a quarter timescale. The highest (lowest) average PNR at hospital wards in the three different types of hospitals appeared in the first (second) month within a quarter timescale. In addition, the Jarque-Bera statistics were used to test the null hypothesis of normality of time series data, and some time series such as real ICE per admission at medical centers and district hospitals, and PNR at acute care wards of regional and district hospitals, were identified to be inconsistent with the normality assumption. These findings validated the application of bootstrap methods to estimate our empirical models. The trends of all variables used in this study can be found in Appendix A, and the median and interquartile range (IQR) are also reported in Table 1.

Table 1. Descriptive Statistics [1].

Panel A: Quarterly Data Description	Mean	Standard Deviation	Median	IQR	Max	Min	JB Stat
Re-emergency-department-visit rate in the same hospital within 3 days after discharge at medical centers $\left(\text{EDV}^{MC} : \%\right)$	2.489	0.139	2.483	0.149	2.807	2.208	0.077
Re-emergency-department-visit rate in the same hospital within 3 days after discharge at regional hospitals $\left(\text{EDV}^{RH} : \%\right)$	2.814	0.170	2.832	0.202	3.199	2.504	0.396
Re-emergency-department-visit rate in the same hospital within 3 days after discharge at district hospitals $\left(\text{EDV}^{DH} : \%\right)$	2.559	0.175	2.539	0.246	2.918	2.241	0.723

Table 1. Cont.

Panel A: Quarterly Data Description	Mean	Standard Deviation	Median	IQR	Max	Min	JB Stat
Unplanned re-admission rate within 14 days after discharge at medical centers $\left(RAD^{MC}:\%\right)$	6.428	0.241	6.467	0.411	6.871	6.103	1.860
Unplanned re-admission rate within 14 days after discharge at regional hospitals $\left(RAD^{RH}:\%\right)$	7.259	0.228	7.239	0.413	7.675	6.947	2.198
Unplanned re-admission rate within 14 days after discharge at district hospitals $\left(RAD^{DH}:\%\right)$	7.460	0.256	7.473	0.303	7.983	6.772	0.705
Inpatient care expenditure per admission at medical centers $\left(ICE^{MC}:USD, Constant\ at\ 2016\ price\ level, USD\ 1 = TWD\ 30\right)$	2629.971	179.855	2589.845	200.537	3078.093	2401.06	6.270 *
Inpatient care expenditure per admission at regional hospitals $\left(ICE^{RH}:USD, Constant\ at\ 2016\ price\ level, USD\ 1 = TWD\ 30\right)$	1826.339	139.494	1795.955	182.638	2146.892	1649.037	4.762
Inpatient care expenditure per admission at district hospitals $\left(ICE^{DH}:USD, Constant\ at\ 2016\ price\ level, USD\ 1 = NTD\ 30\right)$	1679.079	97.236	1645.423	99.390	1943.214	1587.140	13.179 **

Panel B: Monthly Data Description	Mean	Standard Deviation	Median	IQR	Max	Min	JB Stat
Patient-to-nurse ratio at acute care wards of medical centers $\left(PNR^{MC}\right)$	7.436	0.256	7.434	0.388	7.880	6.706	0.809
Patient-to-nurse ratio at acute care wards of medical centers in the 1st month of the observed quarter $\left(PNR_1^{MC}\right)$	7.474	0.251	7.478	0.347	7.866	7.018	1.309
Patient-to-nurse ratio at acute care wards of medical centers in the 2nd month of observed quarter $\left(PNR_2^{MC}\right)$	7.394	0.242	7.375	0.329	7.798	6.788	0.245
Patient-to-nurse ratio at acute care wards of medical centers in the 3rd month of observed quarter $\left(PNR_3^{MC}\right)$	7.439	0.275	7.466	0.386	7.880	6.706	0.930
Patient-to-nurse ratio at acute care wards of regional hospitals $\left(PNR^{RH}\right)$	9.261	0.365	9.365	0.393	10.007	7.649	75.585 **
Patient-to-nurse ratio at acute care wards of regional hospitals in the 1st month of observed quarter $\left(PNR_1^{RH}\right)$	9.292	0.349	9.420	0.387	9.906	8.201	10.223 **
Patient-to-nurse ratio at acute care wards of regional hospitals in the 2nd month of observed quarter $\left(PNR_2^{RH}\right)$	9.205	0.325	9.202	0.507	9.928	8.568	0.288
Patient-to-nurse ratio at acute care wards of regional hospitals in the 3rd month of observed quarter $\left(PNR_3^{RH}\right)$	9.286	0.421	9.372	0.315	10.007	7.649	68.002 **

Table 1. *Cont.*

Panel B: Quarterly Data Description	Mean	Standard Deviation	Median	IQR	Max	Min	JB Stat
Patient-to-nurse ratio at acute care wards of district hospitals $\left(PNR^{DH}\right)$	7.573	0.399	7.602	0.314	8.314	5.943	51.089 **
Patient-to-nurse ratio at acute care wards of district hospitals in the 1st month of observed quarter $\left(PNR_1^{DH}\right)$	7.605	0.392	7.614	0.337	8.314	6.333	13.500 **
Patient-to-nurse ratio at acute care wards of district hospitals in the 2nd month of observed quarter $\left(PNR_2^{DH}\right)$	7.524	0.356	7.541	0.410	8.309	6.733	0.259
Patient-to-nurse ratio at acute care wards of district hospitals in the 3rd month of observed quarter $\left(PNR_3^{DH}\right)$	7.589	0.453	7.669	0.314	8.295	5.943	38.238 **

3.2. Unit Root Tests

It is worth addressing that the PNR, ICQ, and real ICE per admission are time series data that are likely to have the unit root property. As shown in Table 2, the ADF tests with constant and with constant plus trend specifications identified non-stationary time series of real ICE per admission at the three different types of hospitals. In addition, the ADF tests with constant plus trend specification suggest that the time series of the two ICQ indicators were non-stationary except for the 14-day readmission rate at district hospitals. The presence of the unit roots of the 3-day EDV rate (14-day readmission rate) at regional hospitals (medical centers and regional hospitals) was found using the ADF tests with constant specification. Contrarily, the ADF tests with constant and with constant plus trend specifications identified stationary time series of PNR at the three different types of hospitals. These findings suggest that the order of time series data on PNR, the two ICQ indicators, and real ICE per admission is likely to be different at the three different types of hospitals. Since the cyclic components of these time series removed the long-run tendency of time series with zero means, the ADF tests without constant and trend specification were used to test for the unit root property of cyclic components of time series. As we expected, the stationarity of cyclic components of time series for the three different types of hospitals was confirmed. These findings eliminate spurious correlations among all variables used in this research from the unit root property of time series. Therefore, we were able to proceed with the Granger Causality tests with the cyclic components of these variables.

3.3. Granger Causality Tests

Table 3 presents the results of the Granger causality tests under the MF-VAR model for the six causal relationships among ICQ, PNR, and real ICE per admission at the three different types of hospitals during our study period. Mixed frequency data were used for the Granger causality tests. As such, it is vital to understand that the causality running from the low frequency variable to the high frequency variable means causality running from a quarterly variable to a group of three individual monthly variables [40,48,49]. In addition, the asymptotic distribution of the Wald statistic under the null hypothesis of non-causality in the MF-VAR model has a severe size distortion due to a small sample size [40,48,49]. Because of this, p values were generated using the heteroscedasticity-robust parametric bootstrap method introduced by Gonçalves and Kilian [53] with 10,000 replications.

Table 2. ADF Unit Root Tests [2].

Panel A: Quarterly Data

	Mean	Standard Deviation	Constant (C)	Constant+ Trend (T)	Mean	Standard Deviation	Without C+T
			Levels			Cyclical Components	
$\ln(EDV^{MC})$	0.911	0.056	−3.473 *	−3.405	0.000	0.052	−3.952 **
$\ln(EDV^{RH})$	1.033	0.060	−2.329	−3.330	0.000	0.050	−3.874 **
$\ln(EDV^{DH})$	0.937	0.068	−3.247 *	−3.341	0.000	0.060	−3.917 **
$\ln(RAD^{MC})$	1.860	0.038	−2.518	−2.455	0.000	0.033	−2.904 **
$\ln(RAD^{RH})$	1.982	0.031	−2.698	−3.462	0.000	0.025	−3.719 **
$\ln(RAD^{DH})$	2.009	0.035	−3.370 *	−4.306 *	0.000	0.031	−4.250 **
$\ln(ICE^{MC})$	7.873	0.066	0.036	−2.412	0.000	0.025	−4.347 **
$\ln(ICE^{RH})$	7.507	0.074	1.087	−1.824	0.000	0.025	−3.164 **
$\ln(ICE^{DH})$	7.424	0.056	0.676	−1.303	0.000	0.024	−2.221 *

Panel B: Monthly Data

	Mean	Standard Deviation	Constant (C)	Constant+ Trend (T)	Mean	Standard Deviation	Without C+T
			Levels			Cyclical Components	
$\ln(PNR^{MC})$	2.006	0.035	−4.253 **	−4.611 **	0.000	0.027	−5.740 **
$\ln(PNR^{RH})$	2.225	0.041	−4.434 **	−4.596 **	0.000	0.035	−5.397 **
$\ln(PNR^{DH})$	2.023	0.055	−3.434 *	−5.079 **	0.000	0.037	−5.515 **

Panel C: Aggregate Monthly Data

	Mean	Standard Deviation	Constant (C)	Constant+ Trend (T)	Mean	Standard Deviation	Without C+T
			Levels			Cyclical Components	
$\sum_{t=1}^{3} C\_\ln(PNR_t^{MC})/3$	—	—	—	—	0.000	0.057	−5.383 **
$\sum_{t=1}^{3} C\_\ln(PNR_t^{RH})/3$	—	—	—	—	0.000	0.071	−6.482 **
$\sum_{t=1}^{3} C\_\ln(PNR_t^{DH})/3$	—	—	—	—	0.000	0.073	−2.231 *

Table 3. Granger Causality Tests [3].

Panel A: Re-Emergency-Department-Visit Rate in the Same Hospital within 3 Days after Discharge as the Quality of Care Indicator

Types of Hospitals	MF-VAR Model Null Hypothesis			χ2	p Value	LF-VAR Model Null Hypothesis			χ2	p Value
Medical Centers	EDV	≠>	PNR	10.935	0.090 *	EDV	≠>	PNR^A	1.977	0.372
	ICE	≠>	PNR	3.213	0.782	ICE	≠>	PNR^A	2.346	0.309
	PNR	≠>	EDV	16.029	0.014 **	PNR^A	≠>	EDV	3.075	0.215
	ICE	≠>	EDV	3.254	0.776	ICE	≠>	EDV	2.841	0.242
	PNR	≠>	ICE	14.095	0.029 **	PNR^A	≠>	ICE	1.291	0.524
	EDV	≠>	ICE	14.635	0.023 **	EDV	≠>	ICE	7.013	0.030 **
Regional Hospitals	EDV	≠>	PNR	12.035	0.061 *	EDV	≠>	PNR^A	0.520	0.771
	ICE	≠>	PNR	4.706	0.582	ICE	≠>	PNR^A	5.716	0.057 *
	PNR	≠>	EDV	13.365	0.038 **	PNR^A	≠>	EDV	3.121	0.210
	ICE	≠>	EDV	6.021	0.421	ICE	≠>	EDV	3.564	0.168
	PNR	≠>	ICE	18.311	0.005 ***	PNR^A	≠>	ICE	1.871	0.392
	EDV	≠>	ICE	4.700	0.583	EDV	≠>	ICE	0.366	0.833
	RER	≠>	PNR	8.592	0.198	EDV	≠>	PNR^A	0.557	0.757
District Hospitals	ICE	≠>	PNR	4.797	0.570	ICE	≠>	PNR^A	4.162	0.125
	PNR	≠>	EDV	12.614	0.049 **	PNR^A	≠>	EDV	5.049	0.080 *
	ICE	≠>	EDV	2.749	0.840	ICE	≠>	EDV	0.540	0.763
	PNR	≠>	ICE	13.519	0.035 **	PNR^A	≠>	ICE	1.438	0.487
	RER	≠>	ICE	7.127	0.309	EDV	≠>	ICE	5.761	0.056 *

Table 3. Cont.

Panel B:		Unplanned Re-Admission Rate within 14 Days after Discharge as the Quality of Care Indicator						
Types of Hospitals		MF-VAR Model				LF-VAR Model		
		Null Hypothesis		χ2	p Value	Null Hypothesis		χ2	p Value
Medical Centers	RAD	≠>	PNR	8.933	0.177	RAD	≠>	PNR^A	5.054	0.080 *
	ICE	≠>	PNR	6.004	0.423	ICE	≠>	PNR^A	4.763	0.092 *
	PNR	≠>	RAD	7.822	0.251	PNR^A	≠>	RAD	6.941	0.031 **
	ICE	≠>	RAD	8.972	0.175	ICE	≠>	RAD	7.418	0.024 **
	PNR	≠>	ICE	13.079	0.042 **	PNR^A	≠>	ICE	2.848	0.241
	RAD	≠>	ICE	4.386	0.625	RAD	≠>	ICE	1.159	0.560
Regional Hospitals	RAD	≠>	PNR	9.952	0.127	RER	≠>	PNR^A	0.281	0.869
	ICE	≠>	PNR	5.990	0.424	ICE	≠>	PNR^A	3.839	0.147
	PNR	≠>	RAD	8.200	0.224	PNR^A	≠>	RAD	6.799	0.033 **
	ICE	≠>	RAD	8.635	0.195	ICE	≠>	RAD	4.140	0.126
	PNR	≠>	ICE	13.674	0.033 **	PNR^A	≠>	ICE	3.684	0.158
	RAD	≠>	ICE	3.943	0.684	RER	≠>	ICE	2.161	0.339
District Hospitals	RAD	≠>	PNR	13.511	0.036 **	RER	≠>	PNR^A	1.753	0.416
	ICE	≠>	PNR	8.614	0.196	ICE	≠>	PNR^A	4.366	0.113
	PNR	≠>	RAD	4.441	0.617	PNR^A	≠>	RAD	2.971	0.226
	ICE	≠>	RAD	5.582	0.472	ICE	≠>	RAD	1.988	0.370
	PNR	≠>	ICE	12.169	0.058 *	PNR^A	≠>	ICE	1.653	0.438
	RAD	≠>	ICE	2.303	0.890	RER	≠>	ICE	0.765	0.682

Panel A of Table 3 displays the Granger causality tests for the six causal relationships among the 3-day EDV rate, PNR, and real ICE per admission at the three different types of hospitals. In contrast to little significance in the causal relationships identified by the LF-VAR model, the MF-VAR model identified bidirectional causation between PNR and the 3-day EDV rate at medical centers and regional hospitals, and one-way causality running from PNR to the 3-day EDV rate at district hospitals at the 10% (or stricter) significance level. In addition, a causal relationship running from PNR to real ICE per admission was identified for the three different types of hospitals, and another unidirectional causality running from the 3-day EDV rate to real ICE per admission was also detected for medical centers. In addition, Panel B of Table 3 reports results of the Granger causality tests for the six causal relationships among the 14-day readmission rate, PNR, and real ICE per admission at the three different types of hospitals. Although the LF-VAR model identified several causal relationships among the 14-day readmission rate, PNR, and real ICE per admission, previous studies addressed a potential aggregation bias in the statistical inferences of the LF-VAR model [40,47–49]. Therefore, we focused on the results of the Granger causality tests under the MF-VAR model. As indicated in Panel B of Table 3, the MF-VAR model identified one-way causal relationships running PNR to real ICE per admission at the three different types of hospitals. These findings are consistent with the causal linkage running from PNR to real ICE per admission as reported in Panel A of Table 3. Additionally, unidirectional Granger causality running from the 14-day readmission rate to PNR was also identified at district hospitals only.

3.4. Impulse-Response Analyses

Since the causal relationships among PNR, ICQ, and real ICE per admission were verified by the Granger causality tests under the MF-VAR model for Taiwan's NHI system over the period of 2015:Q1–2021:Q4, we further plotted the mixed frequency IRFs to illustrate the propagation mechanism of interdependences between PNR, ICQ, and real ICE per admission across a 12-month period. As indicated in Figure 1, significantly positive (negative) responses of the 3-day EDV rate to a positive PNR shock in the first month of a quarter timespan were identified at the first and eighth (second) month horizons over a 12-month period for regional hospitals (see Figure 1(b1)), and a significantly positive impulse-response relationship between the 3-day EDV rate and PNR in the first month of a quarter timespan was found at the first month horizon over a 12-month period for district hospitals (see Figure 1(c1)).

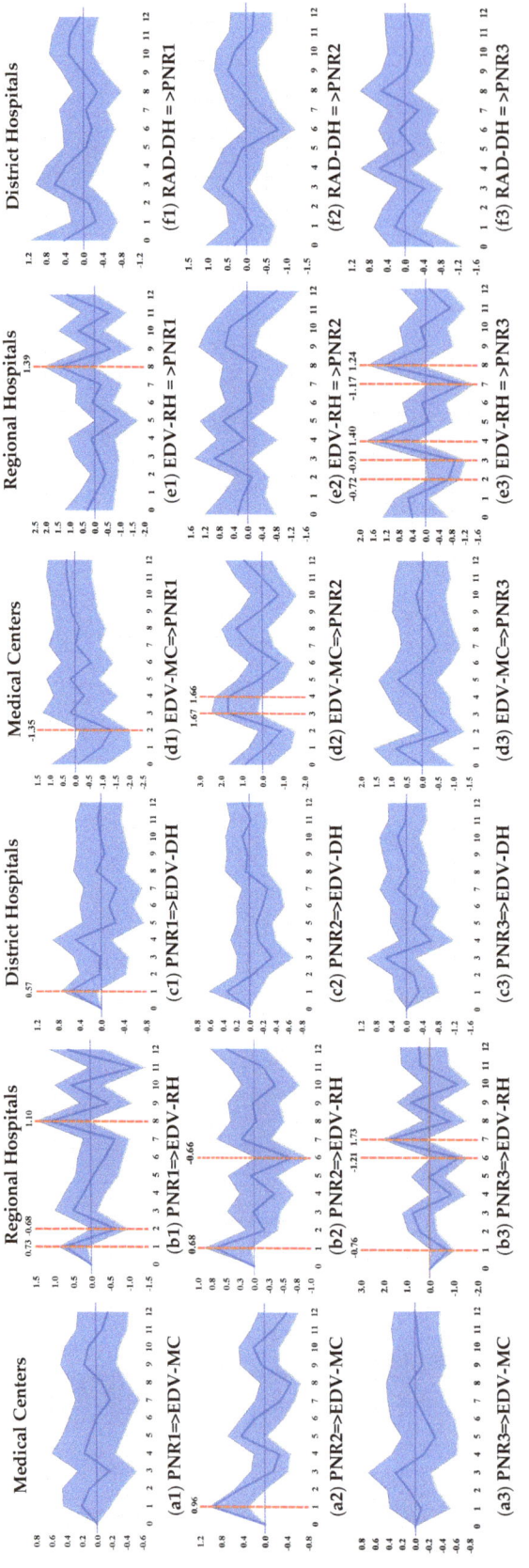

Figure 1. Impulse Response Functions for Quality of Care Indicators and Nurse Staffing Level [4].

The significantly positive effect of PNR in the second month of a quarter timespan on the 3-day EDV rate was found at the first month horizon over a 12-month period for medical centers (see Figure 1(a2)). Nonetheless, the impulse-response relationship between the 3-day EDV rate and PNR in the second month of a quarter timespan was identified as significantly positive at the first month horizon but negative at the sixth month horizon over a 12-month period for regional hospitals (see Figure 1(b2)). Additionally, the responses of the 3-day EDV rate to a positive PNR shock in the third month within a quarter timespan were significantly negative (positive) at the first and sixth (seventh) month horizon over a 12-month period for district hospitals (see Figure 1(b3)). Despite asymmetric impulse-response effects of PNR on the 3-day EDV rate being found, the positive effects of PNR on the 3-day EDV rate dominated the negative effects across a 3-month cycle of a quarter timespan for all three types of hospitals.

As shown in Figure 1(d1,e1), the responses of PNR in the first month of a quarter timespan to a positive shock in the 3-day EDV rate were significantly negative (positive) at the second (eighth) month horizon over a 12-month period for medical centers (regional hospitals). The significantly positive responses of PNR in the second month of a quarter timespan to a positive shock in the 3-day EDV rate were found at the third and fourth month horizons over a 12-month period for medical centers (see Figure 1(d2)). The impulse-response relationship between the 3-day EDV rate and PNR in the third month of a quarter timespan was negative at the second, third, and seventh month horizons, but it was identified to be positive at the fourth and eighth month horizons over a 12-month period for regional hospitals (see Figure 1(e3)). Although a changing impulse-response relationship between the 3-day EDV rate and PNR was identified, as shown in Figure 1(d1,d2,e1,e3), the negative effects of the 3-day EDV rate on PNR were dominated by the positive effect across a 3-month cycle of a quarter timespan for medical centers and regional hospitals. Nevertheless, the impulse-response relationship between 14-day readmission and PNR across a 3-month cycle of a quarter timespan did not generate any significant results for district hospitals.

The impulse-response relationships between PNR and real ICE per admission for the three different types of hospitals are illustrated in Figure 2 in Panels A and B, which, respectively, correspond to the 3-day EDV rate and 14-day readmission rate used to measure ICQ in the estimation of the MF-VAR model. No matter which ICQ indicator was selected, the responses of real ICE per admission to PNR in the second month of a quarter timespan were identified as significantly negative around the third, fourth, and fifth month horizons over a 12-month period for regional hospitals and district hospitals (see Figure 2(b2,c2,e2,f2)). The effects of PNR in the second month of a quarter timespan on real ICE per admission were determined to be significantly negative at the third month horizon and positive at the sixth month horizon over a 12-month period for medical centers (see Figure 2(d2)).

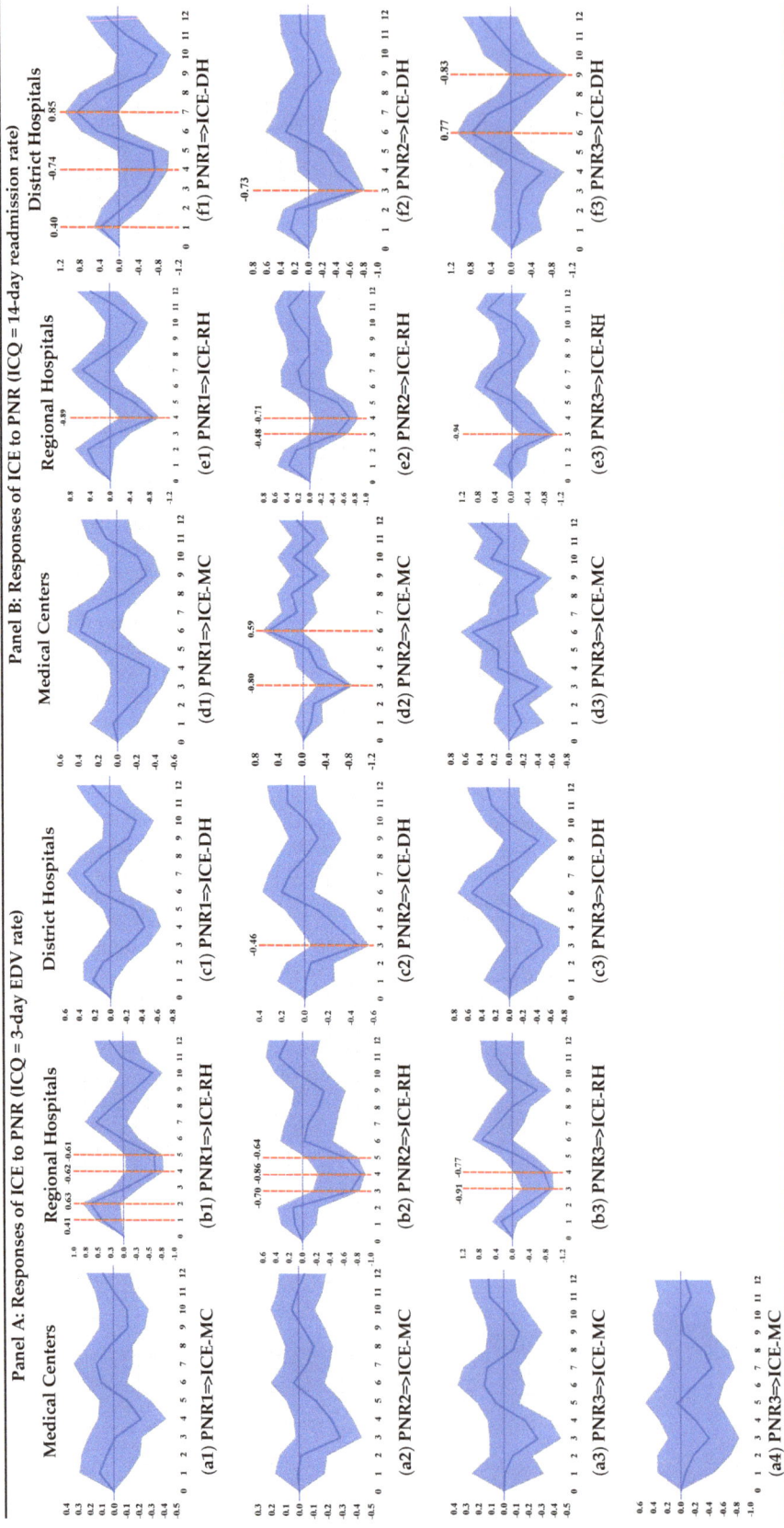

Figure 2. Impulse Response Functions for Inpatient Care Expenditure, Nurse Staffing, and Quality of Care Indicator [5].

The impulse-response relationship between real ICE per admission and PNR in the first month of a quarter timespan was found to be significantly positive around the first and second month horizons and negative around the fourth and fifth month horizons over a 12-month period for regional hospitals (Figure 2(b1,e1)). Figure 2(b3,e3) illustrates a significantly negative impulse-response relationship between real ICE per admission and PNR in the third month of a quarter timespan around the third and fourth month horizons over a 12-month period for regional hospitals. The responses of real ICE per admission on PNR in the first (third) month of a quarter timespan were found to be significantly negative at the fourth (ninth) month horizon and positive at the first and seventh (sixth) month horizons over a 12-month period for district hospitals (Figure 2(f1,f3)). Despite an asymmetric relationship between real ICE per admission and PNR across a 3-month cycle of a quarter timespan being found, the negative effects of PNR on real ICE per admission across a 3-month cycle of a quarter timespan dominated the positive effects for all three types of hospitals.

3.5. Variance Decomposition

Table 4 presents two sets of the forecast error variance decompositions based on whether the 3-day EDV rate or 14-day readmission rate were used to serve as the ICQ indicator in the estimation of the LF-VAR and MF-VAR models. As indicated in Table 4, the proportions of forecast error variance of the ICQ indicator attributed to the PNR within a 3-month cycle of a quarter timespan (i.e., **PNR** = ΣPNR_i) in the MF-VAR model for medical centers are 1.61~4.58 (=21.70/13.46~37.20/8.13), 1.55~3.81(=45.87/29.53~44.06/11.56), and 1.62~3.77 (=46.45/27.73~46.80/12.40) times higher than those attributed to an aggregation of PNR (i.e., PNR^A) in the LF-VAR model in the short-run (h = 2), medium-run (h = 7), and long-run (h = 12), respectively, based on whether the 3-day EDV rate or 14-day readmission rate was chosen to measure ICQ. In addition, the proportions of forecast error variance of the real ICE per admission attributed to the PNR within a 3-month cycle of a quarter timespan (i.e., **PNR** = ΣPNR_i) in the MF-VAR model for medical centers are 1.24~1.36 (=74.07/59.63~73.87/54.34), 1.50~1.65 (=70.93/47.18~71.88/43.48), and 1.60~1.69 (=73.91/46.16~74.71/44.12) times higher than those attributed to the aggregation of PNR (i.e., PNR^A) in the LF-VAR model in the short-run (h = 2), medium-run (h = 7), and long-run (h = 12), respectively, based on whether the 3-day re-EDV rate or 14-day readmission rate was chosen to measure ICQ. Similar results, wherein the MF-VAR model generated a higher explanatory power than the LF-VAR model, could also be found for the relationships among PNR, ICQ, and real ICE per admission for regional hospitals and district hospitals. Therefore, the findings of the forecast error variance decompositions shown in Table 4 indicate that the MF-VAR model has a greater explanatory power than the LF-VAR model in the investigation of interdependences between PNR, ICQ, and real ICE per admission for the three different types of hospitals.

Table 4. Forecast Error Variance Decomposition (%) [6].

Quality	Model	Variable	Horizon	Medical Centers (%)			Variable	Horizon	Regional Hospitals (%)			Variable	Horizon	District Hospitals (%)		
				h = 2	h = 7	h = 12			h = 2	h = 7	h = 12			h = 2	h = 7	h = 12
Panel A: RER as Quality Indicator	LF-VAR	EDV	EDV	86.320.22	63.67	61.75	EDV	EDV	82.96	64.87	58.74	EDV	EDV	88.71	45.95	33.08
			ICE	13.46	6.80	9.52		ICE	7.04	16.37	15.33		ICE	1.79	9.40	20.12
			PNR^A	0.38	29.53	28.73		PNR^A	10.0	18.76	25.93		PNR^A	9.49	44.65	46.79
		ICE	EDV	45.28	30.38	30.51	ICE	EDV	0.81	4.79	7.17	ICE	EDV	0.58	19.57	19.38
			ICE	54.34	26.15	25.37		ICE	57.91	55.43	53.07		ICE	53.66	33.91	35.37
			PNR^A	0.38	43.48	44.12		PNR^A	41.28	39.78	39.75		PNR^A	45.76	46.53	45.25
		PNR^A	EDV	8.13	8.87	10.57	PNR^A	EDV	0.01	9.94	11.55	PNR^A	EDV	0.06	1.19	4.89
			ICE	0.69	11.78	12.15		ICE	7.32	27.75	27.13		ICE	3.86	23.89	25.31
			PNR^A	91.19	79.35	77.27		PNR^A	92.67	62.32	61.31		PNR^A	96.08	74.92	69.80
	MF-VAR	EDV	EDV	78.28	53.24	51.96	EDV	EDV	91.76	62.08	45.48	EDV	EDV	74.44	42.62	36.38
			ICE	0.03	0.88	1.59		ICE	1.80	4.82	8.05		ICE	0.37	1.18	2.41
			PNR=ΣPNR$_i$	21.70	45.87	46.45		PNR=ΣPNR$_i$	6.45	33.11	46.47		PNR=ΣPNR$_i$	25.20	56.19	61.21
			EDV	0.40	16.42	15.23		EDV	2.22	6.22	7.69		EDV	0.60	14.65	5.97
		ICE	ICE	25.72	11.71	10.05	ICE	ICE	47.92	40.84	31.27	ICE	ICE	25.28	78.77	13.03
			PNR=ΣPNR$_i$	73.87	71.88	74.71		PNR=ΣPNR$_i$	49.88	52.94	61.03		PNR=ΣPNR$_i$	74.12	4.76	80.99
			EDV	0.88	1.44	2.23		EDV	9.88	8.52	15.74		EDV	0.72	3.91	3.60
		PNR$_1$	ICE	0.29	1.02	1.39	PNR$_1$	ICE	3.16	8.00	6.56	PNR$_1$	ICE	2.62	2.68	3.64
			EDV	98.84	97.53	96.38		EDV	86.97	83.49	77.71		EDV	94.52	93.40	92.77
		PNR$_2$	ICE	32.33	27.31	29.15	PNR$_2$	ICE	11.67	11.67	9.69	PNR$_2$	ICE	0.00	3.80	4.10
			EDV	0.00	2.83	2.67		EDV	0.30	18.31	14.84		EDV	97.38	91.88	91.80
			PNR=ΣPNR$_i$	67.66	69.85	68.18		PNR=ΣPNR$_i$	88.03	70.01	75.47		PNR=ΣPNR$_i$	0.67	3.88	3.29
		PNR$_3$	EDV	0.13	2.29	2.29	PNR$_3$	EDV	5.23	13.00	16.19	PNR$_3$	EDV	0.00	2.96	3.34
			ICE	0.00	1.29	1.62		ICE	0.70	7.94	4.86		ICE	0.00	0.00	0.00
			PNR=ΣPNR$_i$	99.88	96.43	96.09		PNR=ΣPNR$_i$	94.08	79.07	78.95		PNR=ΣPNR$_i$	99.32	93.16	93.36

Quality	Model	Variable	Horizon	h = 2	h = 7	h = 12	Variable	Horizon	h = 2	h = 7	h = 12	Variable	Horizon	h = 2	h = 7	h = 12
Panel B: URR as Quality Indicator	LF-VAR	RAD	RAD	83.73	73.30	71.73	RAD	RAD	75.56	51.37	46.51	RAD	RAD	89.73	56.37	43.57
			ICE	8.14	15.14	15.87		ICE	12.24	24.29	27.97		ICE	9.58	20.43	27.87
			PNR^A	8.13	11.56	12.40		PNR^A	12.20	24.34	25.51		PNR^A	0.69	23.21	28.56
		ICE	RAD	2.55	19.93	19.43	ICE	RAD	2.08	3.13	3.39	ICE	RAD	0.50	4.00	4.08
			ICE	37.82	32.89	34.41		ICE	66.07	58.67	58.37		ICE	59.39	53.57	53.93
			PNR^A	59.63	47.18	46.16		PNR^A	31.84	38.21	38.23		PNR^A	40.10	42.43	41.99
		PNR^A	RAD	14.55	14.89	14.69	PNR^A	RAD	1.62	1.55	2.18	PNR^A	RAD	0.21	2.76	3.72
			ICE	0.17	29.15	29.28		ICE	3.33	28.30	32.03		ICE	7.04	32.36	35.16
			PNR^A	85.28	55.96	56.04		PNR^A	95.05	70.15	65.78		PNR^A	92.75	64.87	61.12
	MF-VAR	RAD	RAD	60.54	50.90	47.97	RAD	RAD	73.70	45.46	38.00	RAD	RAD	81.99	56.39	48.59
			ICE	2.27	5.03	5.24		ICE	4.72	8.05	12.14		ICE	6.11	15.33	20.14
			PNR=ΣPNR$_i$	37.20	44.06	46.80		PNR=ΣPNR$_i$	21.57	46.49	49.87		PNR=ΣPNR$_i$	11.89	28.29	31.27
			RAD	2.99	16.21	14.00		RAD	7.23	8.59	8.50		RAD	0.67	7.19	10.06
		ICE	ICE	22.94	12.87	12.08	ICE	ICE	56.11	35.53	30.44	ICE	ICE	49.48	32.90	30.98
			PNR=ΣPNR$_i$	74.07	70.93	73.91		PNR=ΣPNR$_i$	36.65	55.87	61.06		PNR=ΣPNR$_i$	49.86	59.90	58.95
			RAD	0.59	6.37	6.66		RAD	16.34	11.66	9.22		RAD	16.46	15.23	15.41
		PNR$_1$	ICE	0.05	5.54	8.03	PNR$_1$	ICE	1.25	9.88	9.43	PNR$_1$	ICE	2.33	9.89	15.41
			EDV	99.37	88.09	85.31		EDV	82.42	78.46	81.35		EDV	81.21	74.88	71.52
		PNR$_2$	RAD	16.47	15.16	12.61	PNR$_2$	RAD	0.02	12.73	10.13	PNR$_2$	RAD	2.50	22.17	21.45
			ICE	0.65	14.33	9.87		ICE	3.62	15.16	13.02		ICE	2.23	11.29	10.76
			PNR=ΣPNR$_i$	82.87	70.51	77.53		PNR=ΣPNR$_i$	96.37	72.11	76.85		PNR=ΣPNR$_i$	95.27	66.54	67.79
		PNR$_3$	RAD	0.17	6.98	7.79	PNR$_3$	RAD	0.91	8.61	9.49	PNR$_3$	RAD	0.48	16.06	15.53
			ICE	0.56	4.28	4.85		ICE	0.07	6.45	5.81		ICE	0.26	5.07	7.37
			PNR=ΣPNR$_i$	99.27	88.74	87.35		PNR=ΣPNR$_i$	99.02	84.93	84.70		PNR=ΣPNR$_i$	99.25	78.87	77.09

4. Discussion

Two unidirectional causal propositions can be justified by looking at the causal relationships among PNR, the two ICQ indicators (i.e., 3-day EDV rate and 14-day readmission rate), and real ICE per admission identified by the Granger causality tests under the MF-VAR model. The PNR leading ICE proposition postulates that PNR leads real ICE per admission, and the EDV leading ICE proposition claims that the 3-day EDV rate leads real ICE per admission. The former proposition was substantiated by data from the three different types of hospitals, and the latter proposition was only verified by data from medical centers. In addition, the Granger causality tests also confirmed a feedback proposition for PNR and ICQ claiming bidirectional causation between PNR and the 3-day EDV rate in medical centers and regional hospitals. Additionally, the PNR leading 3-day EDV rate proposition (stating that PNR leads the 3-day EDV rate) and the 14-day readmission rate leading PNR proposition (asserting that the 14-day readmission rate leads PNR) were corroborated for district hospitals.

In general, four mechanisms activating the vicious cycle of hospital competition are implied by these propositions. First, the PNR origin mechanism suggests that a high PNR (i.e., a poor nurse staffing level) not only worsens the 3-day EDV rate but also reduces real ICE per admission (see Figure 3(a1)). Second, the EDV origin mechanism indicates that a higher 3-day EDV rate influences both real ICE per admission and PNR (see Figure 3(a2)). Third, the EDV rebound mechanism alludes that the 3-day EDV rate results in a higher PNR leading to decreased real ICE per admission (see Figure 3(a3)). Fourth, the readmission rebound mechanism points to the 14-day readmission rate causing a higher PNR which leads to a reduction in real ICE per admission (see Figure 3(a4)). The statistical significances of the signs and paths connecting PNR, the two ICQ indicators (i.e., 3-day EDV rate and 14-day readmission rate), and real ICE per admission (underpinning the four mechanisms described above) were determined based on the impulse-response analyses illustrated in Figures 1 and 2. Several policy implications emerging from this work have merit and are worth being discussed as follows:

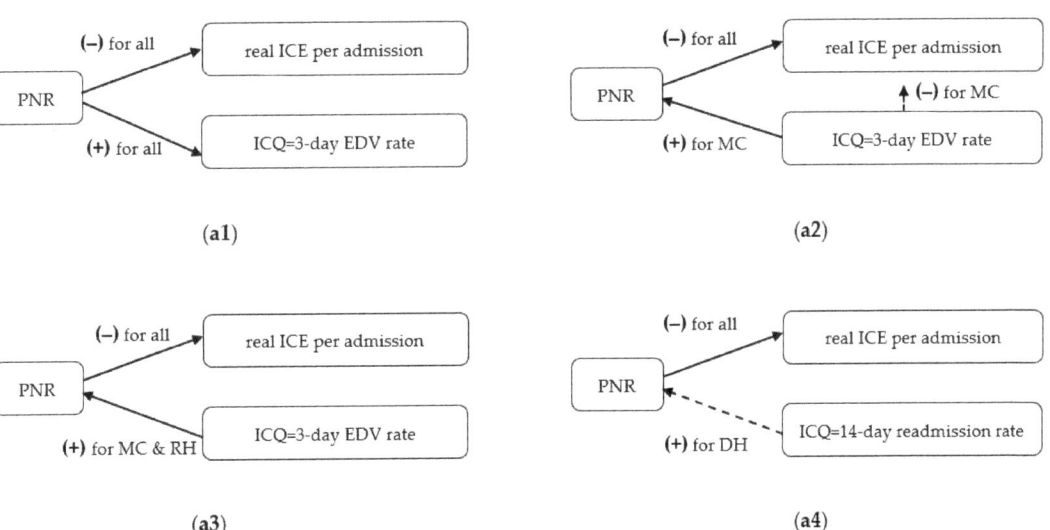

Figure 3. Mechanisms for activating the vicious cycle of hospital competition. (a1) M1: the PNR origin mechanism for the three different levels of hospitals; (a2) M2: the EDV origin mechanism for medical centers only; (a3) M3: the EDV rebound mechanism for medical centers and regional hospitals; (a4) M4: the readmission rebound mechanism for district hospitals [7].

First, as indicated in Figure 3(a1), the PNR origin mechanism was observed in all three different types of hospitals, but the EDV origin mechanism is suitable for medical centers only. The EDV (readmission) rebound mechanism was found in medical centers and regional hospitals (district hospitals). Therefore, the PNR not only qualifies as an important determinant of patient outcomes, but it also serves as both a key factor and mediator influencing real ICE per admission for the three different types of hospitals. In general, a positive impact on PNR increases the 3-day EDV rate but decreases real ICE per admission in all types of hospitals based on the impulse-response analyses over a 12-month period (see Figure 1, Figure 2, and Figure 3(a1)). These findings were consistent with results from previous studies on the relationship between nurse staffing and patient outcomes [1–25,35].

Second, it is important to note that the impulse-response relationship between the 3-day EDV rate and real ICE per admission was not significant based on the impulse-response analyses over a 12-month period. (see Figure 2(a4) and Figure 3(a2)). Therefore, we focus on the two rebound mechanisms for our discussion. As illustrated in Figure 3(a3,a4), we found that the rebound effects running from ICQ to PNR were essentially different between large hospitals (such as medical centers and regional hospitals) and small hospitals (i.e., district hospitals) in terms of the significance of the relationship between ICQ indicators and PNR. As shown in Figure 3(a3,a4), the 3-day EDV rate was found to be a trigger impacting PNR and then influencing real ICE per admission at medical centers and regional hospitals, but the readmission rebound mechanism was not significant in district hospitals based on the impulse-response analyses over a 12-month period (see Figure 1(f1,f3) and 3(a4)). These findings reflect the facts that district hospitals play a minor part in ED care services and that nighttime ED closures (or down-grading to the so-called urgent outpatient centers) are frequently observed in district hospitals due to a lack of sufficient nurses. Such shortages of nurses also lead to hospital bed closures in district hospitals where inpatient care resources are then shifted towards treating chronic rather than acute conditions. Hence, it was reported that the average length of stay ranged from 13~16 days in district hospitals, much higher than that for medical centers (7~9 days), but the mean PNR in district hospitals was very close to that in medical centers (7.572 versus 7.436; see Table 1) during our study period [54].

Third, although the EDV rebound effect was expected to be negative as hospital ad-ministration managerial actions were taken to influence ICQ for the sake of quality-of-care control, a positive rebound effect of the 3-day EDV rate on PNR was identified in medical centers and regional hospitals based on the impulse-response analyses over a 12-month period (see Figures 1 and 3(a3)). According to annual statistics of the medical care institution and hospital utilization reported by Taiwan's Ministry of Health and Welfare, the total number of hospitals decreased from 556 to 478 (of these, the number of medical centers remained stable at around 21~23, while the number of regional hospitals increased from 65 to 74, with a contrasting significant reduction in the number of district hospitals) during our study period of 2015:Q1–2021:Q4 [55]. Moreover, Taiwan's NHIA reported that district hospitals represent over 80% of total hospitals, while approximately 76%~81% of total hospital admissions were contributed by medical centers and regional hospitals under the GBPS of Taiwan's NHI system [55,56]. These statistics suggest that quantity competition for medical centers and regional hospitals is much higher than that for district hospitals, so managerial actions taken for the sake of quality-of-care control in medical centers and regional hospitals are highly likely to be offset by severe quantity competition in the hospital sector of Taiwan's NHI system.

Fourth, the rebound effects of ICQ on PNR from medical centers and regional hospitals will mostly likely counter the adverse effect of hospital competition (see Figure 3(a1,a3)). Considering this along with substantial evidence identifying PNR as one of the crucial determinants of ICQ and real ICE per admission, as indicated in Figure 1, Figure 2, and Figure 3(a1), quality of care maintenance policies (such as directly subsidizing for a lower PNR and the inclusion of a reasonable PNR as a key standard for hospital accreditation) should be enforced in order to reduce adverse effects of higher nurse staffing levels on patient outcomes and quantity competition under the GBPS of Taiwan's NHI system. Special attention should be concentrated on reducing the rebound effects of the 3-day EDV rate on PNR from medical centers and regional hospitals through imposing more substantial quality-of-care control plans and more stringent regulation of seasonal inpatient care volume for medical centers and regional hospitals.

This study makes contributions beyond those of the existing literature on the relationship between nurse staffing and patient outcomes in three respects: First, although the aggregation and omitted variable biases (due to aggregating different frequencies data into single frequency data) have attracted lots of attention regarding the estimation of the nurse staffing and patient outcomes relationship in the healthcare services research field [39], this study, for the first time, adopted the MF-VAR model proposed by Ghysel and his colleagues [47,48] to incorporate different frequencies data into the investigation of the relationships among PNR, ICQ, and real ICE per admission under the GBPS of Taiwan's NHI system over the period of 2015:Q1–2021:Q4. We illustrated that the MF-VAR model is superior to the LF-VAR (i.e., conventional VAR) model in terms of higher explanatory power (See Table 4). Second, this study contrasts with the previous time series research exploring the association between nurse staffing and patient outcomes, in which the causal responses of patient outcomes (nurse staffing) to a nurse staffing (patient outcomes) shock across a period of time were not available. In this study, we not only tested for six causal relationships among PNR, ICQ, and real ICE per admission through the MF-VAR-Granger Causality tests proposed by Ghysel and his colleagues [47,48], but we also estimated the IRFs based on the MF-VAR model. In this way, we were able to capture the dynamic impact of nurse staffing on patient outcomes and on healthcare expenditure for inpatient care service reimbursement across a high frequency timescale (a 3-month cycle of a quarter timespan in this study) over a 12-month period, and four mechanisms potentially triggering the vicious cycle of hospital competition were discussed accordingly.

Third, it is essential to address that the healthcare systems worldwide have been toward public-private mixed (or more private-like) financing systems due to an aging population, diffusion of new technologies, and growth of income [28]. It follows that we observed a common privatization trend in healthcare provision, and, in turn, it created a severer market competition in many publicly financed healthcare systems such as the NHS (e.g., Australia, Belgium, Finland, Iceland, Ireland, Norway, Spain, and United Kingdom) and SHI systems (e.g., Austria, Canada, Korea, and Japan) [26,28]. Although the harmful effects of PNR on patient outcomes were confirmed from previous studies in the NHS [2–4,7,8,10,14–18] and SHI systems [5,9,14–18], most of these studies belonged to the cross-sectional or static-type studies. It follows that these studies failed to identify causality between nurse staffing and patient outcomes, evaluate the propagation mechanism of nurse staffing on patient outcomes, and avoid the potential aggregation biases [2–10,14–18]. Therefore, the methodologies (such as the MF-VAR model, Granger causality test, and impulse-response analyses) used in this study not only generated results echoing the evidence obtained from previous studies [2–10,14–18], but they also amended the disadvantages of the cross-sectional or static-type studies. The methodologies used in this study could be easily performed through inputting publicly reported time series data in cases when individual data are difficult to be collected (e.g., the COVID-19 outbreak period). The empirical results obtained through our empirical models could serve as important information for the surveillance of ICQ under the hospital competition in the publicly financed healthcare system.

This study, nonetheless, has several limitations. First, the potential size distortion due to a small sample size used in this study (i.e., a total of 28 and 84 quarterly and monthly observations) would create invalid inferences, so all results generated from the MF-VAR model were based on the bootstrap method in order to adjust for the size distortion. Second, the cyclical components of time series were used for our MF-VAR model, so inferences obtained from this study are limited regarding the short-run relationships among nurse staffing, patient outcomes, and hospital competition under the GBPS of Taiwan's NHI system. Third, this study belongs to the ecological type of time series analyses. Thus, in order to prevent the ecological fallacy of study [57], our empirical results neither refer to individual patients' decisions in seeking care (such as ED care or inpatient care) after discharge from a hospital nor the hospitals' managerial actions (such as nurse deployment) in response to changes in patient outcomes. We recommend that future studies collect the individual data needed to explore the interactions among hospitals' managerial actions impacting quality of care, the patients' decisions in seeking care, and patient outcomes in response to hospital competition under the GBPS of Taiwan's NHI system.

5. Conclusions

Hospital administrators and healthcare practitioners have long been concerned about the adverse effect of poor nurse staffing on patient outcomes [1–25,35]. The critical force driving inappropriate deployment of nursing staffs at hospitals is hospital (quantity) competition under the GBPS. In this study, we applied the MF-VAR model to investigate the interdependences between nurse staffing, patient outcomes, and hospital competition under the GBPS of Taiwan's NHI system for the first time. Our empirical results from the forecast error variance decomposition yielded higher explanatory power from the MF-VAR model in contrast to the conventional VAR model with single frequency data. The mixed frequency Granger causality tests identified bi-directional causation between nurse staffing and patient outcomes and one-way Granger causality running from nurse staffing to reimbursement to inpatient care services. The impulse-response analyses found positive (negative) effects of PNR on adverse patient outcomes (reimbursement payments for inpatient care services) in all types of hospitals but detrimental effects of adverse patient outcomes on PNR in medical centers (regional and district hospitals) across a 12-month period.

These findings generated from the aforementioned models suggest that nurse staffing is an essential determinant of both patient outcomes and reimbursement payments under the GBPS of Taiwan's NHI system. Therefore, the vicious cycle triggered by hospital (quantity) competition under the GBPS of Taiwan's NHI system works differently in different types of hospitals. Strategic policies (such as directly subsidizing for appropriate nurse staffing levels and the inclusion of the nurse staffing level as a vital standard for hospital accreditation) should be implemented for all hospitals in order to preserve the quality of inpatient care services, and more comprehensive interventions aimed towards switching hospital competition from quantity to quality competition should focus on the harmful effect of adverse patient outcomes on nurse staffing in medical centers and regional hospitals.

Funding: This research was funded by the Ministry of Science and Technology in Taiwan for the research project entitled "Now-casting for the effect of nurse staffing on quality of inpatient care during the COVID-19 pandemic outbreak: Evidence from Taiwan" with Grant No. 110-2410-H-025-012. The APC was funded by the Ministry of Science and Technology and National Taichung University of Science and Technology, Taiwan.

Data Availability Statement: Data are available upon request to the author.

Acknowledgments: The final proof-reading of this study by Lisa Brutcher (at Washington State University, USA) is deeply acknowledged. All errors are mine.

Conflicts of Interest: The author declares no conflict of interest, and the funders had no role in the design of the study; in the collection, analyses, or interpretation of data; in the writing of the manuscript; or in the decision to publish the results.

Appendix A

In order to present these data better, we exhibit the trends of all variables used in this study in Figure A1. Note that Taiwan's NHIA implemented the first stage of the post-acute care intervention program during the period of July 1st 2017~April 10th 2020 [58]. Attributable to this intervention program, we found significant structural changes in the two ICQ indicators and PNR at medical centers and district hospitals during the intervention period. In addition, we also found a sudden drop in PNRs in the three different types of hospitals during the periods of three COVID-19 strike waves (see grey shading area in Figure A1) in Taiwan, corresponding to a sharp fall in the two ICQ indicators and rise in real ICE per admission. These results reflect the fact that inpatient care utilization was largely reduced due to public fear of COVID-19 infection and the promotion of policies discouraging non-urgent healthcare services, and, in turn, a reduction in hospital (quantity) competition and lower PNRs were found. These findings have implications regarding the interdependences between PNR, ICQ, and real ICE per admission under the GBPS of Taiwan's NHI system.

In order to obtain stationary time series of these variables, the cyclic components of these time series were extracted through the Hodrick and Prescott filter method [51]. The cyclic components of all variables with the logarithm transformation in level terms were both de-mean and de-trend time series, which enabled us to accommodate structural changes of those variables discussed in the aforementioned pargagaph. The plots of the cyclic components of all variables are displayed in Figure A2.

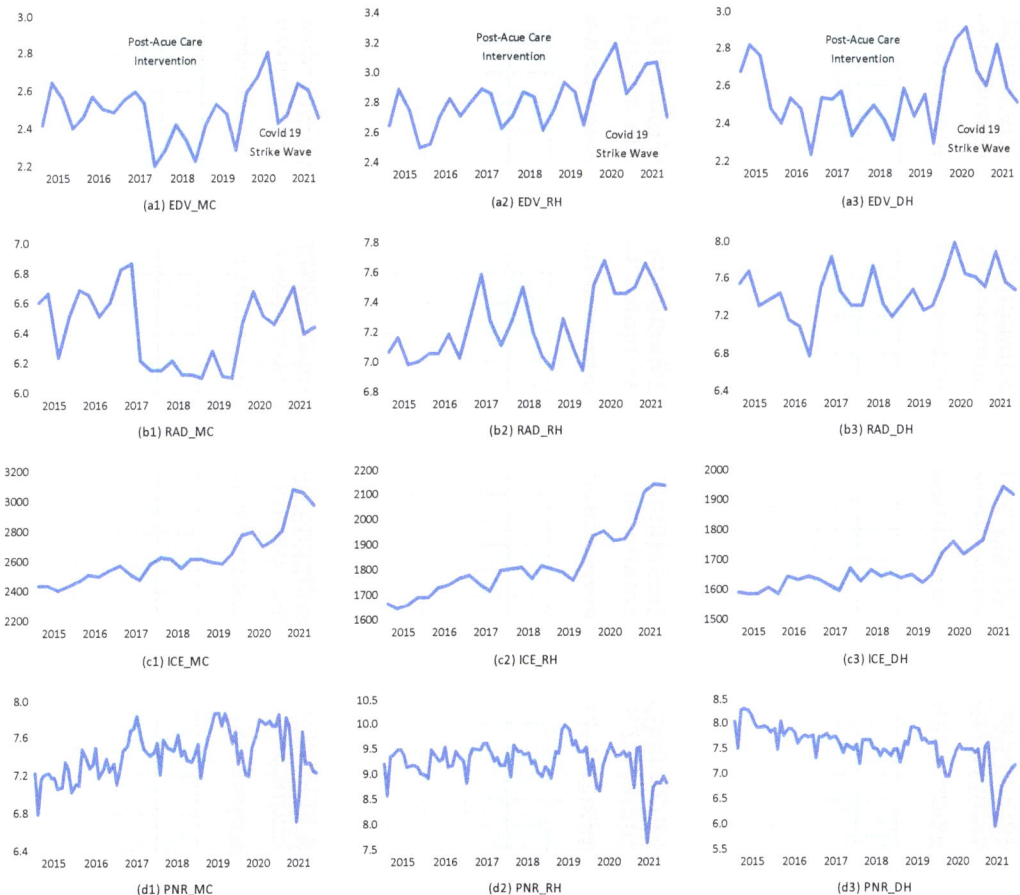

Figure A1. Time plots for all variables used in this study [8].

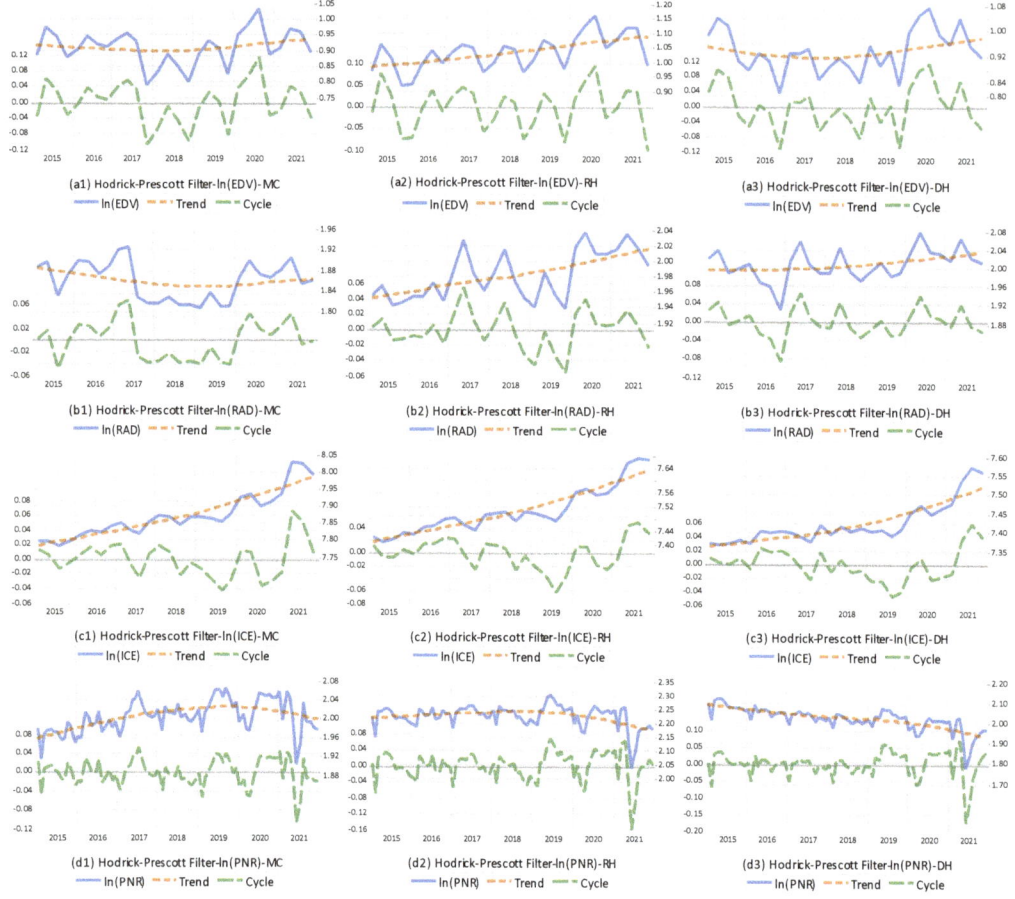

Figure A2. Time plots for all variables transformed by the Hodrick-Prescott filter method [9].

Notes

[1] Inpatient care expenditure per admission was calculated using total inpatient care expenditure divided by total admissions in a specific type of hospital, and it was measured using the 2016 price level (constant 2016 USD). The patient-to-nurse ratio was defined as the mean of number of patients divided by the nurse staffing number within three shifts per day in a specific type of hospital. The quarterly and monthly sample periods start from 2015: Q1 to 2021: Q4 and 2015: M1 to 2021: M12, resulting in a total of 28 and 84 quarterly and monthly observations, respectively. The IQR and JB statistics represent the interquartile range and Jarque-Bera statistics, respectively. "**", "*" denote 1% and 5% significance levels for the rejection of null hypothesis of the normality of time series, respectively.

[2] All variables are defined in the same way as for Table 1. The lag length is selected based on Bayesian Information Criterion (BIC) with the maximal lag as eight. "**" and "*" represent 1% and 5% significance levels, respectively. $\sum_{t=1}^{3} C\_\ln\left(PNR_i^k\right)$, , k = MC, RH, and DH define cyclic components of aggregate monthly PNR.

[3] Quarterly data on cyclical components of quality of care indicators (such as the 3-day EDV rate and 14-day readmission rate), inpatient care expenditure per admission, and monthly data on cyclical components of the patient-to-nurse ratio were used to estimate the MF-VAR model. The monthly data on cyclical components of the patient-to-nurse ratio were aggregated into quarterly data (PNR^A) when the LF-VAR model was estimated. The lag length is selected based on Newey and West's automatic lag selection with the maximal lag as 3 [52]. "PNR$^A \not\Rightarrow$ EDV", for example, represents the null hypothesis of non-causality from PNR^A to RER. The bold font of **PNR** denotes the vector of cyclical components of PNR symbolized by [C_lnPNR1, C_lnPNR2, C_lnPNR3]'. "**PNR** $\not\Rightarrow$ EDV", for example, represents the null hypothesis of joint non-causality from the vector of cyclical

4   Figure 1 plots the impulse response functions (IRFs) for monthly horizons h = 0, 1, 2, ... , 12 based on the MF-VAR model of quarterly data on cyclical components of quality of care indicators (such as the 3-day EDV rate and 14-day readmission rate), inpatient care expenditure per admission, and three individual monthly cyclical components of the patient-to-nurse ratio symbolized by C_lnPNR1, C_lnPNR2, and C_lnPNR3 in a quarter timespan. The Cholesky decomposition with order PNR1, PNR2, PNR3, EDV (or RAD), and ICE is selected. The sample period covers 2015:Q1–2021:Q4. The responses of variable Y (say, EDV) to 1σ shock in X (say, PNR1) at monthly horizon h is written as "PNR1=>RER". MC, RH, and DH represent medical centers, regional hospitals, and district hospitals, respectively. Blue shaded areas denote 90% confidence intervals of IRFs based on the Monte Carlo simulation method with 10,000 replications.

5   Figure 2 plots the impulse response functions (IRFs) for monthly horizons h = 0, 1, 2, ... , 12 based on the MF-VAR model of quarterly data on cyclical components of quality of care indicators (such as the 3-day EDV rate and 14-day readmission rate), inpatient care expenditure per admission, and three individual monthly cyclical components of the patient-to-nurse ratio symbolized by C_lnPNR1, C_lnPNR2, and C_lnPNR3 in a quarter timespan. The Cholesky decomposition with order PNR1, PNR2, PNR3, EDV (or RAD), and ICE is selected. The sample period covers 2015:Q1~2021:Q4. The responses of variable Y (say, EDV) to 1σ shock in X (say, ICE) at monthly horizon h is written as "ICE =>EDV". Blue shaded areas denote 90% confidence intervals of IRFs based on the Monte Carlo simulation method with 10,000 replications. MC, RH, and DH denote medical centers, regional hospitals, and district hospitals, respectively.

6   Notations presented in this table are the same as those used in Table 3. The sum of variance decomposition may not equal 100 due to rounding.

7   The directions of arrows were drawn based on the Granger causality tests. The arrows with bold (dot) lines represent significant (insignificant) paths connecting two target variables based on 90% confidence intervals of the impulse-response effects accumulated across a 3-month cycle of a quarter timespan over a 12-month period. MC, RH, and DH denote medical centers, regional hospitals, and district hospitals, respectively.

8   EDV and RAD represent the 3-day EDV rate and 14-day readmission rate, respectively. ICE is real inpatient care expenditure per admission at the 2016 price level (USD). PNR symbolizes the patient-to-nurse ratio. MC, RH, and DH represent medical centers, regional hospitals, and district hospitals, respectively. Light blue and grey shaded areas show the post-acute care intervention period and COVID-19 strike waves, respectively.

9   All notations used in this figure are the same as for Figure 1. ln(·) represents the natural logarithm transformation.

References

1. Aiken, L.H.; Clarke, S.P.; Sloane, D.M.; Sochalski, J.; Silber, J.H. Hospital nurse staffing and patient mortality, nurse burnout, and job dissatisfaction. *JAMA* **2002**, *2288*, 1987–1993. [CrossRef] [PubMed]
2. McHugh, M.D.; Aiken, L.H.; Sloane, D.M.; Windsor, C.; Douglas, C.; Yates, P. Effects of nurse-to-patient ratio legislation on nurse staffing and patient mortality, readmissions, and length of stay: A prospective study in a panel of hospitals. *Lancet* **2021**, *397*, 1905–1913. [CrossRef]
3. McHugh, M.D.; Aiken, L.H.; Windsor, C.; Douglas, C.; Yates, P. Case for hospital nurse-to-patient ratio legislation in Queensland, Australia, hospitals: An observational study. *BMJ Open* **2020**, *10*, e036264. [CrossRef]
4. Haegdorens, F.; Van Bogaert, P.; De Meester, K.; Monsieurs, K.G. The impact of nurse staffing levels and nurse's education on patient mortality in medical and surgical wards: An observational multicentre study. *BMC Health Serv. Res.* **2019**, *19*, 864. [CrossRef]
5. Rochefort, C.M.; Beauchamp, M.E.; Audet, L.A.; Abrahamowicz, M.; Bourgault, P. Associations of 4 nurse staffing practices with hospital mortality. *Med. Care* **2020**, *58*, 912–918. [CrossRef] [PubMed]
6. Aiken, L.H.; Simonetti, M.; Sloane, D.M.; Cerón, C.; Soto, P.; Bravo, D.; Galiano, A.; Behrman, J.R.; Smith, H.L.; McHugh, M.D.; et al. Hospital nurse staffing and patient outcomes in Chile: A multilevel cross-sectional study. *Lancet Glob. Health* **2021**, *9*, e1145–e1153. [CrossRef]
7. Griffiths, P.; Maruotti, A.; Recio Saucedo, A.; Redfern, O.C.; Ball, J.E.; Briggs, J.; Dall'Ora, C.; Schmidt, P.E.; Smith, G.B.; Missed Care Study Group. Nurse staffing, nursing assistants and hospital mortality: Retrospective longitudinal cohort study. *BMJ Qual. Saf.* **2019**, *28*, 609–617. [CrossRef] [PubMed]
8. Fagerström, L.; Kinnunen, M.; Saarela, J. Nursing workload, patient safety incidents and mortality: An observational study from Finland. *BMJ Open* **2018**, *8*, e016367. [CrossRef]
9. Kim, Y.; Kim, H.Y.; Cho, E. Association between the bed-to-nurse ratio and 30-day post-discharge mortality in patients undergoing surgery: A cross-sectional analysis using Korean administrative data. *BMC Nurs.* **2020**, *19*, 17. [CrossRef] [PubMed]
10. Tvedt, C.; Sjetne, I.S.; Helgeland, J.; Bukholm, G. An observational study: Associations between nurse-reported hospital characteristics and estimated 30-day survival probabilities. *BMJ Qual. Saf.* **2014**, *23*, 757–764. [CrossRef] [PubMed]
11. Liang, Y.W.; Chen, W.Y.; Lin, Y.H. Estimating a hospital production function to evaluate the effect of nurse staffing on patient mortality in Taiwan: The longitudinal count data approach. *Rom. J. Econ. Forecast.* **2015**, *18*, 154–169.

12. Liang, Y.W.; Chen, W.Y.; Lee, J.L.; Huang, L.C. Nurse staffing, direct nursing care hours and patient mortality in Taiwan: The longitudinal analysis of hospital nurse staffing and patient outcome study. *BMC Health Serv. Res.* **2012**, *12*, 44. [CrossRef] [PubMed]
13. Liang, Y.W.; Tsai, S.F.; Chen, W.Y. A longitudinal study of the effects of nurse staffing on patient outcomes for Taiwan acute care hospital. *J. Nurs. Res.* **2012**, *20*, 1–8. [CrossRef] [PubMed]
14. Amiri, A.; Vehviläinen-Julkunen, K.; Solankallio-Vahteri, T.; Tuomi, S. Impact of nursing staffing on reducing infants, neonatal, perinatal mortality rates: Evidence from 35 OECD countries. *Int. J. Nurs. Sci.* **2020**, *7*, 161–169.
15. Amiri, A.; Solankallio-Vahteri, T. Nurse-staffing level and quality of acute care services: Evidence from cross-national panel data analysis in OECD countries. *Int. J. Nurs. Sci.* **2019**, *6*, 6–16. [CrossRef]
16. Ball, J.E.; Bruyneel, L.; Aiken, L.H.; Sermeus, W.; Sloane, D.M.; Rafferty, A.M.; Lindqvist, R.; Tishelman, C.; Griffiths, P.; RN4Cast Consortium. Post-operative mortality, missed care and nurse staffing in nine countries: A cross-sectional study. *Int. J. Nurs. Stud.* **2018**, *78*, 10–15. [CrossRef]
17. Aiken, L.H.; Sloane, D.; Griffiths, P.; Rafferty, A.M.; Bruyneel, L.; McHugh, M.; Maier, C.B.; Moreno-Casbas, T.; Ball, J.E.; Ausserhofer, D.; et al. Nursing skill mix in European hospitals: Cross-sectional study of the association with mortality, patient ratings, and quality of care. *BMJ Qual. Saf.* **2017**, *26*, 559–568. [CrossRef]
18. Aiken, L.H.; Sloane, D.M.; Bruyneel, L.; Van den Heede, K.; Griffiths, P.; Busse, R.; Diomidous, M.; Kinnunen, J.; Kózka, M.; Lesaffre, E.; et al. Nurse staffing and education and hospital mortality in nine European countries: A retrospective observational study. *Lancet* **2014**, *383*, 1824–1830. [CrossRef]
19. Van, T.; Annis, A.M.; Yosef, M.; Robinson, C.H.; Duffy, S.A.; Li, Y.F.; Taylor, B.A.; Krein, S.; Sullivan, S.C.; Sales, A. Nurse staffing and healthcare-associated infections in a national healthcare system that implemented a nurse staffing directive: Multi-level interrupted time series analyses. *Int. J. Nurs. Stud.* **2020**, *104*, 103531. [CrossRef]
20. Wang, L.; Lu, H.; Dong, X.; Huang, X.; Li, B.; Wan, Q.; Shang, S. The effect of nurse staffing on patient-safety outcomes: A cross-sectional survey. *J. Nurs. Manag.* **2020**, *28*, 1758–1766. [CrossRef]
21. Butler, M.; Schultz, T.J.; Halligan, P.; Sheridan, A.; Kinsman, L.; Rotter, T.; Beaumier, J.; Kelly, R.G.; Drennan, J. Hospital nurse-staffing models and patient- and staff-related outcomes. *Cochrane Database Syst. Rev.* **2019**, *4*, CD007019. [CrossRef] [PubMed]
22. Redfern, O.C.; Griffiths, P.; Maruotti, A.; Recio Saucedo, A.; Smith, G.B.; Missed Care Study Group. The association between nurse staffing levels and the timeliness of vital signs monitoring: A retrospective observational study in the UK. *BMJ Open* **2019**, *9*, e032157. [CrossRef] [PubMed]
23. Twigg, D.E.; Kutzer, Y.; Jacob, E.; Seaman, K. A quantitative systematic review of the association between nurse skill mix and nursing-sensitive patient outcomes in the acute care setting. *J. Adv. Nurs.* **2019**, *75*, 3404–3423. [CrossRef] [PubMed]
24. Bobay, K.L.; Yakusheva, O.; Weiss, M.E. Outcomes and cost analysis of the impact of unit-level nursing staffing post-discharge utilization. *Nurs. Econ.* **2011**, *29*, 69–78. [PubMed]
25. Weiss, M.E.; Yakusheva, O.; Bobay, K.L. Quality and cost analysis of nurse staffing, discharge preparation, and post discharge utilization. *Health Serv. Res.* **2011**, *46*, 1473–1494. [CrossRef]
26. National Health Insurance Administration. National Health Insurance: 2021–2022 Annual Report. Executive Yuan, Taiwan. 2022. Available online: https://www.nhi.gov.tw/Content_List.aspx?n=9223A12B5B31CB37&topn=4864A82710DE35ED (accessed on 15 August 2022).
27. Chen, W.Y. On the network transmission mechanisms of disease-specific healthcare expenditure spillovers: Evidence from the connectedness network analyses. *Healthcare* **2021**, *9*, 319. [CrossRef]
28. Chen, W.Y. Does healthcare financing converge? Evidence from eight OECD Countries. *Int. J. Health Care Financ. Econ.* **2013**, *13*, 279–300. [CrossRef]
29. Chen, W.Y.; Chi, C.H.; Lin, Y.H. The willingness-to-pay for the health care under Taiwan's National Health Insurance system. *Appl. Econ.* **2011**, *43*, 1113–1123. [CrossRef]
30. Chen, W.Y. The effect of interdependences of referral behaviors on the quality of ambulatory care: Evidence from Taiwan. *Risk Manag. Healthc. Policy* **2021**, *14*, 4709–4721. [CrossRef]
31. Wong, L. A Guide to Taiwan's Health Industries. Taipei: PricewaterhouseCoopers (PwC). 2020. Available online: https://www.pwc.tw/en/publications/taiwan-health-industries.html (accessed on 15 August 2022).
32. Chen, W.Y.; Lin, Y.H. Hospital non-price competition under global budget payment and prospective payment system. *Expert Rev. Pharm. Outcomes Res.* **2008**, *8*, 301–308. [CrossRef]
33. Lu, M.S.; Tseng, H.Y.; Liang, S.Y.; Lin, C.F. Concept for planning the nurse-patient ratio and nursing fee payment linkage system. *Hu Li Za Zhi* **2017**, *64*, 17–24. [CrossRef] [PubMed]
34. Turton, M. Does Taiwan's nursing problem have a cure? *Taipei Times.* 21 February 2022. Available online: https://www.taipeitimes.com/News/feat/archives/2022/02/21/2003773473 (accessed on 15 August 2022).
35. Jun, J.; Ojemeni, M.M.; Kalamani, R.; Tong, J.; Crecelius, M.L. Relationship between nurse burnout, patient and organizational outcomes: Systematic review. *Int. J. Nurs. Stud.* **2021**, *119*, 103933. [CrossRef] [PubMed]
36. de Cordova, P.B.; Rogowski, J.; Riman, K.A.; McHugh, M.D. Effects of public reporting legislation of nurse staffing: A trend analysis. *Policy Politics Nurs. Pract.* **2019**, *20*, 92–104. [CrossRef] [PubMed]

37. He, J.; Staggs, V.S.; Bergquist-Beringer, S.; Dunton, N. Nurse staffing and patient outcomes: A longitudinal study on trend and seasonality. *BMC Nurs.* **2016**, *15*, 60. [CrossRef] [PubMed]
38. Everhart, D.; Schumacher, J.R.; Duncan, R.P.; Hall, A.G.; Neff, D.F.; Shorr, R.I. Determinants of hospital fall rate trajectory groups: A longitudinal assessment of nurse staffing and organizational characteristics. *Health Care Manag. Rev.* **2014**, *39*, 352–360. [CrossRef]
39. Winter, S.G.; Bartel, A.P.; de Cordova, P.B.; Needleman, J.; Schmitt, S.K.; Stone, P.W.; Phibbs, C.S. The effect of data aggregation on estimations of nurse staffing and patient outcomes. *Health Serv. Res.* **2021**, *56*, 1262–1270. [CrossRef]
40. Liu, Y.H.; Chang, W.S.; Chen, W.Y. Health progress and economic growth in the United States: The Mixed Frequency VAR analyses. *Qual. Quant.* **2019**, *53*, 1895–1911. [CrossRef]
41. Silvestrini, A.; Veredas, D. Temporal aggregation of univariate and multivariate time series models: A survey. *J. Econ. Surv.* **2008**, *22*, 458–497. [CrossRef]
42. National Development Council. Population Projections for the R.O.C. (Taiwan): 2020~2070. Executive Yuan, Taiwan. 2022. Available online: https://www.ndc.gov.tw/en/cp.aspx?n=2E5DCB04C64512CC (accessed on 15 August 2022).
43. Cheng, T.M. Taiwan's Health Care System: The Next 20 Years. Brookings Op-Ed. 2015. Available online: https://www.brookings.edu/opinions/taiwans-health-care-system-the-next-20-years/ (accessed on 15 August 2022).
44. Taiwan Union of Nurses Association. Taiwan Nursing Workforce Statistics. Available online: https://www.nurse.org.tw/publicUI/H/H10201.aspx?arg=8DA73DB09C6642F030 (accessed on 15 August 2022).
45. Huang, C.C.; Lin, S.H.; Zheng, K.W. The relationship among emotional intelligence, social support, job involvement, and turnover intention—A study of nurses in Taiwan. *J. Econ. Bus.* **2019**, *2*, 652–659. [CrossRef]
46. Chin, W.S.; Chen, Y.C.; Ho, J.J.; Cheng, N.Y.; Wu, H.C.; Shiao, J.S.C. Psychological work environment and suicidal ideation among nurses in Taiwan. *J. Nurse Scholarsh.* **2019**, *51*, 106–113. [CrossRef]
47. Ghysels, E. Macroeconomics and the reality of mixed frequency data. *J. Econom.* **2016**, *193*, 294–314. [CrossRef]
48. Ghysels, E.; Hill, J.B.; Motegi, K. Testing for Granger causality with mixed frequency data. *J. Econom.* **2016**, *192*, 207–230. [CrossRef]
49. Motegia, K.; Sadahirob, A. Sluggish private investment in Japan's Lost Decade: Mixed frequency vector autoregression approach. *North Am. J. Econ. Financ.* **2018**, *43*, 118–128. [CrossRef]
50. National Health Insurance Administration. Web of Quality of Care in National Health Insurance. Executive Yuan, Taiwan. 2022. Available online: https://www.nhi.gov.tw/AmountInfoWeb/TargetItem.aspx?rtype=2 (accessed on 15 August 2022).
51. Hodrick, R.J.; Prescott, E.C. Postwar U.S. business cycles: An empirical investigation. *J. Money Credit Bank.* **1997**, *29*, 1–16. [CrossRef]
52. Newey, W.; West, K. Automatic lag selection in covariance matrix estimation. *Rev. Econ. Stud.* **1994**, *61*, 631–653. [CrossRef]
53. Gonçalves, S.; Kilian, L. Bootstrapping autoregressions with conditional heteroscedasticity of unknown form. *J. Econom.* **2004**, *123*, 89–120. [CrossRef]
54. National Health Insurance Administration. Statistics for the Daily Patient-to Nurse Ratio. Executive Yuan, Taiwan. 2022. Available online: https://www.nhi.gov.tw/Content_List.aspx?n=4037A32CDEF1DDCF&topn=CDA985A80C0DE710 (accessed on 15 August 2022).
55. Ministry of Health and Welfare. Statistics of Medical Care Institution & Hospital Utilization. Executive Yuan, Taiwan. 2022. Available online: https://dep.mohw.gov.tw/dos/lp-5099-113.html (accessed on 15 August 2022).
56. National Health Insurance Administration. Business Report for National Health Insurance. Executive Yuan, Taiwan. 2022. Available online: https://www.nhi.gov.tw/Content_List.aspx?n=6A330BB09FB0EA45&topn=23C660CAACAA159D (accessed on 15 August 2022).
57. Robinson, W.S. Ecological correlations and the behavior of individuals. *Am. Sociol. Rev.* **1950**, *15*, 351–357. [CrossRef]
58. Ministry of Health and Welfare. Post-Acute Care Integration Program. Executive Yuan, Taiwan. 2020. Available online: https://www.nhi.gov.tw/Content_List.aspx?n=5A0BB383D955741C&topn=5FE8C9FEAE863B46 (accessed on 15 August 2022).

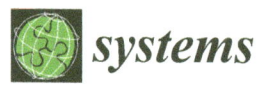

Review

Systems-Oriented Modelling Methods in Preventing and Controlling Emerging Infectious Diseases in the Context of Healthcare Policy: A Scoping Review

Mariam Abdulmonem Mansouri [1,2,*], Leandro Garcia [1], Frank Kee [1] and Declan Terence Bradley [1,3]

1. Centre for Public Health, Queen's University Belfast, Belfast BT12 6BA, UK
2. Ministry of Health, Kuwait City 12009, Kuwait
3. Public Health Agency, Belfast BT2 8BS, UK
* Correspondence: mmansouri01@qub.ac.uk

Abstract: Background: Emerging infectious diseases (EIDs) arise and affect society in complex ways. We conducted a scoping review to explore how systems-oriented methods have been used to prevent and control EIDs. Methods: We used the Joanna Briggs Institute framework for scoping reviews in this study. We included peer-reviewed articles about health care systems preparedness and response, published from 1 January 2000. We considered the World Health Organisation's (WHO) list of prioritised diseases for research and development when choosing the pathogens and only included studies that considered the dynamics between the system's elements. Results: Our initial search yielded 9985 studies. After screening, 177 studies were considered for inclusion in this review. After assessment by two independent reviewers, seven studies were included. The studies were published between 2009 and 2021. Most focused on sarbecoviruses and targeted healthcare policymakers and governments. System dynamics approaches were the most used methods. Most of the studies incorporated the classical epidemiological models alongside systems-oriented methods. The studies were conducted in context of diseases dynamics and its burden on human health, the economy and healthcare systems. The most reported challenge was epidemiological and geographical data timeliness and quality. Conclusions: Systems dynamics approaches can help policy makers understand the elements of a complex system and thus offer potential solutions for preventing and controlling EIDs.

Keywords: emerging infectious diseases; systems thinking; systems approach; systems dynamics; COVID-19; SARS-CoV1; MERS-CoV; healthcare policy; pandemic; outbreak

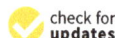

Citation: Mansouri, M.A.; Garcia, L.; Kee, F.; Bradley, D.T. Systems-Oriented Modelling Methods in Preventing and Controlling Emerging Infectious Diseases in the Context of Healthcare Policy: A Scoping Review. *Systems* **2022**, *10*, 182. https://doi.org/10.3390/systems10050182

Academic Editors: Philippe J. Giabbanelli and Andrew Page

Received: 17 August 2022
Accepted: 28 September 2022
Published: 9 October 2022

Publisher's Note: MDPI stays neutral with regard to jurisdictional claims in published maps and institutional affiliations.

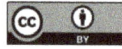

Copyright: © 2022 by the authors. Licensee MDPI, Basel, Switzerland. This article is an open access article distributed under the terms and conditions of the Creative Commons Attribution (CC BY) license (https:// creativecommons.org/licenses/by/ 4.0/).

1. Introduction

Emerging infectious diseases (EIDs) are a group of diseases affecting humans for the first time, or pre-existing diseases that are rapidly spreading in terms of the number of new cases or in new geographical areas [1,2]. The majority of EIDs are zoonotic and at least initially are transmitted from animal sources to humans through spillover [3]. Examples include COVID-19, Ebola virus, Lassa fever, Middle East Respiratory Syndrome coronavirus (MERS-CoV) and monkeypox.

EIDs are complex and not caused merely by the infectious agents themselves. Multiple factors contribute to their emergence, including increased human population size and movement within recent years, increased travel and trade, urbanisation, wars, human behaviour, and climate change [2]. In addition, there is a lack of prior knowledge and limited, if any, immunity to the emerging pathogen, which contributes to additional burden to humans' health and lives.

Preventing and controlling EIDs are important elements of our duties and responsibilities for overall public health preparedness and response. Such responsibilities play out in a complex system with multiple interacting elements and stakeholders [4]. EID preparedness and response must ensure the readiness of the healthcare systems to anticipate and face the threats of a novel pathogen on human health and lives [5]. Readiness also includes healthcare systems resilience and ability to adequately sustain healthcare for patients in need, avoiding delays in diagnosis or treatment during EID emergencies [5].

Systems science can help conceptualize a problem as a perturbation within complex adaptive system [6]. It does so by identifying the components that make up the system and how they are linked, shaping the system's overall form and behaviour [6]. Systems scientists aim to identify leverage points within the system to provide holistic solutions instead of a response to a single aspect of a particular problem [7]. Although a systems science lens and methods have been used in infectious disease research and practice for decades, there is a gap in knowledge of how systems-oriented modelling methods in particular have been and can be used to strengthen healthcare systems' capacity in preventing and controlling EIDs. This scoping review aims to explore how systems-oriented modelling methods have been used to inform healthcare policymakers about healthcare system's preparedness and response to EIDs.

Research Question

The review's main question was: how have systems-oriented modelling methods been used to prevent and control EIDs? We were interested specifically in the preparedness and response of healthcare systems. Further sub-questions were:

- What was the context in which the systems-oriented study was conducted?
- Who were the target population?
- What was the systems-oriented aim?
- What were the main complex-systems features considered?
- What were the system's main elements?
- What were the systems-oriented methods used?
- What challenges related to systems modelling did the authors face?
- Who were the main stakeholder and how were they involved?
- What were the key lessons learned from using the complex systems approach?

Because we were interested in exploring the evidence and lessons to identify the key concepts in this topic, we chose to conduct a scoping review [8].

2. Materials and Methods

A protocol for this review was published in 2021 [9]. Below we outline the relevant steps, updated with any changes that occurred as we developed a deeper understanding of the topic.

2.1. Preparation

We started the scoping review by establishing the research team, which consisted of experts in public health, communicable diseases and systems science. Due to the ill-defined characterisation of EIDs, we decided to use the list developed by the World Health Organisation (WHO) for prioritised EIDs for research and development, which they update according to global circumstances [10].

Before going forward, we searched to find whether any systematic or scoping reviews were published about the same topic. We conducted a comprehensive search in Scopus, Joanna Briggs Institute database, Cochrane database, PubMed and Epistemonikos. To our knowledge, up to the time of starting this review, there were no systematic or scoping reviews that answered our research questions. Therefore, the team agreed on the broad research question and study protocol, including the keyword and databases in this scoping review.

For this scoping review, we followed the Joanna Briggs Institute framework, which is based on previous work from Lavec and colleagues and Arskey and O'Malley's recommendations [8]. Our scoping review consists of six steps: (1) Identify the research questions, (2) Identify keywords and medical subject headings (MeSH) terms, (3) Identify relevant studies, (4) Study selection, (5) Data charting, and (6) Summarise and disseminate the results.

2.2. Identifying Keywords and MeSH Terms

After consulting the subject librarian at the School of Medicine, Dentistry and Biomedical Sciences, Queen's University Belfast, the initial search started on 23 March 2021 in Scopus and Google Scholar to identify keywords, MeSH terms and index terms relevant to the review. The research team agreed on the searched terms (Table 1), which were used across all databases. We searched two databases, PubMed, Web of Science, and Scopus (Appendix A). These databases were selected to allow a broad search for materials in the topic. Additionally, the research team agreed to screen the first ten pages in Google Scholar to identify any relevant studies in grey literature.

Table 1. Keywords used in the searches.

Concept	Search Terms
Systems modelling methods	Complex* systems OR system dynamic* OR agent?based OR stochastic OR network* OR compartmental model* OR multi?agent OR multi-compartment model*
Emerging infectious diseases	Emerging infectious diseases OR coronavirus OR MERS-CoV, COVID-19 OR severe acute respiratory syndrome OR SARS-CoV-2 OR SARS OR Ebola OR zika OR dengue OR Nipah OR pandemic * OR influenza OR outbreak* OR Crimean-Congo haemorrhagic fever OR rift valley fever or "diseases X"* OR Lassa fever

MERS-CoV: Middle East Respiratory Syndrome Coronavirus; SARS-CoV-2: Severe Acute Respiratory Syndrome Coronavirus 2; SARS: Severe Acute Respiratory Syndrome Coronavirus.

All citations were imported into the Endnote X9 citation manager, where they were deduplicated. Next, we imported the selected citations into the web-based systematic review management software, Covidence, for the title and abstract relevance screening and full article selection. During the importation process, Covidence found and removed further duplicated citations.

2.3. Identifying Relevant Studies

Table 2 shows the inclusion and exclusion criteria. Studies were eligible if they investigated an EID in the WHO priority list [10]. After the initial search, we decided to narrow the scope of the review because the number of potential studies was too large. We made the following changes to the protocol in order to achieve this reduced scope. We decided to focus on studies conducted in the context of healthcare policy, those that considered the dynamic relationships between elements of the system (e.g., feedback loops and network effects), and we only included peer-reviewed publications (excluding grey, pre-print and unpublished reports) containing simulation models published on or after 1 January 2000. There were no limits regarding article language, geographic location or country income group of the location of study.

2.4. Study Selection

Title and abstracts were screened to exclude studies that clearly met one or more of exclusion criteria or which did not meet any of the inclusion criteria. In the next stage, a full-text review was conducted on the studies that passed screening to assess them against the eligibility criteria. In both stages, each study was independently assessed by two reviewers. In the case of disagreement, reviewers met to reach consensus.

Table 2. Inclusion and exclusion criteria.

Inclusion Criteria	Exclusion Criteria
Peer-reviewed reports published since 1 January 2000	Abstract-only reports
Studies related to health systems preparedness and response	Studies that do not include healthcare system element
Emerging infectious diseases included in the prioritising diseases for research and development in emergency context list by The World Health Organisation [10]	Studies on non-emerging infectious diseases
Studies conducted to investigate preparedness, prevention and response to EIDs that affect human populations	Studies that do not include the human population
Considered the dynamic relationships between elements of the system (e.g., feedback loops, network effects)	Studies of mathematical models that do not account for dynamic relationships between elements of the system outside the epidemic model
	Seasonal influenza

2.5. Data Charting

We developed a form for data extraction and characterisation that included: authors of the article, year and location of study, context (e.g., disease dynamics, healthcare preparedness and response, resources), target population, complex systems features considered, complex systems-oriented aim, system's elements considered, modelling and analytic methods, reported challenges during modelling and potential solutions, main stakeholders and their involvement in the study, and reported key lessons from the complex systems-oriented approach. The reviewing team discussed and agreed this form. Two independent reviewers tested the form; the reviewing team met to resolve disagreements in the data extraction. The complex systems features considered were based on the list provided by James Ladyman and Karoline Wiesner as follows [11]:

1. Numerosity: complex systems involve many interactions among many components.
2. Disorder and diversity: the interactions in a complex system are not coordinated or controlled centrally, and the components may differ.
3. Feedback: the interactions in complex systems are iterated so that there is feedback from previous interactions on a timescale relevant to the system's emergent dynamics.
4. Non-equilibrium: complex systems are open to the environment and are often driven by something external.
5. Spontaneous order and self-organisation: complex systems exhibit structure and order that arises out of the interactions among their parts.
6. Nonlinearity: complex systems exhibit nonlinear dependence on parameters or external drivers.
7. Robustness: the structure and function of complex system is stable under relevant perturbations.
8. Nested structure and modularity: there may be multiple scales of structure, clustering and specialisation of function in complex systems.
9. History and memory: complex systems often require a very long history to exist and also store information about history.
10. Adaptive behaviour: complex systems are often able to modify their behaviour depending on the state of the environment and the predisposition they make about it.

2.6. Results Summary and Dissemination

The data were aggregated in a single spreadsheet using Microsoft Excel version 16.43 (Microsoft, Redmond, USA) for validation and coding. The rows represented articles, the columns represented the data items extracted to answer the research questions and the cells contained information gathered from the selected articles. We synthesized the results using text and tables and answered each research question and sub-questions set up in the protocol for this scoping review.

3. Results

3.1. Search and Selection of Citations

We initiated this scoping review in March 2021, finding 9985 citations. After deduplication, we screened 9944 titles and abstracts and reviewed 117 full texts. After data characterisation of full-text articles, seven studies [12–18] were included (Figure 1). Many articles were excluded during the title and abstract screening because the keywords used yielded many publications outside the scope of this review or had different study designs that did not address our research question. Reasons for excluding citations at the full-text stage were: studies of mathematical models that did not account for dynamic relationships between elements of the system ($n = 99$), studies that did not include the healthcare policy context ($n = 7$) and abstract only citations ($n = 4$).

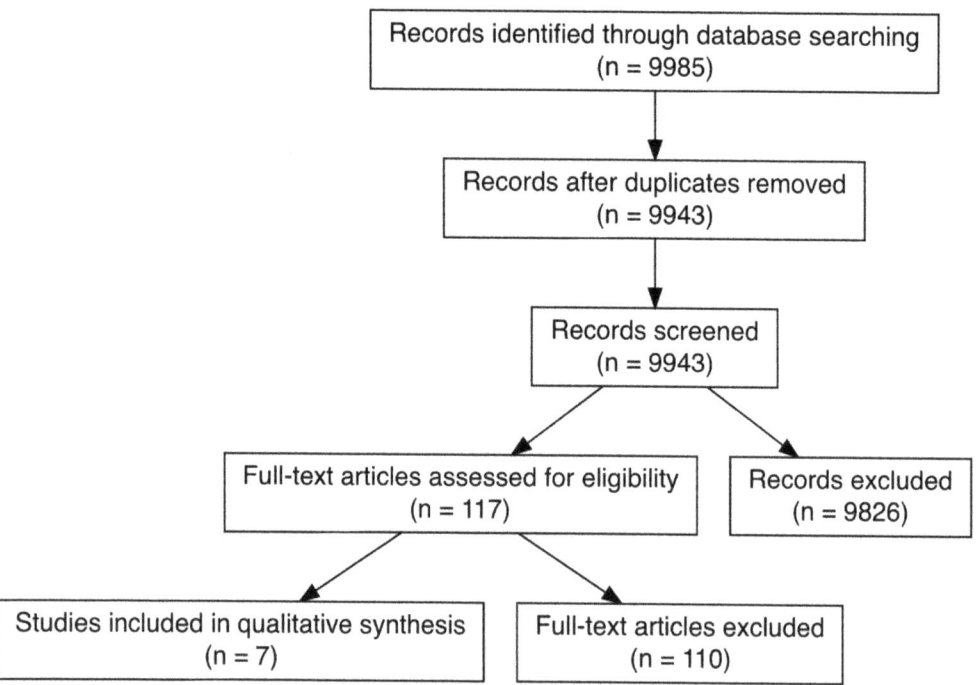

Figure 1. Preferred Reporting Items for Systematic Reviews and Meta-Analysis (PRISMA) flowchart.

3.2. General Characteristics of Included Citations

The general characteristics of papers included in this scoping review are presented in Table 3. All included studies were published between 2009 and 2021, with the majority (5/7) published during the COVID-19 pandemic, in 2020 and 2021.

There were five main stakeholder categories in the included citations. Healthcare policymakers were the main stakeholders, followed by government officials, healthcare demonstrators, politicians, and academics. However, none of the studies reported involvement of stakeholders in the model development or interpretation of the results.

Different systems methods were used in the studies; the most commonly used method was system dynamics. Other methods used once in the studies were dynamic causal modelling, agent-based modelling, total interpretive structural modelling and multilayer complex network.

Table 3. General characteristics of included citations.

Characteristic	Number (n = 7)
Publication year	
2009	1
2017	1
2020	4
2021	1
Publication type	
Journal article	7
Main stakeholders	
Academics Healthcare policymakers	1
Government	3
Healthcare administrators	2
Healthcare policymakers	5
Politicians	2
Systems methods used	
Agent-based modelling	1
Dynamic causal modelling	1
Multilayer complex network	1
System dynamics modelling	3
Total interpretive structural modelling	1
Complex systems feature used	
Adaptive behaviour	6
Disorder	7
Feedback	7
History and memory	0
Nested structure and modularity	6
Non-equilibrium	5
Non-linearity	6
Numerosity	7
Robustness	4
Spontaneous	7

Regarding complex systems features, most studies exhibited most of the features in their modelling. Numerosity, disorder, feedback, and spontaneous order were noted in all included studies. Non-linearity, nested structure and modularity, and adaptive behaviour were displayed in 6/7 of the citations. Non-equilibrium featured in 5/7 of the studies. System history and memory were not seen in any of the models in the included articles.

3.3. Methodological Characteristics of Included Studies

The methodological characteristics of the included studies are presented in Tables 4 and 5. The methodological characteristics that address our research question and sub-questions are as follows:

Table 4. Extracted data: Study Characteristics and Aims.

Study	Publication Year	Country	Disease	Target Population	Aims
Friston [15]	2020	US, Brazil, UK, France, Spain, Italy, Mexico, Belgium, Germany, Canada	COVID-19	Local population of each country investigated	To estimate the duration of population immunity and the latent states and mechanisms that affect the rate of new cases and deaths under the most likely loss of immunity.

Table 4. *Cont.*

Study	Publication Year	Country	Disease	Target Population	Aims
Mutanga [12]	2021	South Africa	COVID-19	National population	To assess the range of systems dynamics modelling ability in forecasting COVID-19 dynamic and investigate the adequacy of government enforced restriction measures to control the pandemic using different "what if" scenarios. To predict the next wave of COVID-19 infection.
Scabini [16]	2020	Brazil	COVID-19	National population	To analyse COVID-19 dynamics in Brazil and to investigate the implications of future actions by the government on the healthcare system
Shin [14]	2017	South Korea	MERS-CoV	Healthcare staff, patients and visitors in hospitals during MERS-CoV outbreak	To investigate the effect of healthcare policy to control MERS-CoV in South Korea on terms of patient care and diseases spread in hospitals.
Silva [18]	2020	Brazil	COVID-19	National population data	To simulate COVID-19 dynamics and the economic impact during different restriction scenarios.
Suresh [13]	2020	India	COVID-19	Healthcare workers (physicians, nurses, health inspectors, paramedics, hospital operation and administrative staff)	To analyse the key factors contributing to the agility of the healthcare system in controlling COVID-19 in the context of available resources during the disease dynamics.
Weixing [17]	2009	China	SARS	Population of Hubei Province	To simulate SARS-CoV-1 spread and evaluate control measures to mitigate further spread of the pathogen.

Table 5. Extracted data: System Features, Methods, Stakeholders and Lessons.

Study	Main Stakeholders	Methods	System's Elements	Challenges and Potential Solutions	Key Lessons
Friston [15]	Policymakers and academics	Dynamic causal modelling	The local population is assigned a state in four distinct attributes (location, infection state, symptoms, and testing). 24 parameters specify aspects associated with state transition probabilities (e.g., the effective number of contacts, transmission strength, the efficacy of tracking and tracing).	Modelling process did not account for geospatial aspects, waves of infection or any interactions with seasonal influenza (no potential solution discussed). Inaccuracy of population demography data. Solution: building a model that accounts to population heterogeneity at a coarse-grained level by using a series of bipartitions of the latent states.	"The rate at which immunity is lost is important because it constrains the onset of any putative second wave." " … the UK might expect a second wave in around January 2021. This is important because there is a window of opportunity in the next few months during which nonpharmacological interventions—especially tracking and tracing—will, in principle, be in a position to defer or delay the second wave indefinitely."

Table 5. Cont.

Study	Main Stakeholders	Methods	System's Elements	Challenges and Potential Solutions	Key Lessons
Mutanga [12]	National authorities	System dynamics model	They divided the national population into stocks (susceptible, exposed, infected, recovered and deceased), with flows between them representing the time in which individuals will move from one stock to the other. The model also contained multiple connected variables (e.g., R0, restriction measures, rate of contacts within the community, diseases duration and rates of individuals moving from one stock to another).	The modellers estimated homogenous population mixing, which might not represent the actual magnitude of COVID-19 spread in South Africa. The authors also mentioned that the national data might be sub-optimal due to the novelty of the pathogen. Solution: to replicate the model using current knowledge of COVID-19 and using a different timeline where data aggregation, including reporting and testing, are more accurate.	The systems dynamics model conducted in the study was proven beneficial to inform policymakers about prediction, prevention and control of COVID-19 with a small yet acceptable error. The study supports lockdown as a measure to prevent healthcare systems from collapsing.
Scabini [16]	Healthcare policymakers and government	Multilayer complex network	The model's layers represent the social interactions/activities between the population, including home, work, transport, school, religious activities and random. The nodes represent people, and the edges are social contacts between the nodes. The epidemic dynamic was also considered. Individuals were categorised as susceptible, infected-asymptomatic, infected-mild, infected-sever, infected-critical, recovered and dead.	The main challenge the authors faced was related to Brazil's geographic and demographic nature. Other challenges included insufficient data and lack of testing. Solution: This study can be repeated in other countries to check if the results are replicated.	The isolation measures in the study are insufficient and could significantly burden the healthcare system and mortality in Brazil. Social distancing is significant to reduce the peak of the pandemic curve. Returning to "normality" would cause a new peak in the pandemic's wave and the need for ICU beds would surpass the country's capacity.
Shin [14]	Health care policymakers and administrators in government and private sectors	System dynamics model	Model A: Stocks represent the susceptible and infected population at emergency rooms and the flow represent the infectious rate. The variables in model A represent types and frequencies of contact between people in the emergency room (ER occupancy rate, number of contacts made in the ER, susceptible contacts at ER, contact between infected and uninfected people at ER, probability of contact with infected patient at ER, total population at ER, patient arrival at ER, number of visitors at ER, number of visitors per patient) and infectivity of MERS. Model B: Stock represents the general ward's susceptible and infected population. The variables represent infectivity of MERS, room occupancy, fractions of rooms with different frequencies, type and probability of contact and visitors.	The author reported a cultural challenge where family members in South Korea are expected to attend to patients even when healthcare staff are available which might lead to an increase in new cases. Solution: To understand the mental model for the studied population and find leverage points for a desirable outcome.	In hospitals, the number of MERS-CoV infections showed no significant difference between single and multiple room occupancy during the low infectivity period. However, it was increased between patients during the high infectivity period. High emergency room occupancy was associated with a higher risk of infection when compared to low occupancy emergency rooms. The number of visitors was directly related to increased infections among inpatients.

Table 5. Cont.

Study	Main Stakeholders	Methods	System's Elements	Challenges and Potential Solutions	Key Lessons
Silva [18]	Politicians, healthcare policymakers	Agent-based model	Agents that make up the society in the model are people and their environment. The agents were grouped into families, business and government. The model contained input parameters (e.g., epidemiology, socioeconomic and demographic) and output parameters.	The scenarios of this study were done on a simulated society; the situation might differ slightly if the author considered confounding factors from real society. Solution: to validate the results by simulating the scenarios for real-world populations.	Lockdown and partial lockdown are best-case scenarios to mitigate the risk of COVID-19 in the context of human lives and health but have a significant impact on the economy. Vertical isolation (isolating infected individuals and high-risk groups) and "Do nothing" approaches had the worst income. The best scenarios were partial isolation (restricting the movement of the agents), using facemasks and social distancing.
Suresh [13]	Healthcare managers and government	Total interpretive structural modelling (TISM)	Factors that make up the agility system in hospitals including building a Rapid Response Team (RRT), leadership support for the RRT, readiness for change, team members' adaptability, strategy fit to match the demand and capacity, accessibility and availability of the required resources, training and development, collaboration and resilience, embracing technology and innovations, multi-tasking and decision making, biomedical waste management, cost-effectiveness, and their interrelationships. Those factors are categorised into five groups according to their influence on the overall hospital agility.	Presenting the interaction of the factors within the model is not very clear at first sight. Solution: feedback back and forth between two factors can be presented with two arrows rather than one.	Using a framework like TISM can help increase agility in the hospitals and improve managers' decision-making when the most influencing factors and their interrelations are mapped and leverage points are explored rather than making decisions based on instinct and experience that might be suitable to the problem at hand. In this paper, the authors indicated that availability of resources, proper training and collaboration, and resilience are key factors in improving agility in hospitals.
Weixing [17]	Healthcare policymakers and government	System dynamics model	They divided the local population into a community, quarantine areas and hospital compartments. Each compartment contains individuals divided into susceptible, latent, infected, recovered and deceased, with flows between them.	The results indicated that most SARS-CoV-1 cases were imported to Hubei from nearby regions. However, events from transportation were not considered in the model. Solution: incorporating modes of transportation in and out of Hubei into future models.	Healthcare in Hubei province is adequate and could control and mintages the risk of SARS-CoV-1. The optimal priority is to quarantine infected patients and reduce the time delay between diagnosis and hospitalisation. Most of the new cases in Hubei were imported from nearby regions.

3.3.1. How Are Systems-Oriented Modelling Methods Used to Investigate How to Prevent and Control Emerging Infectious Diseases (EIDs)?

Among the systems-oriented studies included in this review, six simulated the dynamics of an EID [12,14–18]. The modellers in these studies incorporated the classic susceptible, exposed, infected, recovered (SEIR) epidemiological model alongside systems-oriented modelling which considered the investigated population's environment. Another study, by Suresh et al., did not simulate disease dynamics. Instead the authors used systems methods to examine what factors contributed to the agility of hospitals to face challenges caused by COVID-19 [13]. They derived a five-level system demonstrating factors that supported the agility of hospitals to prepare and respond to EIDs. These factors included a trained rapid response team, effective leadership, strategies for managing resources and cost-effectiveness, readiness to change, adaptability, collaboration and resilience. They also demonstrated in their model how those factors make up the different levels and how the levels are connected.

Three studies used systems methods to predict an upcoming period of growth during an ongoing pandemic or epidemic [12,15,16]. They examined COVID-19 dynamics, population demography and types of public health policies to control the pandemic. Finally, five studies used systems methods to simulate the consequences of non-pharmaceutical public health strategies for controlling EIDs. Shin et al. used retrospective data to simulate how hospital policies affected the dynamics of MERS-CoV in South Korea in emergency rooms and inpatient wards. They took into account the infective status of patients, types of contacts, number of visitors and room occupancy [14]. Silva et al. simulated the effect of policy measures on COVID-19 burden on human health, life and the economy [18]. Magna et al. simulated multiple "what if" scenarios to investigate the "best approach" to control and mitigate the risk of COVID-19. They argued that the best approach for public health policy would be to find measures that would decrease the number of new cases and would be acceptable by the public [12]. Weixing et al., and Scabini et al., used systems methods to evaluate the types and effectiveness of local public health policy to control SARS-CoV-1 and SARS-CoV-2, respectively [16,17].

3.3.2. In What Contexts Were the Systems-Oriented Studies Conducted?

In the included studies, systems-oriented modelling methods were used to investigate how to prevent and control EIDs in the context of diseases dynamics, the burden on human health and life, economic burden and readiness of healthcare systems. All seven studies were conducted in the context of novel coronaviruses preparedness and control. Five studies were on SARS-CoV-2 [12,13,15,16,18], one study on SARS-CoV1 [17] and one study on MERS-CoV [19]. Friston et al., Mutanga et al., and Scabini et al. used the methods to assess the impact of COVID-19 dynamics on the numbers of new cases and deaths [12,15,16]. They did so by simulating scenarios for different local public health interventions. In addition to the epidemiology of the pandemic, Silva et al. included socioeconomic variables to assess the impact of COVID-19 on the economy [18]. Suresh et al. focused on the healthcare setting rather than the national population. Their study focused on the context of the healthcare system to assess its resilience and agility to face challenges related to COVID-19 by identifying and strengthening leverage points. Weixing et al. used compartmental models to assess local SARS-CoV-1 prevention and control measures within a single province [17]. Finally, Shin and colleagues conducted their study in the context of healthcare system policy in preventing and controlling MERS-CoV. They incorporated cultural expectations for patient care into their model and how they affected the spread of MERS-CoV in hospitals [14].

3.3.3. Who Was the Target Population?

All the articles included in this review studied the local population in countries where the studies were conducted. The population scale, however, differed between the studies. Friston et al., and Mutanga et al., used national populations [12,15]. However, while Mutanga and colleagues focused on the population of South Africa [12], Friston and colleagues' study was multinational. involving the US, Brazil, UK, France, Spain, Italy, Mexico, Germany and Canada [15]. Weixing and colleagues conducted their study on the local population of Hubei province in China. They did so to assess the effectiveness of local public health measures and to investigate if new cases were primarily local or imported from other areas in China [17]. Due to the large size, the complex demography of Brazil and challenges with data collection, Scabini and colleagues used the demography of the national population to parameterize a simulated population in their agent-based model, where they built a multi-layered model representing the interactions between individuals and the disease dynamics [16]. The agents represented people in their environment, with input parameters including epidemiology, socioeconomic status, demography and produced epidemiology and economical response variables [18]. Suresh and colleagues used the healthcare population in their study. They included physicians, nurses, health inspectors, paramedics, hospital operation and administrative staff [13]. Shin and colleagues also focused on the healthcare workforce in addition to patients and visitors in South Korean hospitals during the MERS-CoV outbreak.

3.3.4. What Were the Main Complex-Systems Features?

Given the novelty of an EID, all included articles did not exhibit the "history and memory" feature of complex systems. The inclusion of the remaining complex system features is presented in Table 6.

Table 6. Systems feature used in the citations.

First Author	Numerosity	Disorder and Diversity	Feedback	Non-Equilibrium	Spontaneous Order and Self-Organisation	Non-Linearity	Robustness	Nested Structure and Modularity	History and Memory	Adaptive Behaviour
Friston [15]	X	X	X		X	X				X
Mutanga [12]	X	X	X	X	X	X	X	X		X
Scabini [16]	X	X	X	X	X	X	X	X		X
Shin [14]	X	X	X		X	X		X		X
Silva [18]	X	X	X	X	X	X		X		X
Suresh [13]	X	X	X	X	X		X	X		X
Weixing [17]	X	X	X	X	X	X	X	X		X

3.3.5. What Was the Systems-Oriented Aim?

Overall, a systems-oriented approach was used to investigate how to prevent and control EIDs by presenting estimates of projected consequences of different public health policy choices. Friston and colleagues aimed to estimate the duration of effective immunity, to predict the second wave of SARS-CoV-2 and inform policymakers about precautionary and preventive measures [15]. Shin et al., Weixing et al. and Suresh et al., aims were to assess the ability of healthcare systems to respond and control threats related to EIDs [13,14,17]. While Weixing et al., and Shin et al., examined the readiness of the current healthcare system to respond to the threats of an EID, Suresh and colleagues were more focused on what factors make up the network to strengthen the response system to the threats. Finally, for Silva et al., Muntanga et al., and Sacabini et al., the aim was on the readiness of the whole country to face the challenges and burdens caused by SARS-CoV-2 [12,16,18]. The three articles examined the effect of public health measures on the duration of the pandemic wave and provided recommendations for future policies.

3.3.6. What Were the Main Systems Elements?

Overall, the systems elements used in seven articles were attributes of the local population, patients and visitors to hospitals during an EID outbreak and pre-identified key factors that influence healthcare settings' readiness and resilience when faced with an EID.

Five of the included articles used the national population and their environments as systems' elements and employed a version of the classic susceptible, exposed, infected, recovered (SEIR) epidemiological model [12,15–18]. Weixing and colleagues assigned individuals to different compartments (community, quarantine area, and hospitals). Each compartment represented subgroups of susceptible, exposed, infected, recovered and deceased individuals [17]. Mutanga et al. used a stock and flow diagram for their model. They divided the national population into five stocks, namely susceptible, exposed, infected, recovered and deceased (SEIRD), with other model parameters including the reproductive number, rate or contacts within the community, disease duration and the rate at which individuals move from one stock to the other [12]. Similarly, Sabini et al. used a variation of the classical SEIR model. They assigned a stock for the exposed population because they assumed that all exposed individuals were infected. They also divided the infected population into four groups (asymptomatic, mild, severe and critical) in addition to susceptible, recovered and deceased individuals. Friston and colleagues assigned four attributes to the local population (location, infection status, symptoms and testing). They then divided each attribute into smaller compartments representing the state of individuals. They also considered the heterogeneity of exposure, susceptibility and transmission of the local population [15]. In addition to the SEIR model, Silva and colleagues used a compartmental model to represent the elements (agents) activity cycle and a system map to illustrate the economic relations between systems elements [18]. The other two included articles used the local population to focus on healthcare setting as systems elements. Shin et al. used patients, caregivers and visitors during the MERS-CoV outbreak in South Korea as systems elements [14]. They also used stock and flow diagrams to assess the spread of infection in the emergency room and hospital wards [14]. Suresh and colleagues took a different approach. After identifying the key leadership and managerial factors that support the agility of hospitals to combat COVID-19, they used these factors as the elements [13].

3.3.7. What Were Systems-Oriented Methods Used?

The most commonly used systems simulation method among the included articles was systems dynamics. Other methods included causal dynamic modelling, agent-based modelling, Total Interpretive Structural Modelling and multilayer complex network methods. In addition, all articles included a variation of a classical, SEIR epidemic model. Three used systems dynamics methods. Weixing et al., and Shi et al., started with a simple conceptual model for SASR-CoV1 and MERS-CoV. Later, they created systems dynamic models accounted for disease dynamics in the context of their study populations [14,17]. In contrast, Mutanga and colleagues did not present a conceptual model. However, their systems dynamics model is similar to that of Weixing and Shi. It included the SEIR model and different variables representing the COVID-19 situation in South Africa [12]. Friston and colleagues used dynamic causal modelling. Their approach focuses on probability densities rather than disease dynamics. For example, rather than assuming an individual is either infected or recovered, an individual can be infected and asymptomatic [15]. Silva and colleagues employed an agent-based model, focusing on individuals (agents) in a closed simulated society, with a variety of socioeconomic and epidemiological parameters, in order to run different "what if" scenarios simulating different health policies [18]. Finally, Suresh and colleagues used the Total Interpretive Structural Modelling approach. After performing a literature review to identify factors that influence hospital agility to face COVID-19, they collected and analysed responses from healthcare workers, created a matrix from these responses and finally created a graph presenting the disclosed factors and how are they are connected [13]. Sabino and colleagues used the multilayer complex network method, extending the SEIR model to include multilayers representing social interactions in Brazil [16].

3.3.8. What Challenges Related to Systems-Modelling Did the Authors Face?

In four articles, the authors mentioned challenges, related to data collection and data accuracy in building the models. Friston et al.'s and Mutanga et al.'s main challenge was data collection and accuracy during an ongoing pandemic [12,15]. Friston and colleagues also mentioned that cross-infection with other diseases like influenza contributes an extra challenge in the modelling process [15]. In addition to inaccuracy in disease dynamic data, Scabini and colleagues faced other challenges because of Brazil's geography and demography, which can compound data inaccuracies [16]. Weixing and colleagues reported challenges related mainly to the data collection environment. They used retrospective hospital data relating to patients and visitors during the SARS-CoV1 outbreak in Hebei province in China and mentioned errors in time recording of visits [17]. Shin et al., Silva et al., and Suresh et al. did not report any challenges.

3.3.9. Who Were the Main Stakeholders? Moreover, How Were They Involved?

The main stakeholders were healthcare policymakers, governments and politicians. All the studies were conducted to provide evidence-based recommendations to these stakeholders to inform national public health policies aimed at reducing the burden of EIDs by preventing, controlling, and mitigating their risk to the local population. However, none of the stakeholders had any role in developing the models included in the articles or the interpretation of the results.

3.3.10. What Were the Key Lessons Learned from Using the Complex Systems Approach?

Three of the included articles mentioned lessons learned during the systems model development process. Overall, the main lesson was that there was always room for model improvement when appropriate data are available. Additionally, there was a desire to account for parameters that go beyond disease dynamics, like social, demographic, or economic aspects, which would provide a more holistic perspective on what is going on during an EID. For example, Friston et al., and Scabini et al. stated that their models could be improved by including and/or stratifying the demographic groups by age and ethnicity. The latter also suggested incorporating the clinical presentation of the diseases within the model [15,16]. Silva and colleagues stressed the importance of considering the population's social interactions and economic status to provide a better representation of the pandemic effects on the investigated population [18]. Weixing et al., Shin et al., Mutanga et al., and Suresh et al. did not report or indicate any lessons learned while building their models.

4. Discussion

Our review indicates that systems-oriented modelling methods used in the context of preparedness and response in the face of EIDs can be valuable in identifying healthcare policy approaches and actions for preventing and controlling EIDs. Most of the included studies focused on disease dynamics within the context of the multiple linked elements of the complex systems generating EID threats in a particular population, providing the basis for running simulations of different "prevention" scenarios. Other studies' contexts included healthcare resilience, resource allocation and the economic impact of EIDs.

A variation of the classical SEIR epidemiological model was used in most of the studies, showing that systems methods are not meant to replace classical epidemiological methods. Instead, they can complement evidence provided by other methodological approaches, providing opportunities for original research and potential collaborations between epidemiologists and systems scientists. Systems-oriented modelling differs from classical mathematical modelling in its focus and approach to problem-solving. Instead of analysing a particular problem, systems modellers mainly focus on systems' elements and their connections. By simulating real-world problems, systems modellers can make clear to policy makers the feedback loops affecting outcomes in the system and thus make tangible recommendations about where solutions might lie [19,20]. Another difference is that not all systems-oriented methods involve mathematical modelling, but rather may point qualitatively, in diagrammatic form initially, to causal loops affecting the outcomes [21–23]. In addition, systems modellers can incorporate multiple sub-systems, which build bridges between different stakeholders, including healthcare policymakers, governments, the private sector, healthcare workers and society. This can be useful in examining and improving healthcare system resilience during a public health crisis posed by EIDs threats [22]. Hence, systems methods can offer a birds-eye view of healthcare systems and their links to connected systems within a society, eschewing a reductionist approach policy and its implementation [24].

The main challenges reported by the authors while using a systems approach to prevent and control EIDs were related to the availability and accuracy of epidemiological data. Data availability and accuracy are constrained by EIDs' novel nature, by environmental factors, and by the geography or demography of the studies' locations and populations. These factors lead to imprecision in observed data which might hinder model calibration.

However, Cassidy and colleagues argued that systems methods are less affected by this issue than classical mathematical methods [25]. Moreover, methods to assess the impacts of these uncertainties in the models' results can explore the sensitivity to these effects and help prioritize which aspects of the models or their inputs would benefit the most from more accurate and timely data.

All included studies focused on sarbecoviruses, with the first study published in 2009. However, in addition to sarbecoviruses, the WHO also prioritizes other EIDs for research and development [10]. Our review sheds light on how systems approaches can be used for future research and practice on these diseases. Moreover, the global community has learned from the current COVID-19 experience that the consequences of an uncontrolled EID are more extensive than previously imagined and can lead to a significant burden not only on human health but also on the economy and how society functions. Thus, it is necessary to use a holistic approach for problem-solving when it comes to EIDs, to which systems science can contribute.

The main lesson learned from our review is that systems methods are adaptable and informative. Besides the possibility of systems modellers to further develop existing models when clinicians have deeper understanding of an EID and/or more data are available, there is an added value in considering the dynamic relationship between systems elements and/or other features of complex systems. Moreover, incorporating socioeconomic and demographic data to diseases dynamics in systems models can provide a more holistic presentation of the magnitude and burden of an EID, which in turn helps in producing more specific recommendation to a particular situation or a population.

Our review noted some limitations of systems-oriented methods. The model development process and validation were not transparent in all the included studies, making it challenging for researchers to reproduce the results [25,26]. In addition, the models varied in depth and detail and the reporting style was inconsistent across studies. These limitations are expected because systems methods have only been used recently in EID prevention and control research. With more adaptation of systems methods in EIDs and healthcare policy research, there is a need for clear guidelines in terms of visualisation, transparency and reporting style to enhance reproducibility [25]. Other limitations of systems methods in healthcare policy are their inability to represent all the spill-over phenomena in a healthcare system and the (deliberate and necessary) oversimplification that is inherent to the modelling process [26].

Limitations and Strengths

The main limitation of our review is that due to the volume of COVID-19 research reported during the current pandemic, relevant literature may have been published since our original search. Due to the lead time between searches and reporting a review, there is a need in a rapidly changing situation such as the COVID-19 pandemic to strike a balance between keeping the searches up-to-date and sharing the findings at a point at which they are useful. It is possible that some reports used systems-oriented modelling methods but did not allude to it in their title, abstract or keywords/descriptors.

As for the strengths of this review, we performed a comprehensive search using agreed-upon keywords (with the support of a subject librarian) linked to the WHO list of EID for research and development and followed the Joanna Briggs Institute guidelines for scoping reviews [8,10], guided by a protocol that was reviewed by the research team and peer reviewed [9]. Additionally, we maintained transparency on the need to narrow the scope of the review due to time limitations arising from university regulations governing doctoral studies. Additionally, the reviewing process was done by two independent reviewers.

5. Conclusions

Systems methods can be used to prevent and control EIDs in many ways. The value of systems methods in preparedness and response of healthcare systems to EIDs have been increasingly appreciated because they account for the complexity of this group of diseases.

A range of methods was identified, they were used either alone or in combination with other epidemiological methods. Finally, we conclude that systems methods may help in designing policies to improve healthcare system resilience in response to EIDs.

Recommendations for Future Research

Since systems science is multidisciplinary, we encourage collaboration between researchers from different disciplines to prevent and control EIDs. Teams comprising systems scientists, epidemiologists, systems engineers and social scientists can build systems models to provide a deeper understanding of the EID threat to societies. COVID-19 was prominent in the studies that were included in this review. Systems-oriented methods take account of context, and models and interventions designed in one context might not be helpful in the contexts of different diseases, places or times, for example. As of now there is relatively limited evidence available from the practical application of systems-oriented methods in EID control, and we therefore encourage systems researchers and policymakers to evaluate and report their past and future experiences of implementing systems-oriented methods in EIDs prevention and control.

Author Contributions: Conceptualization, M.A.M., D.T.B., L.G. and F.K.; Methodology, M.A.M., D.T.B., F.K. and L.G.; formal analysis, M.A.M.; Writing—original draft preparation, M.A.M.; Draft review and editing, D.T.B., L.G. and F.K.; Supervision, D.T.B., L.G. and F.K.; project administration, M.A.M. All authors have read and agreed to the published version of the manuscript.

Funding: This research received no external funding.

Data Availability Statement: The search strings from each database are mentioned in Appendix A.

Acknowledgments: This scoping review is part of Ph.D. studies for MAM, funded by Kuwait Civil Commission Service. However, the organization has no role or influence in the review's design or conduct. Also, we acknowledge the contribution of Maha Ahmed Abdeldayem for her contribution in the reviewing stage of the scoping review and Richard Fallis, the medical librarian at Queens University Belfast for his contribution during the planning phase.

Conflicts of Interest: The authors declare no conflict of interest.

Appendix A. Keywords Search across Databases

Appendix A.1. PubMed 23/3/21, 1905 Results

(Emerging-infectious-disease*[Title/Abstract] OR coronavirus[Title/Abstract] OR MERS-CoV[Title/Abstract] OR COVID-19[Title/Abstract] OR severe-acute-respiratory syndrome[Title/Abstract] OR SARS-CoV-2[Title/Abstract] OR SARS[Title/Abstract] OR Ebola[Title/Abstract] OR avian-influenza[Title/Abstract] OR zika*[Title/Abstract] OR dengue[Title/Abstract] OR nipah[Title/Abstract] OR pandemic*[Title/Abstract] OR outbreak* OR Crimean-Congo-haemorrhagic-fever[Title/Abstract] OR rift-valley-fever [Title/Abstract] OR disease-X [Title/Abstract] OR lassa-fever[Title/Abstract])

AND

(complex* near/2 system*[Title/Abstract] OR system-dynamic*[Title/Abstract] OR agent-based[Title/Abstract] OR stochastic[Title/Abstract] OR compartmental-model*[Title/Abstract] OR multi-agent[Title/Abstract] OR multi-compartment-model*[Title/Abstract] OR network near/2 analys*[Title/Abstract])

Appendix A.2. Web of Science 23/3/21, 1880 Results

(

TI=("Emerging infectious disease*" OR coronavirus OR MERS-CoV OR COVID-19 OR "severe acute respiratory syndrome" OR SARS-CoV-2 OR SARS OR Ebola OR "avian influenza" OR zika* OR dengue OR nipah OR pandemic* OR outbreak* OR "Crimean Congo haemorrhagic fever" OR "rift valley fever" OR "disease X" OR "lassa fever")

OR

AB=("Emerging infectious disease*" OR coronavirus OR MERS-CoV OR COVID-19 OR "severe acute respiratory syndrome" OR SARS-CoV-2 OR SARS OR Ebola OR "avian influenza" OR zika* OR dengue OR nipah OR pandemic* OR outbreak* OR "Crimean Congo haemorrhagic fever" OR "rift valley fever" OR "disease X" OR "lassa fever")
)
AND
(
TI=(complex* W/2 system* OR "system dynamic*" OR "agent based" OR agent-based OR stochastic OR "compartmental model*" OR "multi agent" OR multi-agent OR "multi compartment model*" OR "multicompartment model*" OR "multi-compartment model*" OR network W/2 analys*)
OR
AB=(complex* W/2 system* OR "system dynamic*" OR "agent based" OR agent-based OR stochastic OR "compartmental model*" OR "multi agent" OR multi-agent OR "multi compartment model*" OR "multicompartment model*" OR "multi-compartment model*" OR network W/2 analys*)
)

Appendix A.3. Scopus 23/3/21, 9230 Results

(
TITLE-ABS(Emerging infectious disease*) OR TITLE-ABS(coronavirus) OR TITLE-ABS(MERS-CoV) OR TITLE-ABS(COVID-19) OR TITLE-ABS(severe acute respiratory syndrome) OR TITLE-ABS(SARS-CoV-2) OR TITLE-ABS(SARS) OR TITLE-ABS(Ebola) OR TITLE-ABS(avian influenza) OR TITLE-ABS(zika*) OR TITLE-ABS(dengue) OR TITLE-ABS(nipah) OR TITLE-ABS(pandemic*) OR TITLE-ABS(outbreak*) OR TITLE-ABS(Crimean Congo haemorrhagic fever) OR TITLE-ABS(rift valley fever) OR TITLE-ABS(disease X) OR TITLE-ABS(lassa fever)
)
AND
(
TITLE-ABS(complex* W/2 system*) OR TITLE-ABS(system dynamic*) OR TITLE-ABS(agent?based) OR TITLE-ABS(stochastic) OR TITLE-ABS(compartmental model*) OR TITLE-ABS(multi?agent) OR TITLE-ABS(multi?compartment model*) OR TITLE-ABS(network W/2 analys*)
)

References

1. Nandi, A.; Allen, L.J.S. Probability of a zoonotic spillover with seasonal variation. *Infect. Dis. Model.* **2021**, *6*, 514–531. [CrossRef] [PubMed]
2. World Health Organization ROfS-EA. A brief guide to emerging infectious diseases and zoonoses. *WHO Reg. Off. South-East Asia* **2014**, *1*, 1–2.
3. McArthur, D.B. Emerging infectious diseases. *Nurs. Clin. N. Am.* **2019**, *54*, 297–311. [CrossRef] [PubMed]
4. Lee, V.J.; Aguilera, X.; Heymann, D.; Wilder-Smith, A.; Bausch, D.G.; Briand, S.; Bruschke, C.; Carmo, E.H.; Cleghorn, S.; Dandona, L.; et al. Preparedness for emerging epidemic threats: A Lancet Infectious Diseases Commission. *Lancet Infect. Dis.* **2020**, *20*, 17–19. [CrossRef]
5. (CDC) CfDCaP. Division of Preparedness and Emerging Infections (DPEI). 2021. Available online: https://www.cdc.gov/ncezid/dpei/eip/index.html (accessed on 21 April 2022).
6. Meadows, D.H. *Thiniking in Systems*; Earthscan: London, UK, 2009.
7. Meadows, D. Leverage Points: Places to Intervene in a System. 1999. Available online: https://donellameadows.org/archives/leverage-points-places-to-intervene-in-a-system/ (accessed on 26 May 2021).
8. Joanna Briggs Institute. Joanna Briggs Institute Reviewer's Manual. 2019. Available online: https://wiki.joannabriggs.org/display/MANUAL/11.1+Introduction+to+Scoping+reviews (accessed on 21 April 2022).
9. Mansouri, M.A.; Kee, F.; Garcia, L.; Bradley, D.T. Role of systems science in preventing and controlling emerging infectious diseases: Protocol for a scoping review. *BMJ Open* **2021**, *11*, e046057. [CrossRef] [PubMed]

10. WHO. *Prioritizing Diseases for Research and Development in Emergency Contexts*; WHO: Geneva, Switzerland, 2021. Available online: https://www.who.int/activities/prioritizing-diseases-for-research-and-development-in-emergency-contexts (accessed on 26 May 2021).
11. Ladyman, J.; Wiesner, K. What Is a Complex System? Yale University Press: New Haven, CT, USA; London, UK, 2020.
12. Mutanga, S.S.; Ngungu, M.; Tshililo, F.P.; Kaggwa, M. Systems dynamics approach for modelling South Africa's response to COVID-19: A "What if" Scenario. *J. Public Health Res.* **2021**, *10*, 8. [CrossRef] [PubMed]
13. Suresh, M.; Roobaswathiny, A.; Lakshmi Priyadarsini, S. A study on the factors that influence the agility of COVID-19 hospitals. *Int. J. Healthc. Manag.* **2021**, *14*, 290–299. [CrossRef]
14. Shin, N.; Kwag, T.; Park, S.; Kim, Y.H. Effects of operational decisions on the diffusion of epidemic disease: A system dynamics modeling of the MERS-CoV outbreak in South Korea. *J. Theor. Biol.* **2017**, *421*, 39–50. [CrossRef] [PubMed]
15. Friston, K.J.; Parr, T.; Zeidman, P.; Razi, A.; Flandin, G.; Daunizeau, J.; Hulme, O.J.; Billig, A.J.; Litvak, V.; Price, C.J.; et al. Effective immunity and second waves: A dynamic causal modelling study. *Wellcome Open Res.* **2020**, *5*, 204. [CrossRef] [PubMed]
16. Scabini, L.F.S.; Ribas, L.C.; Neiva, M.B.; Junior, A.G.B.; Farfán, A.J.F.; Bruno, O.M. Social interaction layers in complex networks for the dynamical epidemic modeling of COVID-19 in Brazil. *Phys. A Stat. Mech. Appl.* **2021**, *564*, 125498. [CrossRef] [PubMed]
17. Weixing, W.; Yanli, L.; Jinjin, Z. System dynamics modeling of SARS transmission—A case study of Hebei Province. In Proceedings of the 2009 International Conference on Management and Service Science, Beijing, China, 20–22 September 2009.
18. Silva, P.C.L.; Batista, P.V.C.; Lima, H.S.; Alves, M.A.; Guimarães, F.G.; Silva, R.C.P. COVID-ABS: An agent-based model of COVID-19 epidemic to simulate health and economic effects of social distancing interventions. *Chaos Solitons Fractals* **2020**, *139*, 110088. [CrossRef] [PubMed]
19. Lanza, F.; Seidita, V.; Chella, A. Agents and robots for collaborating and supporting physicians in healthcare scenarios. *J. Biomed. Inform.* **2020**, *108*, 103483. [CrossRef] [PubMed]
20. REALKM. The Mathematics of Modeling: Differential Equations and System Dynamics [Systems Thinking & Modelling Series]. 2017. Available online: https://realkm.com/2017/11/28/the-mathematics-of-modeling-differential-equations-and-system-dynamics-systems-thinking-modelling-series/ (accessed on 29 July 2022).
21. Bradley, D.T.; Mansouri, M.A.; Kee, F.; Garcia, L.M.T. A systems approach to preventing and responding to COVID-19. *eClinicalMedicine* **2020**, *21*, 100325. [CrossRef] [PubMed]
22. Kontogiannis, T. A qualitative model of patterns of resilience and vulnerability in responding to a pandemic outbreak with system dynamics. *Saf. Sci.* **2021**, *134*, 105077. [CrossRef]
23. Sahin, O.; Salim, H.; Suprun, E.; Richards, R.; MacAskill, S.; Heilgeist, S.; Rutherford, S.; Stewart, R.A.; Beal, C.D. Developing a preliminary causal loop diagram for understanding the wicked complexity of the COVID-19 pandemic. *Systems* **2020**, *8*, 20. [CrossRef]
24. Klement, R.J. Systems thinking about SARS-CoV-2. *Front. Public Health* **2020**, *8*. [CrossRef] [PubMed]
25. Rahmandad, H.; Sterman, J. Reporting guidelines for simulation-based research in social sciences. *Syst. Dyn. Rev.* **2012**, *28*, 396–411. [CrossRef]
26. Cassidy, R.; Singh, N.S.; Schiratti, P.-R.; Semwanga, A.; Binyaruka, P.; Sachingongu, N.; Chama-Chiliba, C.M.; Chalabi, Z.; Borghi, J.; Blanchet, K. Mathematical modelling for health systems research: A systematic review of system dynamics and agent-based models. *BMC Health Serv. Res.* **2019**, *19*, 845. [CrossRef] [PubMed]

MDPI
St. Alban-Anlage 66
4052 Basel
Switzerland
www.mdpi.com

Systems Editorial Office
E-mail: systems@mdpi.com
www.mdpi.com/journal/systems

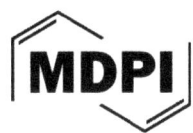

Disclaimer/Publisher's Note: The statements, opinions and data contained in all publications are solely those of the individual author(s) and contributor(s) and not of MDPI and/or the editor(s). MDPI and/or the editor(s) disclaim responsibility for any injury to people or property resulting from any ideas, methods, instructions or products referred to in the content.

www.ingramcontent.com/pod-product-compliance
Lightning Source LLC
LaVergne TN
LVHW070411100526
838202LV00014B/1433